The
ELECTRONIC
HEALTH RECORD

for the
Physician's Office

for SimChart® for the medical office

Julie Pepper, BS, CMA (AAMA)

Medical Assistant Instructor
Chippewa Valley Technical College
Eau Claire, Wisconsin

Second Edition

ELSEVIER

ELSEVIER

3251 Riverport Lane
St. Louis, Missouri 63043

THE ELECTRONIC HEALTH RECORD FOR THE PHYSICIAN'S OFFICE:
FOR SIMCHART FOR THE MEDICAL OFFICE, SECOND EDITION   ISBN: 978-0-323-51146-9

Notices

Knowledge and best practice in this field are constantly changing. As new research and experience broaden our understanding, changes in research methods, professional practices, or medical treatment may become necessary.

Practitioners and researchers must always rely on their own experience and knowledge in evaluating and using any information, methods, compounds, or experiments described herein. In using such information or methods they should be mindful of their own safety and the safety of others, including parties for whom they have a professional responsibility.

With respect to any drug or pharmaceutical products identified, readers are advised to check the most current information provided (i) on procedures featured or (ii) by the manufacturer of each product to be administered, to verify the recommended dose or formula, the method and duration of administration, and contraindications. It is the responsibility of practitioners, relying on their own experience and knowledge of their patients, to make diagnoses, to determine dosages and the best treatment for each individual patient, and to take all appropriate safety precautions.

To the fullest extent of the law, neither the Publisher nor the authors, contributors, or editors, assume any liability for any injury and/or damage to persons or property as a matter of products liability, negligence or otherwise, or from any use or operation of any methods, products, instructions, or ideas contained in the material herein.

Previous edition copyrighted 2015.

Library of Congress Cataloging-in-Publication Data

Names: Pepper, Julie, author. | Preceded by (work): DeVore, Amy. Electronic
    health record for the physician's office.
Title: The electronic health record for the physician's office for SimChart
    for the medical office / Julie Pepper.
Description: Second edition. | St. Louis, Missouri : Elsevier, [2018] |
    Includes index. | Preceded by The electronic health record for the
    physician's office : with SimChart for the medical office / Amy M.
DeVore.
    c2015.
Identifiers: LCCN 2016057561 | ISBN 9780323511469 (pbk. : alk. paper)
Subjects: | MESH: Electronic Health Records--organization & administration|
    Practice Management, Medical--organization & administration | Database
    Management Systems
Classification: LCC R858 | NLM WX 175 | DDC 610.285--dc23 LC record available at
    https://lccn.loc.gov/2016057561

Executive Content Strategist: Jennifer Janson
PSE Content Development Manager: Ellen Wurm-Cutter
Senior Content Development Specialist: Rebecca Leenhouts
Publishing Services Manager: Jeff Patterson
Project Manager: Lisa A. P. Bushey
Designer: Bridget Hoette

Printed in Canada.

Last digit is the print number: 9 8 7 6 5 4 3 2 1

ACKNOWLEDGMENTS

To my husband Jeff: I could not do what I do without your unwavering support. Thank you for putting up with all that goes into writing a textbook.

PREFACE

It is so important for students entering the workforce to be well prepared for the challenges found there. For those students hoping for a career in health care, it is imperative that they have an understanding of electronic health records and how those records impact patient care and reimbursement.

The Electronic Health Record for the Physician's Office, Second Edition, can provide the instructional tools needed to facilitate student learning of the electronic health record process. Both theory and hands-on activities are included in this textbook. Administrative, clinical, and billing applications are discussed, and scenario-based activities provide real-world situations that the students will encounter in the workforce. Critical-thinking and problem-solving skills will be developed as students work through the content and are reinforced with the chapter review activities, including terminology review, Workplace Applications, and EHR in Review sections.

This textbook uses SimChart for the Medical Office, but its concepts are broad enough to cover most electronic health record software available to health care facilities. Students who complete the activities found in *The Electronic Health Record for the Physician's Office* should be able to transfer their knowledge to other EHR software. Although the screens may look different, the basic functions are the same. Working with SimChart for the Medical Office and this textbook, students will have an advantage over those who have not had a detailed exposure to electronic health records. After completing the course using *The Electronic Health Record for the Physician's Office, Second Edition,* students will feel prepared and confident working with an EHR.

The web-based software allows student to access the product wherever they have internet access. This is important for the changing instructional environment. This text can accommodate traditional classrooms, as well as hybrid and online courses. The accessibility of the software allows students more practice, repetition, and opportunities for exploration.

ORGANIZATION

This textbook is organized in a work-text format and is designed to combine both theory and practice throughout each chapter. Common tasks and features of EHR software are explained one step at a time using examples and screenshots from SimChart for the Medical Office. EHR exercises then follow, allowing students a hands-on opportunity to apply the previously learned concepts.

DISTINCTIVE FEATURES

- *Trends and Applications* give students real-life examples of how EHR systems are being used to improve health care and how they may be used in the future.
- *Critical Thinking Exercises* appear throughout each chapter and provide students with thought-provoking questions to enhance learning and stimulate discussion.

- *Review of Paper-Based Office Procedures* provides a reference for students that walks them through how tasks are completed when the health care facility is using paper-based procedures instead of electronic.
- *CMS Documentation Guidelines* gives students additional information on what CMS expects for documentation in either a paper-based or EHR system.

LEARNING AIDS

- Well-developed *Learning Objectives* follow the organizational flow of each chapter. They are also summarized at the end of each chapter for student review.
- *Key Terms* are listed and defined at the beginning of each chapter and are bolded where they appear in the text. The key terms are also available in a glossary at the back of the book for quick reference.
- A variety of *Chapter Review Activities* are available at the end of each chapter, allowing students to assess their knowledge of the material. Activities include key terms review, matching, true/false, and additional opportunities to practice with the software.
- *EHR Exercises* allow for the application of the theory presented with step-by-step instructions for the completion of the activity. They are integrated throughout each chapter, providing students an opportunity to practice with actual software and reinforce key concepts. **Important note:** The EHR Exercises increase in difficulty based on the knowledge gained, and some depend on the successful completion of previous exercises. Therefore the EHR Exercises should be completed in the order in which they appear in the text.

NEW TO THIS EDITION

- Enhanced content coverage and mapping to support preparation for the Certified Electronic Health Records Specialist (CEHRS) examination
- Grading rubrics for all SCMO application activities
- Entry point for all SCMO application activities
- CEHRS Examination preparation tools on Evolve

ANCILLARIES

Evolve Resources, with TEACH Instructor Resources and Student Resources, provides instructors and students with supplemental features that complement this textbook. The website also allows students and instructors to stay current with trends, developments, and news of the electronic health record.

For the Student

- Direct access to SimChart for the Medical Office
- Mock CEHRS Examination

For the Instructor

- **Answer Keys** provide answers to the EHR Exercises, *Critical Thinking Exercises,* and *Chapter Review Activities.*
- **ExamView test bank** offers instructors test items for a wide variety of examination styles.
- **Correlation guides** map content to CAAHEP, ABHES, and CEHRS blueprint.
- **Grading rubrics** are provided for all SCMO application activities.

- **TEACH Instructor Resources** for each chapter are available on the Evolve site, including the following:
  - Lesson Plans provide instructors with customizable lesson plans for each chapter.
  - PowerPoints provide instructors with talking points, thought-provoking questions, and unique ideas for lectures.
  - Student Handouts are available for use in class and as study tools for students.

CONTENTS

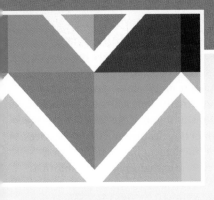

1

Introduction to Electronic Health Records

Assignment
Quiz

CHAPTER OBJECTIVES

1. Explore the history and current use of patient health records, their importance to individuals' health, and their contribution to the healthcare system.
2. Become familiar with the content of a typical electronic health record (EHR).
3. Explain who documents in the medical record.
4. Discuss ownership of the health record.
5. Describe the basic functions and advanced clinical decision support (CDS) features of EHR software.
6. Define *practice management software* and explain how it is used with the EHR system.
7. Describe advantages of EHR systems.
8. Describe disadvantages of EHR systems.
9. Identify the roles of various healthcare professionals in implementing an EHR system.
10. Investigate various professional organizations aimed at promoting the use of EHR systems.

KEY TERMS

account ledger Lists services provided, payments made by the patient, reimbursement received from the patient's insurance company, adjustments, and outstanding amount owed.

audit A review of employee activity within the EHR system, including an examination of which files were accessed or modified, when, and why.

chief complaint The patient's stated primary reason for seeking treatment.

clinical decision support (CDS) A set of patient-centered tools embedded within EHR software that can be used to improve patient safety, ensure that care conforms to pub- lished protocol for specific conditions, and reduce duplicate or unnecessary care and its associated costs.

computerized provider order entry (CPOE) An EHR func- tion that allows a provider or provider-appointed licensed healthcare professional or credentialed medical assistant to enter the ordered medications and tests using an automated format; CPOE can reduce prescribing errors, delays, and du- plication and can simplify inventory and billing processes.

continuity of care A key aspect of quality that encompasses planning and coordination of care, communication among members of the healthcare team, and accessibility and transportability of information.

copayment A fixed sum of money, dictated by the insurance company, that is paid by the patient, usually at the time medical services are rendered.

day sheet A register for all daily business transactions such as patient services, payments, and adjustments; also called a *day journal.*

documentation The process of recording data about a patient's health history and status, including clinical observations and progress notes, diagnoses of illnesses and injuries, plans of care, patient education and self-care instructions given, vital signs taken, physical assessment findings, laboratory and imaging test results, medical treatments prescribed or administered, surgeries performed and outcomes; the term can also refer to the chronologic record that results from such data entry.

electronic health record (EHR) A computerized patient health record that allows the electronic management of a patient's health information by multiple healthcare providers and stores the patient's contact information, legal documents, demographic data, and administrative information; the term can also refer more broadly to a system that manages such records.

electronic transcription Data entry into the EHR using handwriting recognition, voice recognition, electronic sentence building, scanning, and other means.

encounter A documented interaction or visit between a patient and healthcare provider.

interoperability The ability of separate EHR systems to share information in compatible formats.

Meaningful Use (MU) Part of the federal EHR Incentive Program. If providers can show that they have implemented and are using EHRs in specified meaningful ways, they will receive financial incentives from the government.

Office of the National Coordinator for Health Information Technology (ONCHIT) Division of the Office of the Secretary, within the Department of Health and Human Services. Coordinates the effort to implement health information technology and the electronic exchange of health information.

patient information form A form used to gather data about the patient, including basic demographic information, medical insurance data, and emergency contact.

practice management software (PMS) Software used in a medical office to accomplish administrative (nonclinical) tasks, including entry of patient demographics, record-keeping for insurance and other billing transactions, appointment scheduling, and advanced accounting functions.

structured data entry Documentation using controlled vocabulary via preloaded data, drop-down menus, radio buttons, and sentence builders.

superbill/encounter form An itemized form used to document services provided to the patient and the diagnoses for the services. Also the main source of information used to create the insurance claim.

third-party payer A party other than the patient, spouse, parent, or guardian who is responsible for paying all or part of the patient's medical costs, typically the insurance company.

WHAT IS A MEDICAL RECORD?

History of Medical Records

Nearly as long as there have been physicians, there have been medical records. A patient medical record is a complete physical collection of an individual's healthcare information. Chunyu Yi, who was born in China in approximately 200 BCE, is one of the first physicians known to have kept records on the patients he treated. His written observations of patient signs and symptoms are one of the first known forms of patient documentation. A hospital in Damascus, Syria, built in 706 CE, was perhaps among the first in history to adopt the widespread use of medical records.

Medical records and death ledgers were kept during the plagues that swept through Europe during the fourteenth and seventeenth centuries. In the United States during the Civil War era, soldiers' medical records documented "nervous disease" (later known as shell shock and now posttraumatic stress disorder), as well as injuries suffered in combat and infectious diseases contracted in the crowded, unsanitary military camps. Between 1892 and 1954, medical records were created for most of the 12 million immigrants who passed through Ellis Island, eager to begin their new lives in America. The record served as proof that the person had been deemed able-bodied and free of communicable diseases, such as tuberculosis and smallpox, which would have prompted quarantine or deportation.

Of course, medical records haven't always been used in positive ways. Nazi physicians often kept meticulous records on each "patient" forced to participate in their gruesome, cruel experiments. Between 1932 and 1972, researchers documented the signs, symptoms, and complications of syphilis in the records of hundreds of African American men during the infamous Tuskegee syphilis experiment. The men were denied proper care and allowed to suffer long after penicillin was found to be a highly effective treatment for syphilis.

These researchers, fortunately, represent an exception to the generally high standard of conduct upheld by members of the medical and scientific communities. Researchers studying human immunodeficiency virus/acquired immunodeficiency syndrome (HIV/AIDS), for example, have used retrospective (that is, backward-looking) studies of medical records in several ways. First, they were able to confirm that HIV/AIDS was, in fact, a new infectious disease. Second, by studying who had contracted the disease (for example, through sexual behaviors, infants of infected mothers, and patients with hemophilia who had used contaminated blood products), they were able to determine how HIV is transmitted. Finally, they were able to track the spread of the disease within various population groups and geographic areas. At first all this research was done by studying the paper medical records of individual patients. However, the process of tracking the incidence and prevalence of this disease and others has become easier as more and more data have been digitized. Of course, in the United States and other developed countries, healthcare providers are required by law to report new cases of HIV/AIDS (and other communicable diseases) to the Centers for Disease Control and Prevention (CDC). The person's identity is held in strict confidence.

As you can see, the medical record has been used throughout history to benefit individual patients and to advance medical knowledge through research. Of course, there was the occasional country physician who never saw a need to keep records beyond those in his own head because he treated the same families in the same small communities generation after generation. However, failing to document a patient's care is no longer an option. Federal laws have been put in place that require all patient care to be documented in a medical record. Although paper records can still be found, the vast majority of healthcare providers are documenting patient care in an **electronic health record (EHR)**. In the following sections, we will explore documentation stored in the EHR and the person responsible for maintaining it.

Content of the Electronic Health Record

Each patient has his or her own health record in the provider's office. This record tells the patient's health story. It is the source document for providers and the documentation that provides evidence of care. Complete documentation in these records is vital to ensuring the highest level of care. The complexity of one's own health history is too overwhelming to memorize. Can you imagine trying to care for thousands of patients by memory? Impossible, and not an effective way to manage health. It's been said, "If it isn't documented, it never happened." Every patient **encounter** with the medical office must be tracked. Medical documentation of the events is the easiest and most effective way, and it's required by law. Therefore, maintaining the accuracy of the medical record is one of the most important duties of the healthcare staff. The contents of the medical record may vary slightly from office to office, but most records contain the types of documents in the following list. Note, however, that there is some overlap among the categories—an insurance form, for example, is both an administrative and a legal document, and it may contain health information as well.

Clinical Information

The medical record is the primary source of information about the patient's medical history, such as immunization records, operative reports, and progress notes. This information is gathered mostly during patient encounters with the provider. Over time, the stored clinical data are used to predict risk for disease, compare measurements and values against one another, and determine what is or is not effective for treatment of illness or other health problems. The more complete this record is, the better the care the provider can offer. Clinical information includes the following:

- Medication list (Fig. 1.1)
- Allergies list
- Immunization records
- Laboratory reports
- Pathology reports
- Surgical reports

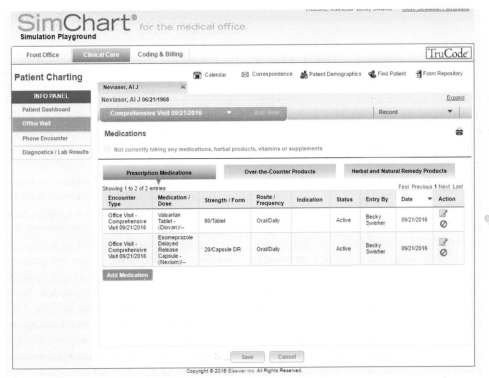

FIG. 1.1 SCMO Medications list.

- Hospital records
- History and physical assessment findings
- Risk assessment
- Preventive services
- Progress notes
- Vital signs and growth charts
- Imaging test results, such as radiographs and magnetic resonance imaging (MRI) films

Administrative Information

In addition to providing clinical information, the medical record enables the administrative staff to perform front office activities such as maintaining appointments, storing patient contact information, and creating patient correspondence. Administrative tasks also include the necessary coding and billing processes that keep the office doors open. Medical insurance policies are changing regularly, which makes gathering and storing current payer information important. Administrative information includes the following:

- Patient demographics
- Name of emergency contact person
- Patient correspondence
- Referral and consultation letters
- Prior authorizations
- Insurance information, copies of insurance cards
- Health Insurance Portability and Accountability Act (HIPAA) 5010 claims status
- Billing account ledgers
- Superbills/encounter forms
- Day sheets
- Appointment history
- Diagnosis and procedure codes

Legal Documents

The complete medical record is considered a legal document, as federal law requires that providers document patient care. In addition, a patient medical record may be used during court proceedings for malpractice suits. Thorough, accurate documentation helps prove what, when, and why care was provided. For example, a complete record will show what information was provided to the patient and what decisions the patient or the patient's family made concerning care options based on that information. Thus proper documentation is important to protect the practice as well as to ensure that the patient receives high-quality care.

Within a medical record there are legal forms. Some, such as do not resuscitate (DNR) orders, may need to be accessed quickly so the medical team knows how to proceed in an emergency; others are used to document consent and treatment options. Legal forms include the following:

- Medical records releases
- Consent forms (Fig. 1.2)
- HIPAA forms (Notice of Privacy Practices acknowledgment)
- Advance directives (living will, DNR, healthcare power of attorney)
- Disclosure logs

WHO DOCUMENTS IN THE MEDICAL RECORD?

Physicians, nurse practitioners, physician's assistants, nurses, and clinical and administrative medical assistants all document information in the patient's medical record. All aspects of the patient encounter must be recorded in the medical record, including the following: patient health history, **chief complaint**, clinical observations, diagnoses, tests that are ordered, and treatment plans. The patient's information is documented in chronologic order, including all new information or changes to the patient's health. The process of the documentation could include handwritten, dictated, **structured data entry**, or scanned-in patient information.

In the past, some healthcare providers preferred to handwrite their notes. Caution had to be taken to ensure the notes were clear, complete, and easy to read. Handwritten notes helped the provider avoid paying for transcription services, thereby reducing costs for the practice during the period of paper-based records. With the implementation of electronic systems, providers may choose to dictate a patient encounter directly into the medical record with the aid of voice recognition software. This is a computerized system that automatically converts voice into text as the provider speaks directly into a microphone. The error-free implementation of this software takes time because the software must be trained to recognize the idiosyncrasies of individual voices. Many medical software systems are moving from narrative-type notes to templates and structured data entry. These data are selected from a fixed field or database by utilizing drop-down menus and radio buttons and make documentation from a mobile device easier to perform. Structured data also provide standardization across all medical records in the system and allow for graphing of the data, or for finding research data. Using these methods of documentation eliminates the need for a staff member to file provider documentation in the record or to transcribe recorded information into the record.

Many different staff members within the provider's office contribute to the patient medical record. First, the administrative medical assistant, receptionist, or other member of the front-office staff records important basic data about the patient in preparation for consultation with and examination by the provider. This information is gathered using a **patient information form** (Fig. 1.3). The receptionist may be responsible for documenting Notice of Privacy Practices (NPP) acknowledgments, chief complaint, **copayments**, requests for prescription refills, and authorization to release medical records or obtain records from other providers, as well as for recording no-shows or cancellations of patient appointments.

The next documenter will generally be the clinical medical assistant, who accompanies the patient to the examination room, records weight and vital signs, and notes preliminary clinical information, such as an expanded chief complaint including a history of the present illness (the duration and context of the chief complaint), medications including over-the-counter and herbal supplements, and any known allergies.

Once the medical assistant has prepared the patient for the provider's examination or consultation, the provider sees the patient and documents the examination findings, plan of care,

WALDEN-MARTIN
FAMILY MEDICAL CLINIC
1234 ANYSTREET | ANYTOWN, ANYSTATE 12345
PHONE 123-123-1234 | FAX 123-123-5678

General Procedure Consent

Patient Name: _____   **Date:** _____

The Doctor has discussed with you your condition and the recommended surgical or medical procedures to be performed. This discussion was intended to ensure that you had the opportunity to receive the information necessary to make a reasoned and informed decision whether or not to consent to the procedure. This document is written confirmation of the discussion and contain some of the more significant medical information discussed.

1. Based on this discussion, I understand the following condition may exist in my case:

2. I understand the procedure proposed for treating or diagnosing my condition is:

3. I have been informed of the purpose and reasonable expected benefits of the proposed procedure, the possibility of success or failure, major problems of recuperation, the reasonably anticipated consequences if the procedure is not performed, and the available alternatives.

4. I understand that all surgical and therapeutic procedures involve some risks including pain, scarring, bleeding and infection.

5. I am aware that in the practice of medicine, other unexpected risks or complications not discussed may or may not further acknowledge that no guarantees or promises have been made to me concerning the results of any procedures. Although the benefits are judged to outweigh the risks, should any complications occur, any one of them could be permanent. I hereby voluntarily give my authority and consent to the doctor to perform the proposed procedure described above.

6. I have been given the opportunity to ask questions about my condition, alternative forms of treatment, risk treatment, the procedure to be used, and the risks and hazards involved. I believe I have sufficient information to give this informed consent.

I understand I have read and fully understand the contents of this form, that the disclosures referred to above were made to me and that all blanks and statements requiring insertion or completion were filled in before I signed my name below.

Patient Signature: _____   **Date:** _____

If a patient is a minor or unable to give consent,
Signature of person authorized to consent for patient: _____

Relationship to Patient: _____

FIG. 1.2 SCMO General Procedure form.

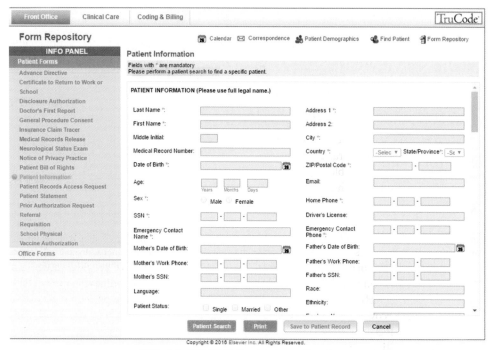

FIG. 1.3 SCMO Patient Information form.

and any other observations made during the patient encounter. The provider is the main documenter of the patient record, and all additions to the patient medical record should be signed and approved with his or her signature. Many different healthcare providers may have documentation responsibilities, including the following:

- Primary care physician
- Physician's assistant
- Nurse practitioner
- Physical or occupational therapist
- Social worker
- Specialist
- Surgeon
- Medical biller

Each of these providers may contribute to the patient medical record in different ways. For example, the physical therapist's correspondence will document the treatment plan and progress, whereas the primary care physician is responsible for coordinating all aspects of the patient's care. The medical biller may need to document the patient's insurance information and authorization numbers as well as file appeal letters and abstract data for claims submission.

WHO OWNS THE MEDICAL RECORD?

Patient medical records are considered the property of the individuals who created them. For example, a provider in a private practice owns the records created in his or her own practice. Records created at a hospital or a long-term care facility are the property of the institution. However, the patient controls the *information* within the medical record. In other words, the patient has a legal right to access or view a copy his or her own medical information at any time by signing a medical

release form; however, the original copy of the record never leaves the facility that owns it. The patient also has the right to request restricted access, request amendments to errors, and obtain a list of disclosures (who has viewed or received the information).

A medical practice may legally charge a fee for copying a medical record. This charge is based on the cost of preparation and production of the medical record. A provider cannot withhold copies of the medical record if a patient has an unpaid balance on his or her account.

CRITICAL THINKING EXERCISE 1.1

Sherry Macken is a patient at the office where you work. She plans to move out of state and insists on taking her original (paper) patient medical chart with her. The office manager refuses to release the record to her. Ms. Macken has just faxed a letter threatening to involve her brother-in-law, a personal injury lawyer whose ad appears on the back cover of the local phone book, if she does not receive her records within 1 week. Who legally owns the medical record, and how can this patient's situation be resolved amicably?

One exception to the patient's right to view his or her medical records is called the *doctrine of professional discretion*. This principle states that a provider can exercise his or her best judgment when deciding whether to share progress notes and clinical observations with a patient who is being treated for mental or emotional disturbances. The doctrine of professional discretion is intended to protect mentally or emotionally ill patients from any additional harm that viewing their medical records could cause. For example, fragile patients who are depressed or suicidal may be upset to read the practitioner's assessment of their unstable condition.

THE ELECTRONIC HEALTH RECORD

Traditionally, information pertaining to the patient's care in the medical office has been maintained using a paper-based chart. However, advancements in technology and government programs have caused a shift from paper-based records to digital ones. The EHR, simply put, is a patient medical record in an electronic format. Ideally, the EHR can exchange data freely with other computer systems, such as those of other healthcare providers, pharmacies, hospitals, laboratories, and insurance companies, creating one central EHR that is easily accessible to authorized parties yet secure from those who do not have the right to see it.

Transitioning from Paper to Electronic Records

The Bush administration first declared 2004 to 2014 "the decade of health information technology [HIT]" and established the Office of the National Coordinator for Health Information Technology (ONCHIT). The Obama administration continued to endorse and promote the universal use of certified EHR and computerized provider order entry (CPOE) in the Recovery Act of 2009 and the Affordable Care Act. These programs focus on improving coordination of care, reducing duplicative testing, and rewarding hospitals and providers for keeping patients healthier.

The transition of health information from paper-based records to electronic media has been slow but has had a dramatic increase over the past several years. A nationwide survey conducted by DesRoches and colleagues showed that as of 2007 to 2008, only 17% of practices had adopted an EHR system. Data from the CDC's National Center for Health Statistics in 2014 reveal encouraging trends, with an implementation rate of 74.1% for physicians' offices with 47.8% sharing patient health information electronically with other ambulatory providers or hospitals. Government programs offering financial incentives for EHR adoption have surely contributed to this trend.

The ONCHIT has established requirements for EHR certification as part of the American Recovery and Reinvestment Act (ARRA). EHR vendors are evaluated on a set of core and menu objective measures. The Meaningful Use (MU) incentive program is a payment incentive program made available for eligible professionals (EPs) or physicians who implement and use their EHR technology in a meaningful way. EHR usage must meet specific requirements. These are organized into three stages of core and menu objectives. The main goals of the MU program are:

- Improve quality, safety, and efficiency and reduce health disparities
- Engage patients and family
- Improve care coordination, and population and public health
- Maintain privacy and security of patient health information

The MU program is divided into three stages. The goal was to allow a slow but meaningful implementation of electronic technology. In 2011 to 2012, stage 1 of MU was made available. This stage was referred to as data capture and sharing. Under the policy, providers must successfully complete stage 1 requirements before continuing to stage 2. Stage 2, advance clinical processes, is under way and will continue throughout 2014 to 2017. This stage builds on the established objectives to increase use and evaluation. For example, under stage 1

requirements, EPs are required to document demographics as structured data for more than 40% of patients. The stage 2 requirement increases that value to 50% of all patients. As these requirements have providers scrambling to get their data in order and new workflow under way, the implementation date for stage 3, improved outcomes, has been pushed back to 2018. It is hoped that this will give providers enough time to understand how their data monitoring is affecting patients and give EHR vendors enough time to be compliant under the strict stage 3 requirements expected to be announced. Beginning in 2015 all EPs were required to demonstrate 10 objectives and measures:

1. Protect electronic health information created or maintained by the certified health record technology (CEHRT).
2. Use clinical decision support (CDS) to improve performance on high-priority health conditions.
3. Use computerized provider order entry for medication, laboratory, and radiology orders directly entered by any licensed healthcare professional who can enter orders into the medical record per state, local, and professional guidelines.
4. Generate and transmit permissible prescription electronically (eRx).
5. Health Information Exchange—The EP who transitions the patient to another setting of care or provider of care refers the patient to another provider of care and provides a summary care record for each transition of care or referral.
6. Use clinically relevant information from CEHRT to identify patient-specific education resources and provide those resources to the patient.
7. The EP who receives a patient from another setting of care or provider of care or believes an encounter is relevant performs medication reconciliation.
8. Patient electronic access—Provide patients with ability to view online, download, and transmit their health information within 4 business days of the information being available to the EP.
9. Use secure electronic messaging to communicate with patients on relevant health information.
10. Public Health Reporting—The EP is in active engagement with a public health agency to submit electronic public health data from CEHRT, except where prohibited, and in accordance with applicable law and practice.

EASING THE TRANSITION 1.1   Will E-prescribing Solve the Problem of Medication Errors?

Medication errors due to handwritten prescriptions were one of the driving forces behind the development of e-prescribing and the reason why it was one of the very first requirements of Meaningful Use. An estimated 1.5 million medication errors occur each year, thousands of which can be attributed to sloppy script. Hespan can be mistaken for Heparin, or Norcuron can look like Narcan. In fact, the manufacturer of the Alzheimer's drug Reminyl changed the drug's name because two people died after being given the diabetes drug Amaryl.

Continued

EASING THE TRANSITION 1.1   Will E-prescribing Solve the Problem of Medication Errors?—cont'd

The problem goes beyond drug names, though. Hurriedly written 2's can look like 7's, or 0's can resemble 6's, leading to dosage errors. Abbreviations are another source of peril. For example, the abbreviation "qhs" on a prescription, which means "taken at the hour of sleep [bedtime]," can look like "qhr," which means "taken every hour." Seven thousand deaths each year are attributable to these kinds of medication errors.

A number of solutions have been proposed for the problem. The Institute for Safe Medication Practices (ISMP) publishes a continually updated list of sound-alike medications and a list of dangerous abbreviations, symbols, and dose designations, along with suggested alternatives. The ISMP recommends, for example, that "nightly" be substituted for "qhs." In addition, safety advocates urge prescribers to write a brief description of the diagnosis, such as "for Alzheimer's," directly on the prescription as an additional cross-check for the pharmacist to confirm that he or she is dispensing the right medication. Patients, too, should take an active role in preventing errors by checking prescription labels, reading the leaflets or product inserts accompanying their prescriptions, and consulting with the pharmacist if the pills they're given are a different size, shape, or color from those previously dispensed for the same prescription.

But is e-prescribing (computerized provider order entry [CPOE]) the real solution to poor penmanship? The answer is a qualified yes. After all, typewritten drug names and dosages are always legible. The VA, which has converted entirely to EHR systems, issues more than 230 million prescriptions a year and claims an accuracy rate of nearly 100%. The VA checks hospital patients' prescriptions against a bar code on their wristbands to make sure that the drug being dispensed will not react adversely with the patient's other medications. By using built-in clinical decision support tools, the EHR system makes sure the drug is compatible with the patient's diagnosis. The system also produces automatic warnings if the dosage entered is beyond the range normally prescribed.

According to an annual survey on EHR systems conducted by the American Academy of Family Physicians, physicians are enthusiastic about e-prescribing, ranking it as one of the top five advantages of EHR systems. However, the e-prescribing function isn't foolproof. A study published in the *Journal of the American Medical Association (JAMA)* found that the use of EHR systems actually facilitated 22 new kinds of prescribing errors unrelated to legibility. For instance, the prescriber can still click on the wrong medication when selecting from an alphabetical list, or choose, say, a tablet instead of the liquid formulation of a drug. Another kind of error occurred when prescribers viewed a pharmacy inventory on the screen (indicating, for instance, that the 200-mg tablets of a given medication were in stock) and mistook it for prescribing guidelines that help physicians determine the customary dosage of a drug. Because it may take as many as 20 screens to view a single patient's medications, errors also occurred in failing to discontinue a previously prescribed drug when a replacement drug is ordered. A medication can even be prescribed to the wrong patient when one prescriber fails to log off the system at a shared computer terminal.

Nevertheless, the advantage of an electronic system over paper in reducing medication errors is undeniable. Even the aforementioned *JAMA* study concluded that EHR systems are less subject to error caused by sound-alike drug names and mistaken dosages. The report also concluded that the CPOE systems built in to EHR systems are able to reduce under- and overprescribing and can easily be linked to drug interaction warnings and clinical decision support systems that help ensure accuracy. Although we should be aware that e-prescribing is not a cure-all and has generated unexpected kinds of errors, we must acknowledge that it nevertheless represents a dramatic advance toward the goal of keeping patients safe.

What Is the Difference Between an Electronic Health Record and an Electronic Medical Record?

As the concept of the EHR evolved over time, a distinction was sometimes made between the terms *EHR* and *electronic medical record (EMR)*. The EMR was said to be an electronic patient record created and maintained by a medical practice or hospital, whereas the EHR was said to be an interconnected aggregate of all the patient's health records, culled from multiple providers and healthcare facilities. In other words, the EMR was said to be a component of the EHR. In practice, however, the line between these terms has blurred to the point that they are now used virtually interchangeably, although there has been a shift toward EHR as the preferred term. This makes sense. After all, the purpose of converting records from paper to an electronic format is ultimately to create a single record for each patient that allows providers and facilities to update, access, and share information efficiently. Using the term *EHR* reflects the healthcare industry's optimism that this goal will be met in the foreseeable future, whereas continuing to make a distinction between the terms perpetuates the idea that each medical practice maintains its own records. In this text, we will refer to electronic patient records, whether created by a medical practice or by a hospital or other facility, as EHR systems.

Electronic Health Records Software

A variety of EHR software systems are on the market. In order for a provider to qualify for MU incentives, he or she must select software that has been tested by an Accredited Testing Laboratory and certified by an ONC-Authorized Certification Body (ONC-ACB) to meet the criteria specified by the Department of Health and Human Services (HHS). Although the systems still may not be compatible, this standardization of functionality is a necessary first step toward becoming interconnected.

Most EHR systems have the same basic functionality, with differences in task execution, navigation, workflow, and so forth. Because their fundamental features are similar, the user can adapt to different systems with little difficulty. SimChart for the Medical Office (SCMO) is a web-based EHR that has real functionality used in physicians' offices and outpatient facilities while giving students a safe academic learning environment. Its features are demonstrated throughout this text.

Basic Functions

Commercial EHR systems have the following fundamental capabilities:

- Progress notes
- Documentation using free text, predefined clinical templates, or user-defined clinical templates
- Provider review of incoming laboratory data and reports
- Patient correspondence
- Storage of office forms (incident reports, inventory, petty cash, release of information)
- Images and report attachment function
- Electronic signature insertion
- Prescription (CPOE) templates that provide dosage, suggest alternatives, list prices, and cross-check prescriptions for drug interactions, patient allergies, and availability in the formulary

- Fax and messaging functions to transmit prescriptions directly from the EHR to the patient's pharmacy
- Reminders that the patient is due for a screening or other health maintenance test or procedure
- Vital signs data capture
- Patient portal
- Importation of laboratory data from an outside or in-house laboratory, using industry-standard formats
- Automatic flagging of abnormal data and test results
- Intraoffice messaging and email functions
- Summary and print functions

Clinical Decision Support

An advanced feature called clinical decision support (CDS) allows providers to tailor the care of an individual patient by making sure it adheres to published guidelines for the patient's specific diagnoses. Clinical decision support tools allow providers to do the following:

- Ensure that the patient's care complies with established screening recommendations for the diseases for which he or she is at risk (colon cancer or glaucoma, for instance). EHR systems analyze patient data, such as age and gender, in order to produce automated reminders for mammograms, Pap tests, colonoscopies, diabetic retinopathy examinations, immunizations, and other screening tests and procedures.
- Plan treatment in accordance with evidence-based treatment guidelines (for heart failure or hepatitis, for example). The practitioner can make more accurate and timely diagnoses with the aid of advice automatically generated by the EHR system based on the patient's clinical data.
- Generate patient data reports and summaries.
- Complete documentation templates specific to the patient's diagnosis, such as knee pain or kidney disease.
- Perform database searches to identify patients who meet specific criteria, such as those within a particular age range who have a given diagnosis, in order to ensure that they are receiving the recommended care and screening. For example, it is recommended that pregnant women with diabetes be closely monitored for diabetic retinopathy for 1 year postpartum because pregnancy can accelerate the development of this ophthalmologic complication. The provider could query the EHR database to produce a list of women in the practice with diabetes who have given birth within the past year and who have not received a diabetic retinopathy screening in 3 months or longer. These patients could then be contacted and immediately referred to a retina specialist.

The CDS tools work, however, only if providers take advantage of them. A statewide study of Massachusetts providers found that fewer than half of them whose EHR systems offered CDS actually used it. Furthermore, if information is not entered properly, some CDS functions are less effective. For example, one practice decided to use its EHR system to identify all female patients ages 50 to 65 who had not had a mammogram in a year or longer. Because of data that had been entered in an improper format, 15% of patients who met those criteria were not found during the initial search.

In addition, providers may ignore system-generated advice either because they're busy or because they prefer to rely on their own judgment and experience. Some practices may not even install this function, especially if there is no financial incentive for delivering care in conformity with established protocols.

Proponents of the advanced tools say that CDS allows them to focus more on patient communication skills and on their ability to make critical decisions. Instead of spending all of their time trying to memorize treatment protocols, providers are able to focus on the patient examination and the needs of the individual. On December 11, 2013, legislators introduced the Excellence in Diagnostic Imaging Utilization Act of 2013, which requires the use of clinical guidance tools (CDS tools) when ordering diagnostic testing. Along with this act is the requirement that any provider who wishes to receive Meaningful Use Incentive Program dollars implement at least one CDS element (or rule) for patients. Under the requirement, the clinical decision support can help providers:

- Share best practices regarding the treatment and diagnosis of disease
- Reduce the amount of testing ordered by physicians and then denied by insurance companies
- Improve clinical outcomes and reduce the number of misdiagnoses
- Reduce costs from unnecessary testing
- Improve patient safety

CRITICAL THINKING EXERCISE 1.2

During Dr. Martin's visit with Mr. Hickman, he discovers that the patient has gained 22 pounds since his visit 4 months ago and that his triglycerides are high. Dr. Martin wants to check the recommended adult dosage of the cholesterol-lowering drug he intends to prescribe; calculate the patient's body mass index (BMI) based on his height and weight; and give Mr. Hickman a patient education brochure explaining the link between physical inactivity, being overweight, and type 2 diabetes. Which of these functions can he accomplish using his practice's EHR system? How would Dr. Martin go about gathering this information? How might the use of CDS tools help manage Mr. Hickman's diagnosis?

Practice Management Software

The EHR lies at the heart of the modern digital medical office, but most medical practices choose to kick it up a notch by using a fully integrated EHR and practice management system, such as that offered in SCMO. Practice management software (PMS) allows electronic management of the business side of the practice. It allows efficient handling of all front-office administrative procedures, including entering patient demographics, tracking billing and insurance information, scheduling appointments, and processing payments for patient visits. Let's take a look at what integrated practice management software has to offer.

Patient Demographics #6

Practice management software compiles all of a patient's demographic information—socioeconomic data such as age, sex, marital status, education, occupation, language, race, and

FIG. 1.4 SCMO Patient Demographics screen.

ethnicity—within the EHR. When patients present to the provider's office, they are asked to fill out a **patient information form** that asks them to provide their identifying and contact information, including name, home and work addresses, phone numbers, email address, and Social Security number. Some questions about clinical issues, such as reason for visit, and administrative matters, such as insurance information, are included on the form as well. The Patient Demographics tool in the SCMO stores all of the information on three tabs: Patient, Guarantor, and Insurance (Fig. 1.4).

Billing and Insurance Information

It should be determined who is legally responsible (the guarantor) for the patient's account. If the patient is over the age of 18, he or she is most likely the guarantor. In the case of minors, it would be the patient's parent or guardian. It is important to obtain the guarantor's name, address, and date of birth.

The patient's health insurance card(s), if he or she is insured, should be reviewed at each visit and scanned into the system if different from the previous visit. Information found on the insurance card includes the type of medical insurance (for example, workers' compensation or Medicare), subscriber (person responsible for paying the premium) insurance carrier, claims submission address and phone number, policy and group numbers, and required copayment. A copayment is the amount of money a patient is contracted to pay out of pocket at each visit. Fig. 1.5 shows sample insurance cards.

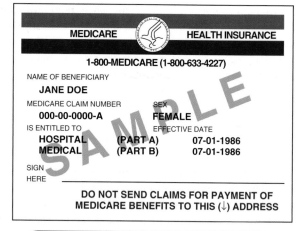

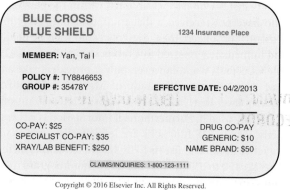

FIG. 1.5 Sample insurance cards. (**Top**, From Bonewit-West K: Today's medical assistant, ed 3, St. Louis, 2016, Elsevier.)

Appointment Scheduling

Patients who need to see a healthcare provider are usually asked to make an appointment—a specific time and date reserved to meet with the healthcare professional (physician, physician's assistant, or nurse practitioner). The healthcare professional will examine the patient and consult with him or her about the chief complaint. Depending on office policy, the patient may be scheduled in a variety of ways. The most common method of appointment scheduling is a fixed schedule, according to which the patient is asked to appear in the office at a specific date and time. Typical fixed appointments range from 10 to 20 minutes for acutely ill established patients to 1 hour for new-patient visits. An established patient is one who has been seen by a member of the healthcare team within the past 3 years. A new patient is one who has not been seen in the past 3 years by any member of the office. Electronic appointments integrated into the EHR allow quick search of available appointments, easy rescheduling, documentation of cancellations, and quick links to the patient's clinical record. (We talk more about these functions in Chapter 4)

Advanced Accounting Procedures

Patient accounting is important to the success of the healthcare practice. Accounting procedures performed by practice management software include creation and management of patient statements, generation of day sheets, and completion of insurance claims in the HIPAA 5010 claim format. An **account ledger** is a document that contains a responsible payer's name (guarantor), patient's identifying and contact information, services provided, payments made, insurance reimbursements received, account adjustments, and balance owed. A day sheet, or day journal, is a register of daily business transactions (Fig. 1.6). The day sheet is a system of checks and balances for the office as it prepares to make deposits into the bank. The account ledger and day sheet are both ways of documenting patients' financial information.

After the patient's financial information has been documented for the medical office, a claim must be submitted to a **third-party payer** if the patient is covered by a health insurance policy. A third-party payer is someone other than the patient, spouse, parent, or guardian who is responsible for paying all or part of the patient's medical expenses. In most cases, the third party is a health insurance company. HIPAA 5010 is a standard electronic format that speeds claims processing for physicians and suppliers (Fig. 1.7).

Most certified EHR systems can perform these functions. The billing functionality of the EHR is discussed in greater detail in Chapter 6.

ADVANTAGES OF ELECTRONIC HEALTH RECORDS #6 (main headings)

Improved Quality and Continuity of Care

With complete and immediate access to patient records, providers can provide better and faster treatment, raising the level of both medical care and personal attention from the healthcare team. With the integration of the EHR with outside facilities and the increased use of digital imaging, laboratory and diagnostic imaging results are made available much more quickly. Multiple providers and healthcare workers are able to access and view the EHR at one time, allowing for a more efficient workflow in all aspects of the medical office.

One of the most important ways in which an EHR can improve quality is by ensuring continuity of care. Contemporary healthcare—and the fast pace of modern life in general—requires complex patient histories to be documented quickly and accurately. Providers must be able to plan and coordinate care efficiently in order to ensure high quality of care and avoid duplication of services. To do so they must be able to communicate with each other promptly, without waiting for phone calls to be returned or copies to be made and faxed. Ideally, patients should be able to move from one physician to another—for a second opinion, for example—without having to visit or call physicians, hospitals, imaging centers, and labs to collect their records on paper or film.

Let's look at a few situations in which this kind of continuity is especially important.

Managing Patients with Chronic Conditions

First, continuity of care is critical when multiple specialists must plan and coordinate the treatment of a patient with a serious chronic condition like Parkinson's disease, hepatitis C, or prostate cancer. Specialists must be able to communicate laboratory findings, medications prescribed, operative notes, and other information within a hospital, assisted living center, hospice, or other healthcare setting. In addition, the patient's primary care provider must be able to track, organize, store, and retrieve the information so that the patient will receive competent follow-up when treatment ends. The physician will want to know, for instance, how many treatment cycles are planned, which tests have been performed, whether the patient has any new mobility restrictions, what medications have been prescribed, and whether the patient has experienced confusion, memory loss, sexual dysfunction, or other side effects.

Disaster Preparedness and Response

Continuity of care is also crucial for effective disaster preparedness and response. The advantage for an emergency department or field triage unit of gaining immediate access to a person's medical record is obvious. The more victims whose records can be accessed at or near the time and place of a disaster, the better. But the benefit of EHR systems extends beyond this immediate need. Electronic records are generally backed up by a secure web-based system and thus can be retrieved even when the computers at a medical practice or hospital are destroyed by fire, flood, or other means. In fact, more and more EHR systems are being offered completely over the Internet to their subscribers. In this respect, EHR systems are actually more durable than paper records. We learned much from Hurricane Katrina in 2005. Victims whose care had been received and documented electronically through the Veterans Health Administration (VA), for instance, received better, more timely care than those whose paper records were destroyed in the hurricane and its aftermath. The benefits of EHR systems continue to be seen

WALDEN-MARTIN
FAMILY MEDICAL CLINIC
1234 ANYSTREET | ANYTOWN, ANYSTATE 12345
PHONE 123-123-1234 | FAX 123-123-5678

Day Sheet - 09/21/2016 01:52 pm

				Column A	Column B	Column C	Column D	Column E
DATE	PATIENT NAME	PROVIDER	SERVICE	CHARGES	PAYMENT	ADJMT	NEW BALANCE	OLD BALANCE
09/21/2016	Ella Rainwater	-Select-	99212	$ 32.00	$ --	$ --	$ 32.00	$ --
09/21/2016	Robert Caudill	-Select-	82962	$ 32.00	$ --	$ --	$ 32.00	$ --
09/21/2016	Casey Hernandez	-Select-	99212	$ 32.00	$ 25.00	$ --	$ 7.00	$ --
09/21/2016	Casey Hernandez	-Select-	94640	$ 49.22	$ --	$ --	$ 56.22	$ 7.00
09/21/2016	Robert Caudill	-Select-	99213	$ 43.00	$ --	$ --	$ 43.00	$ --
			TOTALS:	$ 188.22	$ 25.00	$ 0.00	$ 170.22	$ 7.00

Daily Posting Proof	
Column E	$ 7.00
Plus Column A	$ 188.22
Subtotal	$ 195.22
Minus Column B	$ 25.00
Subtotal	$ 170.22
Minus Column C	$ 0.00
Equals Column D	$ 170.22

Accounts Receivable Proof	
Accts. Receivable Previous Day	$ 2300.00
Plus Column A	$ 188.22
Subtotal	$ 2488.22
Minus Column B	$ 25.00
Subtotal	$ 2463.22
Minus Column C	$ 0.00
Accts. Receivable End of Day	$ 2463.22

Deposit Proof	$ 25.00
Total receipts must equal total of payments (Column B).	

FIG. 1.6 SCMO Day Sheet.

in subsequent events as well. As part of the Hurricane Sandy preparation in 2012, hospitals were able to plan for patient care by contacting patients and having generators in place to operate their systems. Less valuable health information was lost because more records were being kept electronically. Reflection of these events has revealed three health IT must-haves during natural disasters: on-site safety, off-site data, and accessibility. All of these are possible with EHR systems.

Increased Efficiency

An EHR system makes patient information readily available to healthcare providers and support staff. Providers who use the EHR include physicians, nurse practitioners, physician's assistants, nurses, medical assistants, laboratory technicians, administrative assistants, medical records management personnel, medical coders, and medical billing specialists. Using the EHR saves time. Instead of hunting down a misfiled chart in a large

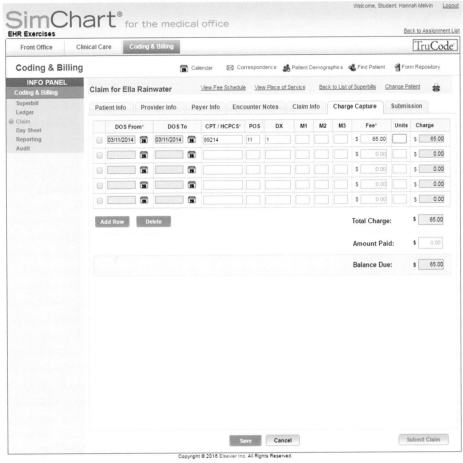

FIG. 1.7 SCMO HIPAA 5010

file room or conducting an archaeologic dig through the pile on Dr. Martin's desk, the EHR puts the patient record right at your fingertips. There are fewer paper reports and correspondence that need to be filed, and those that do come in will simply be scanned into the EHR. Time that was wasted in the past can now be used to perform other duties in the office. In addition, much less office space is required to store the records, providing extra space for examination rooms, offices, medical equipment, and other uses.

Improved Documentation

Documentation provides legal evidence of competent patient care and serves as an invaluable research tool. **Electronic transcription** using structured data entry (drop-down menus and automatic sentence builders) eliminates the need for handwritten notes, which tend to be riddled with errors (Fig. 1.8). These structured data entry tools allow the provider or other documenter to select from preconstructed options (templates) or choices within a record or document. By stringing these choices together, progress notes, letters, medication lists, and other documentation can be accomplished electronically. Forcing the documenter to use selected choices within the screen's template eliminates the need to free-key the work and can be used more easily when working with mobile devices.

This form of data entry essentially eliminates illegible handwriting and incomplete notes. Illegible handwriting can lead to errors in reporting, diagnosis, treatment, and billing procedures. However, in earlier EMR systems, using this tool was sometimes more time consuming than documenting on paper. One physician found that it took more than a minute and a half and 17 clicks on yes/no and drop-down menu choices to document one patient's back pain diagnosis. Yet it took just 41 seconds to handwrite his documentation for the same diagnosis into the patient's paper chart. Certified EHR systems have recognized this inconvenience and worked to make documentation more user friendly.

The EHR also can link records electronically. This is useful in patient education, allowing providers to compare test results or graph a comparison of patient weight and blood pressure.

Electronic documentation reduces data entry errors and helps ensure a complete patient record. Documentation that is clear, complete, accurate, and legible is extremely important to the success of the EHR and to the medical practice.

Why Document Properly?

1. To facilitate communication among healthcare providers.
2. To avoid delay of reimbursement or denial of claims because medical necessity of services provided has not been proved.

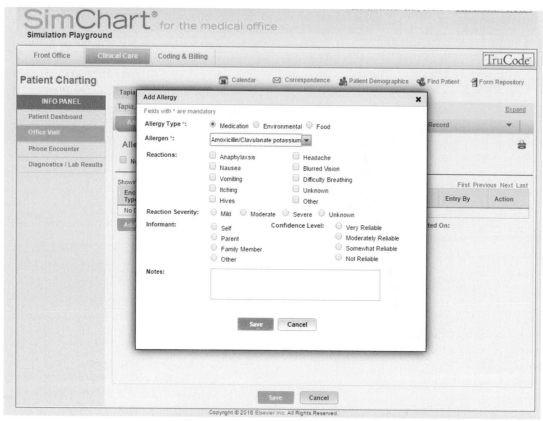

FIG. 1.8 SCMO Add Allergy Screen

3. To comply with insurance companies' and accreditation companies' enforcement of documentation guidelines for healthcare facilities.
4. To aid the work of investigators and regulators when legal issues arise, including subpoenas of medical records in court cases and state investigations.
5. To protect the practice in case a malpractice suit is brought.
6. To establish evidence of care.

Easier Accessibility at the Point of Care

The EHR is intended to make patient information more accessible to healthcare providers. The availability of the EHR is limited only by privacy and security measures. As we know, patients don't get sick only during regular office hours. An injured or acutely ill patient may present to the emergency department at 3 AM. The availability of an interconnected EHR allows the medical team to access the patient's health history immediately. Having the entire health record at their fingertips gives medical personnel a broad, accurate picture of the patient's health status and decreases delays in initiating care.

Better Security

User names and passwords increase security and allow only authorized individuals to access patient medical records. The system administrator will determine how much access a user has. A physician is going to have much more access to the EHR than an appointment scheduler. That access is attached to the user name. Passwords are used to allow access to the EHR system.

HIPAA requires that users change their passwords periodically. It is very important to keep your user name and password private so that no one else can log in as you. Tracking or **auditing** user access reveals a history, like a trail of breadcrumbs, of who has accessed the record, what users have viewed, and who modified any given patient record. Auditing is usually performed by a member of office management and can be done to determine whether an employee has accessed information inappropriately. Violating a patient's privacy is illegal under HIPAA and is grounds for immediate termination of employment.

Reduced Expenses

As discussed earlier, an EHR system eliminates the need for most transcription, which can cost an office thousands of dollars each year. Records are stored electronically, dramatically reducing the need for paper storage facilities. Using an EHR system also reduces duplication of services, such as tests that have already been performed at another facility. Using CDS functionality, EHR systems can also flag any tests ordered that might be unnecessary given the patient's diagnosis and clinical data.

Improved Job Satisfaction

Once an EHR system has been adopted and fully implemented within an office, most say they would never go back to paper. A 2012 EHR user satisfaction survey conducted by the American Academy of Family Physicians reported that 75% of physician users were happy with their EHR system (total sample size of 3088).

Providers

Those directly involved in patient care, such as physicians and nurse practitioners, feel more confident that they are delivering high-quality care after an EHR system is implemented. For example, if a drug is recalled from the market, every patient in the practice to whom that drug has been prescribed can be identified by executing a simple computer search that takes just seconds. The patients can then be quickly notified, and either a prescription for a substitute drug can be called in to the patient's pharmacy (whose phone number is listed in the EHR), or an appointment can be scheduled. In fact, the VA used clinical data, such as laboratory values, stored in patients' EHR systems to identify chronic kidney disease in one-third of those with diabetes even though they had no symptoms. Small practices can conduct this kind of analysis on a smaller scale. They can also deliver better quality at the point of care.

A survey of Massachusetts physicians showed that those whose practices had adopted EHR systems were less likely to feel demoralized about the state of the medical profession, reported significantly more positive views about how computers might affect healthcare quality, and were far more likely to believe that computers have a positive effect on communication with their patients.

Staff

Support staff, too, feel better able to manage a busy practice when an EHR system is in place. The software provides neat, standardized forms on which to record phone messages and transmit them to providers. A logical, built-in workflow allows prescription refills to be handled safely and efficiently. Laboratory reports, results of imaging studies, and similar data are handled in a consistent fashion. Letters to patients can be expedited using customizable templates. Staff members say they spend less time chasing charts, clarifying prescription orders for pharmacies, and performing billing, coding, and transcription tasks. Communication with providers requires fewer interruptions during patient appointments, which makes everyone happier—including the patients.

Improved Patient Satisfaction

Patients appreciate the increased efficiency an EHR system offers. A 2013 survey by the Employee Benefits Research Institute revealed that 82% of Americans say they believe they receive better quality of care from a provider who uses EHRs. When the medical office uses an EHR system, patients tend to have greater confidence that their messages will be returned quickly and that their call-in prescriptions will be refilled promptly. Patients appreciate having access to their health information via a patient portal, ease of appointment scheduling, and receiving test results. Office visits are more productive because the provider can access the data he or she needs just by tapping on the screen of a tablet PC. The provider no longer has to retrieve a file or book to look up dosages and no longer has to thumb through the patient's chart looking for stray information.

A study by Johnson and colleagues concluded that computerized documentation had a positive effect on interaction between providers and parents during pediatric visits. In particular, providers using EHR systems posed more open-ended questions and had a conversational style that was more patient centered than that of providers who were not using electronic documentation. A study by Ventres and colleagues found that patients as well as providers liked EHR systems that can be displayed on a flat-screen computer monitor with a mobile arm, so that providers can discuss the information in the patient's own charts. Most providers preferred to alternate between entering data and interviewing the patient, creating a collaborative provider-patient-computer interaction. The authors of the study observed that the EHR becomes a reliable "third party" in the provider-patient conversation.

DISADVANTAGES OF ELECTRONIC HEALTH RECORDS

Of course, any technologic advance comes with a downside, and EHR systems are no exception. Let's take a look at some of the kinks that still need to be worked out, as well as some disadvantages of EHR systems that are likely to remain permanently.

Lack of Interoperability

Compatibility standards have not yet been universally applied to ensure that systems can interact with, or "talk to," one another. This capability is known as interoperability. The concept is similar to the interoperability of some computer operating systems and is one of the core functions of certified electronic health record technology. Certified EHR systems are compatible with specific laboratory, pharmacy, and hospital networks. However, not all EHR systems are compatible with one another. When information is received in an incompatible format, it must be hand-keyed into the record, or the appropriate template must be filled out. One small practice found that it took 13 mouse clicks just to enter mammography data for one patient.

This lack of uniformity has become a real dilemma both for individual patients and for the U.S. healthcare system as a whole. If a hospital uses a different EHR system from that of a patient's primary care provider, the patient's health records may not be available to the hospital, or vice versa. Let's say a patient experiences a bowel perforation. Emergency personnel at the trauma center request a list of medications from the patient's provider. The list has to be faxed to the trauma center and then keyed in to the patient's record there because the provider's EHR system can't communicate with the hospital's EHR interface. As the patient is treated, his or her operative summary, progress notes, radiographs, and psychiatric consultation reports must be snail-mailed to his or her primary care provider.

As you can see, EHR systems reduce paperwork within an office, but until they become interoperable, communication among various treating healthcare providers, pharmacies, and allied healthcare workers will be limited. The healthcare system must solve the interoperability problem because it increases costs, decreases efficiency, introduces opportunities for error (when information is rekeyed), and discourages small providers from adopting EHR systems.

Cost

One of the chief barriers to adopting an EHR system is the steep start-up cost in terms of both time and money. Nearly 70% of all interactions between physicians and patients occur in practices that have four physicians or fewer. These practices are small businesses that, just like any other, must control costs, weigh the benefits of capital investment (such as an EHR system), and decide how staff time will be spent.

Financial Investment

The medical office must buy the software system or subscribe to an EHR vendor to record and store patient charts. The cost of EHR implementation depends on the type of system being used. A recent survey shows that healthcare organizations can expect to spend up to $70,000 per provider. Customizing the EHR for a particular medical office is very costly. In addition, hardware upgrades may be necessary to accommodate the new software.

The cost of these investments is borne by the practice, yet insurance companies and other third parties may benefit most from the upgrades. Grants and incentives may be available to offset the cost. The Meaningful Use legislation offers federal incentives to providers who use EHRs in specified meaningful ways. Disincentives to remain with paper charting have entered the mix, too. By federal law, a reimbursement penalty of 1% to 5% is in place for providers who do not successfully demonstrate meaningful use of an EHR for their Medicare patients.

Many providers are concerned that they could purchase one system, only to have it become obsolete if another platform becomes the standard. It is important for providers to purchase only EHR systems listed on the Certified Health IT Product List (CHPL). Many practices have been waiting for the bugs to be worked out and for interconnectivity to improve. However, publication of the CHPL seems to have been a tipping point, after which the conversion to EHR systems began to gather momentum. Those who had been wavering apparently have begun to feel more secure about making the investment and are being required to do so to maintain current reimbursement levels.

Time

Additional costs include the expense of lost productivity while staff members are training instead of doing their normal jobs and the price of paying for the training sessions, although the latter are often provided free by the software company as a purchasing incentive. Finally, converting all charts to the electronic format is costly and time consuming because it takes staff away from their normal jobs and limits the number of patients who can be seen during the transition. All information in a patient's paper chart must be entered into the EHR before the electronic system can be used for that patient. Depending on whether a phased implementation is used, this process can divert resources from patient care and office support functions for weeks or even months.

Employee Resistance

Employees who have been part of the medical office for an extended time may resist the conversion to an EHR. They may be concerned that the EHR is difficult to use and may not be familiar with computer technology. Providers may feel as if they are doing "busywork" that they used to be able to delegate to staff. Those who plan to retire within 5 or 10 years will endure all the pain of the transition but have many fewer years during which to gain from the system's implementation.

The EHR changes the way the administrative and clinic processes are done in the office. Job responsibilities and duties often need to be modified. For example, the role of the file clerk changes dramatically. No longer will this staff member have to pull charts or file documents. Everything is done digitally. Perhaps this person will take on new duties, such as importing documents from other providers and facilities or focusing on maintenance of the EHR system.

The medical staff, including physicians, will have to take additional steps and time to ensure that proper documentation is done. This can distract EHR users from patient care as they try to learn the new technology.

EASING THE TRANSITION 1.2   Generation Gap: Training the Office "Dinosaur"

Your practice has finally decided to adopt an EHR system, and everyone in your practice is pumped with excitement about making the switch—well, nearly everyone. One of the senior physicians, Dr. Crabtree, refuses to take part, insisting that he'll continue to maintain paper records for his patients.

This scenario is familiar in just about every office that has exchanged paper charting for the great unknown of electronic records. In fact, businesses of all kinds are faced with the problem of workers who are uncomfortable using new technology. Some of these late adopters seem to take a certain pride in remaining "dinosaurs." But does adopting an EHR system have to lead to generational skirmishes, with seniors on one side and everyone else on the other?

The term "computer literacy"—which is really too vague to be useful—has given way to the idea of "networked workers." A networked or wired worker is likely to take advantage of electronic devices, such as cell phones, laptop computers, and tablet PCs, both at home and at work. According to data from the Pew Internet and American Life project, 86% of American workers use the Internet or email at least occasionally. Nearly half of all employed Americans have worked from home using a computer. But only about half of working adults ages 60 to 69 go online. (This proportion is growing, but only because aging Baby Boomers, who tend to be avid networked workers, are entering the 60+ age group.)

Older healthcare personnel—physicians, nurses, and office workers alike—may perceive computerized health records systems as complex, inflexible, or even unnecessary. They may have heard horror stories from their adult children and others about having their hard drives wiped out or becoming the victims of phishing scams. Researchers at Fidelity Investments have coined the term "cautious clickers" to describe the computer behavior of older generations. They move from screen to screen with extreme hesitation, fearing that one false click will crash the system or that they won't remember how to get back to where they were. They linger over instructions and become frustrated trying to scroll and navigate windows and screens.

So how can the networked workers bring the late adopters on board? Here are a few tips on winning over the Dr. Crabtree in your office:

1. Avoid teasing your reluctant convert. The person may already feel left out or be embarrassed by a lack of computer skills, and rubbing it in won't help. Offer a separate training session for employees with varied levels of computer comfort.

2. Remind Dr. Crabtree how much he relies on older technologies that were once considered cutting edge—calculators, cell phones, and medical imaging devices such as MRI machines, for instance.

Continued

EASING THE TRANSITION 1.2 **Generation Gap: Training the Office "Dinosaur"—cont'd**

3. Appeal to Dr. Crabtree's sense of fairness and teamwork. If he refuses to use the technology, others will have to take up the slack. And besides, using the EHR system makes it easier for other physicians to cover for him when he is out of the office.

4. Offer to provide additional training as he learns to use the system. If possible, have someone who knows the software shadow him for a couple of days—or longer—to mentor him as he gets his feet wet. Reassure him that he can come on in—the water's fine!

5. Explain how an EHR system can enhance the quality of patient care with CDS tools by sending automatic cancer screening reminders, matching cardiac patients with American Heart Association treatment protocols, and so on. With patients' permission, let Dr. Crabtree observe another physician to see how EHR systems can be displayed on-screen and used as a partner, of sorts, during consultations.

6. Keep your language simple, and avoid using acronyms, abbreviations, and computer terminology that might confuse him. For example, don't assume Dr. Crabtree knows what it means to IM, to download an image, or to execute a search. Remember that he probably won't understand what things like drop-down menus and dialog boxes are.

7. Figure out what motivates your unwired colleague and appeal to his self-interest. For example, if Dr. Crabtree often stays late at the office, show him how the EHR system will allow him to work from home. If he has 11 grandchildren, remind him how easy it will be to stay in touch with them once he learns to use email and share files. Computer skills are transferable, after all!

8. Above all, be patient! The Fidelity researchers found that it takes people older than age 55 nearly 50% longer than their younger counterparts to complete a given computer task. It's likely that any of us would have the same hesitation and apprehension if we'd been born a few decades earlier. A little genuine understanding goes a long way.

Regimentation

The standardization built in to almost any computer program cannot accommodate idiosyncrasies. Providers who formerly had different ways of handling their charting must suddenly adapt to a regimented system that pigeonholes tasks. Despite evidence indicating potential improvements in quality of care, some providers complain that EHR systems rely too heavily on check boxes and quantitative data rather than on descriptive terms and narrative. They believe that the need to standardize documentation takes the art out of the science of medicine.

One older internist, referring to the electronically prepared reports he receives from other providers, lamented the lack of any evidence of the provider's reasoning or the patient's emotions, saying that the templates produce "a skeleton of data without the meat." This concern was echoed by participants in a study by Ventres and colleagues. They worried that EHR notes lack narrative depth, creating "cookie cutter" charts and forcing them to practice "cookbook medicine." However, other providers who took part in the study noted that the built-in clinical protocols gave them a quick and effective way to apply evidence-based algorithms to individual patients. Perhaps as systems evolve and as providers adapt to using them, EHR interfaces will offer more opportunities to enter descriptive data, and providers will be more willing to take advantage of these features.

CRITICAL THINKING EXERCISE 1.3

Dr. Gregorio is in practice with his daughter, a new physician, who is urging him to make the switch from paper to electronic records. The elder Dr. Gregorio believes his modest practice is too small to require such a system. Besides, he argues, his patients find it reassuring to see him take notes on paper. The younger Dr. Gregorio thinks it's her father, not his patients, who are reluctant to change. How could you encourage the two Dr. Gregorios to purchase an EHR system? What do you think would be the pros and cons of purchasing the system for a small practice?

Security Gaps

With the implementation of HIPAA, interest in protecting patient security and privacy has been heightened. A patient's medical records must remain confidential. However, it may be possible for individuals to penetrate EHR systems despite security precautions and then sell, release, or change confidential information. This has some patients worried about how safe and confidential their electronic medical records really are. Security standards are outlined by HIPAA and the Health Information Technology for Economic and Clinical Health (HITECH) Act; both work to streamline methods of implementation. Power outages, viruses, backup procedures, and computer freezes and crashes pose other safety and security concerns for medical offices using EHR systems. System security is one important step to proving compliance with the Meaningful Use program, and providers must prove that standard and compliance programs are in place (see Chapter 3).

SECURITY CHECKPOINT 1.1 **Celebrity Health Records Become Tabloid Fodder: Should You Care?**

Checkout-line tabloids are willing to pay big bucks to snoop into celebrities' personal lives, and their health records have become more vulnerable now that they can often be accessed electronically on the networks of healthcare institutions that employ thousands of people. The health records of Britney Spears, George Clooney, Maria Shriver, Tom Cruise, Brad Pitt, and Michael Jackson have allegedly been subject to recent privacy invasions. Spears's records, for instance, may have been viewed without her consent when she gave birth to her first child and when she was hospitalized for a psychiatric evaluation. In 2013 six Cedars-Sinai Medical Center employees were fired for inappropriately accessing the patient record of Kim Kardashian's stay while giving birth to her daughter.

To avoid such situations, celebrities often check in to the hospital using aliases. However, Spears's own name was reportedly restored on her file when she left the hospital, apparently in an effort to keep her health information in one record. Other high-profile people, such as politicians, check in under aliases as well. Even so, employees at New York-Presbyterian Hospital allegedly tried to gain unauthorized access to Bill Clinton's health records when he had cardiac surgery in 2004. The records of crime victims whose names have been in the news also have been viewed improperly.

In all of these cases the hackers or would-be hackers are on the inside. They are people with legitimate access to the institution's computer system and perhaps to certain patients' records, but not to the records of the VIPs whose records they're trying to peek at. In 2008 a former employee of UCLA Medical Center was indicted for selling confidential health information in exchange for a mere $4600. The hospital discovered that at least 31 celebrities' records had been accessed without authorization, and at least a dozen employees have

Continued

SECURITY CHECKPOINT 1.1   Celebrity Health Records Become Tabloid Fodder: Should You Care?—cont'd

been fired for letting curiosity or greed get the better of them. These breaches are prohibited by HIPAA, a law intended to protect the privacy of all patients in the United States. Civil and criminal penalties can be imposed for violating the law.

High-profile patients have just as much right to medical privacy as the rest of us, but why should we be concerned?

Every time another well-publicized privacy breach occurs, we lose a little more confidence that our own records are safe from prying eyes. According to a 2013 Health Information Trends Survey, 12.3% of us admit to having withheld information from our physicians for fear it will end up on TMZ someday—or at least in the hands of a nosy coworker, neighbor, or relative. This percentage is higher among those who are in worse health, and when our physicians don't have a complete picture of our health status, the care they're able to provide suffers.

The lack of widely available and interoperable electronic records, in turn, hampers public health surveillance of diseases such as cancer, hepatitis, and influenza. (Researchers are exempt from HIPAA and may access patients' health information as long as their identities are kept confidential.) Such monitoring is important because it allows agencies like the CDC to spot patterns, such as an increase in the incidence of tuberculosis. It was just such public health surveillance that helped scientists recognize HIV/AIDS as a new disease in the early 1980s. If electronic records had been available then, it's likely the pattern would have emerged sooner, spurring prevention efforts and research into treatments.

In addition, researchers use EHR systems to find and recruit participants for clinical trials. For example, a researcher might search an EHR database to determine how many men ages 25 to 34 use chewing tobacco. The researcher can then ask each patient's provider to notify him that he is eligible for the study. An EHR system can even be customized so that when he visits his provider, every man in the correct age range is asked about his use of smokeless tobacco. Researchers can also cross-check chewing tobacco use against clinical data recorded in the EHR, such as blood pressure, to look for an association between tobacco use and high blood pressure.

These are just some of the ways in which EHR systems improve public health. For you as an individual patient, having an EHR promotes your health in a host of ways. For example, you're less likely to suffer an adverse drug reaction due to a drug dosage error when your provider is prescribing medications electronically. However, media hype about high-profile privacy violations tends to get us all wondering who might want to take a gander at our records—and that's bad news for everyone's health.

ROLE OF THE HEALTHCARE PROFESSIONAL USING THE ELECTRONIC HEALTH RECORD

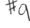
#9

The EHR has many users within the healthcare environment and will have an effect on all areas of the medical office. Physicians, nurses, physician's assistants, medical assistants, and medical coders and billers all must use or be exposed to the EHR. Although learning new software may be difficult and time consuming, it is important to keep patient care front and center at all times. Having certain basic skills can help you use an EHR effectively:

- **A working knowledge of medical terminology and anatomy and physiology.** The healthcare staff is responsible for documenting the patient's health history and status. Proper documentation of the patient's medical care is much easier

for those who are familiar with medical terminology and have a solid grasp of how the body works. The EHR user also has to interpret information already documented in the patient chart, and many providers use an alphabet soup of medical abbreviations. Therefore, the ability to decipher medical information will continue to be one of the main job duties of the healthcare staff.

- **Basic typing and computer skills.** Ventres and colleagues found that the ability to type was crucial to effective use of the EHR system. The providers in this study also noted that the ability to type is key to limiting transcription costs in their practices. Although free text writing is not the primary method of documentation within the patient medical record, some narrative data entry is required. The ability to type also eases navigation through the system.

- **Organizational skills.** The physician's office is busy and hectic most of the day. Patients are coming in and out of the office, the telephone is constantly ringing, and the stack of "to-do's" piles up on the desk. It's important for the healthcare staff to remain calm and properly manage their time and responsibilities. The EHR can help organize an office by keeping all of the patient data in one place, but it also takes time and work to keep the records updated. Strong organizational skills are required to ensure patients' care and office workflow are managed effectively on busy days.

- **Interpersonal skills.** The genuine desire to work with people is a requirement for anyone in the medical field. The healthcare staff should always demonstrate a positive, warm, caring attitude toward their patients and coworkers. These skills include maintaining eye contact during communication, speaking slowly and clearly, and listening carefully. All staff members must show respect at all times during patient encounters and with one another. It is important to remember that navigating an EHR is a learning process for everyone, and not all individuals will catch on at the same time. Patience and a helpful personality are the key to keeping staff morale at its highest.

Duties and Workflow

The modern healthcare worker must possess basic skills and attributes when using the EHR. Many medical care facilities may require or prefer their employees to be cross-trained in various areas of the medical office. *Cross-training* means being able to perform more than one duty or skill across various task areas. Cross-training is especially helpful in a healthcare environment when a coworker calls in sick or is otherwise unable to perform his or her typical duties. Along with cross-training, the healthcare provider should demonstrate flexibility and the ability to multitask. The implementation of new EHR software takes time and patience. The healthcare worker may become frustrated with the additional work and new way of performing daily tasks, but must remember to keep the patients' care the top priority.

#10

Administrative

The adoption of an EHR system affects many of the administrative duties within the medical office. Medical office personnel will need to adapt to these changes to ensure a smooth transition from paper-based records to EHR systems. The EHR is purchased in a generic format and must be customized to fit a given office. Doing so represents a large chunk of the administrative work in a medical office. Some of the other administrative tasks include:

- Reception (front office) duties
- Appointment scheduling
- Electronic chart creation
- Inactive chart purging
- Gathering and entering patient information
- Creating patient correspondence
- Maintaining email communications
- Providing patient instructions
- Coordinating patient care (including setting up patient referrals, treatments, procedures)

Clinical

The EHR is a great way to coordinate a patient's care and to document the record of treatment. The EHR can be customized to ensure that all components of the patient visit are well documented. As discussed, some of the clinical information that may be documented using the EHR includes patient history, vital signs, progress notes, laboratory requisitions, prescriptions, and test results.

Billing and Coding

Fully integrated EHR and practice management systems allow the user to review the clinical documentation while preparing claims for submission. Data from patient demographics and the Superbill are populated into the insurance claim. The EHR aids in billing and coding tasks in the following ways:

- Submission of Superbills/encounter forms
- Creation of billing statements
- Assignment of procedural and diagnostic codes
- Linking of procedural and diagnostic codes for reimbursement
- Auditing
- Organizing office finance (day sheets, deposit slips, and patient account ledgers)
- Generating prior authorization forms
- Monitoring the submission and follow-up of claims (insurance claim tracers)

PROFESSIONAL ORGANIZATIONS

Learning should be lifelong, especially in a constantly changing environment like healthcare. Current healthcare trends, like the International Classification of Diseases (ICD) 10, HIPAA policy, and patient engagement, are a main focus of professional organizations to help their members be skillfully competent in their job duties. Depending on your chosen field, you will want to become a member of one or more professional organizations. Many professional organizations offer discounted student memberships. All of the professional organizations listed here have one thing in common: They all aim to provide an up-to-date, informed approach to healthcare. These organizations have a wide variety of membership benefits, including the following:

- Offer certification examinations at a discounted rate
- Provide a wide range of continuing education unit (CEU) opportunities
- Provide a forum for networking with other professionals in your field of study
- Publish newsletters and magazines dealing with current issues and trends in healthcare
- Offer discounts on publications
- Sponsor conferences, workshops, and web-based activities

With the advent of EHR systems, professional organizations are focusing on helping members adapt to the new technology and on research regarding its implementation in their medical offices. Professional publications such as the *Journal of AHIMA,* published by the American Health Information Management Association; *Healthcare Business Monthly,* published by the American Academy of Professional Coders; and *CMA Today,* offered by the American Association of Medical Assistants (AAMA) regularly include articles and links related to the development and use and evaluation of EHR systems.

American Health Information Management Association

The American Health Information Management Association (AHIMA) is the leading professional organization made up of health information management (HIM) professionals. AHIMA has more than 71,000 members who are dedicated to the effective management of personal health information. Originally established in 1928 as the American Association of Record Librarians, AHIMA works to improve the quality of medical records for the diagnosis and treatment of health conditions. This professional organization is committed to advancing the HIM profession in critical topics such as privacy and security, medical coding, EHR systems, reimbursement, and compliance. AHIMA continues to develop new opportunities in an increasingly electronic and global environment through leadership in advocacy, education, certification, and lifelong learning. For more information, go to www.ahima.org.

American Academy of Professional Coders

The American Academy of Professional Coders (AAPC) was founded in 1988 in an effort to elevate the standards of medical coding by providing certification, ongoing education, networking, and recognition. The AAPC has a membership base of 126,000 worldwide. AAPC certifications focus on a variety of disciplines. These disciplines encompass the physician's office, represented by the Certified Professional Coder (CPC); the hospital outpatient facility, represented by the Certified Professional Coder–Hospital (CPC-H); and payer perspective coding, represented by the Certified Professional Coder–Payer (CPC-P). Specialty credentials are offered in evaluation and management, auditing, general surgery, obstetrics and gynecology, emergency medicine, and cardiology. The AAPC offers continuing education through local chapters, workshops, a monthly newsmagazine (*Healthcare Business Monthly*), publications, and conferences. More information can be found at www.aapc.com.

American Association of Medical Assistants

The American Association of Medical Assistants (AAMA) is a professional organization for medical assistants searching for professional development, continuing education, approved programs, and certification information. The AAMA is vital to the accreditation process of medical assistant training programs and publishes a bimonthly journal called *CMA Today*. As far back as 2007, the Occupational Analysis of the CMA AAMA identified the use of computers and electronic equipment in the medical office as one of its key competencies. This skill is only becoming more and more important. You can further search the AAMA at www.aama-ntl.org.

American Medical Technologists

The American Medical Technologists (AMT) is a nonprofit certification agency and professional membership association representing more than 60,000 individuals in allied healthcare. Established in 1939, AMT provides allied health professionals with professional certification services and membership programs to enhance their professional and personal growth. The AMT publishes *AMT Events,* a quarterly magazine offering educational articles and professional development opportunities. For more information regarding the registered medical technologist, go to www.americanmedtech.org.

CHAPTER SUMMARY

- Patient health records were used as early as 200 BCE to document treatment of patients and to record signs and symptoms of illness. These records serve as important tools for research and have been traditionally paper-based records. Emerging technology is moving these documents into a digital form.
- The patient health record is a collection of an individual's healthcare information. It includes both patient information (demographics and insurance information) and clinical data (immunization records, operative reports, office notes, and so on). In addition, the patient medical record can be an important resource in legal actions and financial reimbursement matters. Attention must be paid to ensure the patient medical record is accurately maintained by all healthcare staff.
- Documentation is the process of recording data about a patient's health history and status or about the chronologic record that results from such data entry. Taken together, it is a legal document and a key component of an EHR. Documentation may include clinical observations and progress notes, diagnoses of illnesses and injuries, plans of care, patient education and self-care instructions given, vital signs taken, physical assessment findings, laboratory and imaging test results, medical treatments prescribed or administered, surgeries performed, and outcomes.
- The patient medical record or patient chart is the property of its creator. For example, if a physician's office creates the patient medical record, the record itself is the property of the physician's office. Control of the information within the medical record belongs to the patient. A patient may request a copy of his or her medical record or view its contents by signing a release.
- The Meaningful Use incentive program has greatly influenced the adoption of EHRs. The main goals of the MU program are: improve quality, safety, and efficiency and reduce health disparities; engage patients and family; improve care coordination and population and public health; and maintain privacy and security of patient health information. This is being accomplished in three stages and involves 10 objectives and measures.

- Basic functions of EHR software include documentation using electronic transcription, provider review of incoming laboratory data and reports, electronic prescribing, transcription, and automatically generated clinical flags and reminders. Clinical decision support is an advanced feature of EHR software. This function comprises a set of tools that can improve patient safety, ensure that care conforms to established clinical guidelines for specific conditions, and reduce unnecessary care, duplicated services, and their associated costs.
- Practice management software is used for administrative duties in the medical office and is commonly an integrated part of the EHR. It can be used to enter patient demographics and insurance information, schedule appointments, and perform advanced accounting functions.
- The advantages of using an EHR system include improved quality and continuity of care, increased efficiency, improved documentation, easier point-of-care accessibility, better security, reduced expenses, improved job satisfaction for providers and staff, and improved patient satisfaction.
- The disadvantages of using an EHR system include lack of interoperability, a high cost of initial investment in time and money, resistance from some employees, regimentation as a result of using standardized templates to document patient care, and security gaps attributable to the electronic availability of confidential patient information.
- Factors such as length of response time and ease of correcting mistakes influence a practice's adoption of EHR systems.
- The roles of healthcare professionals change with the implementation of the EHR. Administrative, coding, billing, and clinical duties must all be refined to ensure a smooth transition from paper-based to electronic records systems.
- Membership and active involvement in professional organizations promote the use of EHR systems and broaden opportunities for valuable continuing education.

CHAPTER REVIEW ACTIVITIES

Key Terms Review
Match the following key terms with their definitions.

1. CPOE
2. Electronic transcription
3. Copayment
4. Interoperability
5. Ledger
6. Chief complaint
7. Structured data entry
8. HIPAA 5010
9. Day sheet
10. Practice management software

a. The ability of electronic systems to share information in compatible formats

b. The patient's stated primary reason for seeking treatment

c. Screen that contains the amount owed and other billing details

d. An EHR function that facilitates automated prescribing

e. A fixed sum of money usually paid at the time medical services are rendered

f. An electronic format that speeds the claims process for physicians and suppliers

g. A register of business transactions for a single day

h. Data entry using structured data entry or voice recognition

i. Documentation that utilizes drop-down menus, radio buttons, and sentence builders

j. Used for administrative tasks such as appointment scheduling and billing

True/False
Indicate whether the statement is true or false.

1. _____ An audit is performed by the office manager to investigate whether appropriate employees have viewed the contents of a high-profile patient's chart.
2. _____ The medical record contains legal documents but is not itself a legal document.
3. _____ The medical assistant's typical duties will be modified with the implementation of the EHR.
4. _____ Clinical decision support tools are effective only if the provider chooses to use them.
5. _____ An EHR system can help the provider and medical staff plan and coordinate care for a patient with a chronic illness.
6. _____ Automated sentence building is a means of electronic transcription.
7. _____ Reduced productivity is to be expected for a period of time during the conversion to an EHR system.
8. _____ Communication among various treating healthcare providers, pharmacies, and allied healthcare workers will be limited until EHR interoperability has been achieved.
9. _____ It is possible for individuals to penetrate EHR systems despite security precautions.
10. _____ EHR systems make it unnecessary for office staff to be familiar with medical terminology.
11. _____ Most EHR systems hold the ability to handle clinical and administrative functions without purchasing separate practice management software.
12. _____ Professional organizations offer continuing education for the core skills of their discipline and do not have any opportunities for learning about the EHR.

Workplace Applications
1. Jamie is considering becoming a member of a professional organization but is unsure of the benefits. He's a new medical assistant in a practice with five physicians, and he hopes to become the office manager at a larger practice someday. To which professional organization should Jamie belong? What services does this organization provide that will help Jamie achieve his goals?
2. Kathy works for a pediatrician's office that is beginning the EHR implementation process. She has been asked to research the different systems available and general start-up cost. Create a list of functions the EHR should have specific to the practice's large pediatric office. What are the general start-up costs of EHR systems?
3. During an EHR training session you are leading for staff, one of the members states that she is upset with the new EHR requirements and the changes to her job duties. How can you ease her fears and help her understand the need for EHRs?

2

Overview of SimChart for the Medical Office

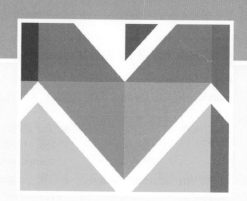

CHAPTER OBJECTIVES

1. Describe the medical assistant's role in promoting electronic health records.
2. Find and use the Student Resources available for SimChart for the Medical Office.
3. Understand how to view and submit assignments in SimChart for the Medical Office.
4. Access the SimChart for the Medical Office Simulation Playground and navigate across modules.
5. Identify common buttons and other recurring elements in SimChart for the Medical Office.
6. Explain the difference between active and closed records.
7. Create new patient records in SimChart for the Medical Office.
8. Discuss the appropriate use of the Internet in the physician's office.

KEY TERMS

active patient An established patient who has seen the provider or another provider in the billing group within the past 3 years.

button An element of the user interface on which the user can click to execute a command, such as save, confirm, cancel, or exit.

check box A specialized type of button that toggles on (checked) and off (unchecked). Check boxes are often used when more than one response might be appropriate (as in "Check all that apply"), but sometimes they should be interpreted to mean yes or no (as in a check box next to the caption "OK to mail?").

closed patient record The record of a patient who will not be returning to the medical office or who has not been seen in the past 10 years.

default A preselected value or setting that will be used unless the user specifies a substitute by overriding the preselected choice.

field Space allocated on a form for specific numeric or text data.

inactive patient An established patient who has not seen the provider or another provider in the billing group for 3 or more years.

radio button A specialized type of button on a software interface that toggles on (round button visible) and off (blank circle). Radio buttons tell the user that only one response is appropriate because two radio buttons can't be depressed at the same time.

retention period The amount of time patient records must, by law, be maintained by the medical office.

THE MEDICAL PRACTICE GOES DIGITAL

According to the U.S. Department of Labor, electronic health record (EHR) systems are good for business—at least when it comes to medical assisting. As standards of interoperability have been adopted and financial incentives for EHR use have become more attractive, adoption of EHR systems has reached a tipping point. The major accrediting bodies for medical assistant programs are requiring that students learn and use EHRs as part of the curriculum. This has helped make medical assisting one of the fastest-growing professions in the United States.

According to the 2015 Medical Assisting Compensation and Benefits Report of 8112 respondents, 64% of medical assistants work in primary care practice, while another 30% work with medical or surgical specialty offices. Tech-savvy medical assistants are in great demand, often commanding higher salaries and landing positions in the most desirable practices.

As EHRs have become more common in physicians' offices, healthcare personnel have come to appreciate its potential to streamline office management and improve patient care (Box 2.1). A comprehensive EHR can be used to schedule patients, establish and maintain health records, ensure continuity of care, improve communication, document clinical work, and perform billing and coding functions. Medical assistants are in the unique situation of being trained in all aspects of the medical office. This means that medical assistants should be proficient in all aspects of the EHR. If you're just getting your feet wet, don't worry—you have plenty of time to learn. The Glossary for Computer Novices located at the end of this chapter is a great place to start.

In this chapter we will be taking a look at the basics of EHR systems. Although you'll be using SimChart for the Medical Office (SCMO), you won't be wasting your time if you end up working in an office that uses a different software application. Using SCMO is sort of like familiarizing yourself with the controls of a vehicle—once you have that experience under your belt, you will feel comfortable behind the wheel of any car.

SCMO simulates the real-life application of the EHR. It is a primary care office with multiple providers. You will also get to know a variety of the office's existing patients like sweet Norma Washington, independent Celia Tapia, and accountant Al Neviaser, just to name a few. You can also add new patients, which we will do a little later in this chapter.

BOX 2.1   Digital Basics for Computer Novices

Today, there's a PC in every cubicle and a mobile device in every hand. You can download an "app" for any game, food diary, or pregnancy predictor (just to name a few) you desire. Information is at our fingertips, and patients expect their physician's office to be just as connected. After all, healthcare is also one of the most high-tech businesses in America. Recent federal legislation has had many medical offices jump on the EHR bandwagon. This means that the office staff has had to learn the EHR system, and not everyone is ready for

that change. It may take a generation, says John Hsu, an anesthesiologist who has written about the problem, before computer-phobic healthcare personnel are replaced by more tech-savvy workers. And therein lies a key factor—the human factor—in resistance to EHR adoption, says Hsu.

Invariably, some staff members will plead computer illiteracy and expect to be let off the hook when an EHR is introduced to the practice. A physician may want to retain his own paper files, or a longtime staff member might somehow expect to float outside the system—take vitals, say, and let someone else enter them into the EHR. But allowing parallel paper and electronic systems to exist beyond the transitional period is like having one person in a design studio creating illustrations on mat boards while the other six graphic artists use Photoshop.

Compromise may be a good thing, but it's not what's needed when a clinician or staffer tries to opt out of converting to the EHR. Strong leadership and a heavy dose of enthusiasm will generally carry the day. Owen O'Neill, a champion of his practice's EHR, was both delighted and astonished to watch physicians in his group with only rudimentary computer skills become versatile EHR users. These computer converts tend to take advantage of more of the EHR's features, O'Neill notes, perhaps because they participated in additional training. With that in mind, be sure everyone on your staff is familiar with the computing terms and concepts outlined in the Glossary for Computer Novices at the end of this chapter.

From Hsu J: Why hasn't EHR been adopted faster? Gerson Lehman Group: November 26, 2008. Available at www.glgroup.com/News/Why-hasnt-EHR-been-adopted-faster-29330.html, Accessed 03.01.09

CRITICAL THINKING EXERCISE 2.1

Consider your own experience with medical office technology. If you've had experience using an electronic appointment book or a full-blown EHR, how has it helped you and your patients? If you haven't, think about other ways in which technology has been useful to you—in school, for example, or in a job outside the medical field. How do you think a person's attitude toward technology influences that of the people they work with?

CRITICAL THINKING EXERCISE 2.2

Review the Glossary for Computer Novices, located at the end of this chapter. Which computer terms are new to you? How would the computer concepts apply to the medical setting? Other than EHRs, in what type of scenarios could you use the computer to enhance patient care?

ACCESSING SCMO THROUGH EVOLVE

1. From the main menu of your computer, open Mozilla Firefox. (Evolve and SCMO are compatible with most browsers, but Chrome or Mozilla Firefox works best.)
2. Go to http://evolve.elsevier.com/enrollcourseid.
3. Enter the course ID in the field (provided by your instructor) and click Submit (Fig. 2.1).
4. A pop-up window asking you to log in or create a new account will appear. If you are a returning user, enter your Evolve username and password and click Login. If you are new to Evolve, enter your name, email, desired password, and institution information (if applicable) and click Continue.
5. If you have a 12-character access code, type it into the field provided and select Apply. Note: Access codes may only be used once. If you do not have an access code, SimChart for the Medical Office is available for purchase.

6. Next, select Redeem/Checkout. (Note: You may be prompted to update your account information at this point. Ensure that it is still accurate before continuing.)
7. Check the box to accept the Registered User Agreement.
8. Click Submit.
9. Your enrollment confirmation will appear on the next page. A confirmation email will additionally be sent to your instructor to inform him or her of your enrollment. If you are a new user, your Evolve username and password will also be emailed to you.
10. Click the Get Started link to get to your course located in the My Evolve area. Visit and bookmark http://evolve.elsevier .com/student for future logins.

GETTING COMFORTABLE WITH ELECTRONIC HEALTH RECORDS SOFTWARE

SCMO is a type of Software as a Service (SaaS), which is a software licensing and delivery model. The software is housed in a central location and is accessed via the Internet. SCMO is able to function in a variety of locations, such as a medical office, classroom, laboratory, home—basically anywhere you have Internet access. The EHR system includes Front Office, Clinical Care, and Coding & Billing modules to provide real-life application in a safe learning environment. All users have their own access into the system, so you do not need to worry about any of your work showing up on someone else's screen or about your work affecting someone else's work. All of your data are specific to you, so feel free to explore. This includes spending time looking around, becoming familiar with the available resources, and examining the EHR functions and tools of the Simulation Playground. As with any new skill, practice makes perfect.

Resources for SCMO

SCMO has a robust number of resources to help you get the most from the system. You can access these from the Evolve page. The link for Student Resources is found on the left-side info panel, listed under Course Content (Fig. 2.2).

Here's a summary of some of the items you will find listed in SCMO Student Resources:
Getting Started:
- Quick Tips for Students

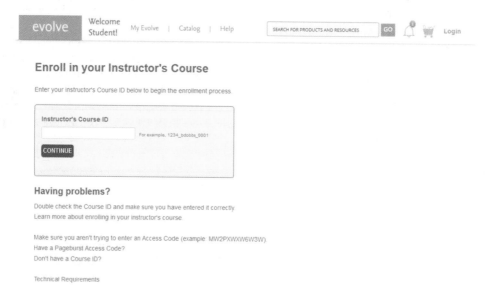

FIG. 2.1 Evolve Course Enrollment screen.

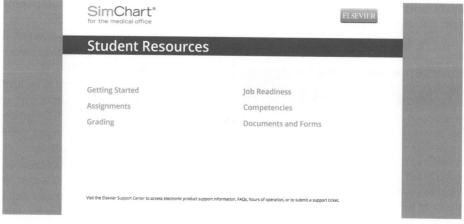

FIG. 2.2 Student Resources link.

- Modules
- Simulation Playground
- Student FAQ
- Glossary
- Info Panel Guide
- Medical Office Workflow
- Using the Encoder
- TruCode User Guide

Assignments:
- Assignments List
- Assignments Overview
- Submitting Assignments

Grading:
- Grading Overview

Job Readiness:
- Student Portfolio Tips
- Job Readiness Skills
- Student Success
- Showcasing Experience

Competencies:
- Competencies Overview
- ABHES Accreditation Manual, 17e
- CAAHEP Competency Standards

Documents and Forms
- CMS 1500 Claim Form
- CMS 1500 Claim Form Instructions
- CMS 1500 Claim Form Change Log

SCMO ASSIGNMENT VIEW

When you enter SCMO from the Evolve portal, you will be directed to the Open Assignments page. From this page you can access the EHR Simulation Playground. This is a practice environment that allows you to explore a fully functioning EHR and to familiarize yourself with the features and workflows available. As within the rest of the system, you can save work, print, return to previous entries, and build patients all in this practice setting.

The Open Assignments grid within the Assignment page (Fig. 2.3) displays assignments released by your instructor. This grid displays the assignment title, module, estimated duration (approximately how long it should take to complete the assignment), and status of an assignment. Once you click on the assignment title, you will enter the assignment portal, which contains:
- Case: An EHR case study with listed objectives and attachments (if needed to complete the assignment)
- Competencies: A list of any accreditation competencies covered in the assignment
- Post-Case Quiz: A series of content questions related to the assignment
- Additional Resources

You can toggle back and forth between these sections but must click the Start Assignment button in the bottom right corner of the Case section to start the simulation portion of an assignment. The information found in the Case section can be printed by clicking on the Print button at the bottom of the page. The Front Office calendar is the default landing page for all assignments. From this view you must use the details in the Assignment Description to determine how to complete the tasks in an assignment. This information can be viewed and/or printed when you are in the simulation by clicking on the orange Assignment Details tab on the right side of the screen. The assignment title displays at the top of the screen in black text, distinguishing this environment from the Simulation Playground environment. Once you complete your EHR activity, click the Back to Assignment link to the left of the View Assignment Description link in order to save your work. At this point you can submit your assignment for grading, if your instructor does not require that you complete the Post-Case Quiz, by clicking on the Submit Assignment button in the

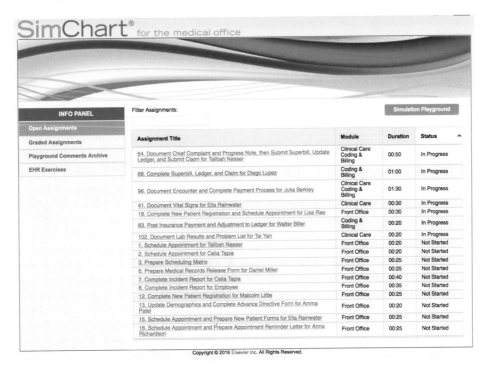

FIG. 2.3 Open Assignment table screen.

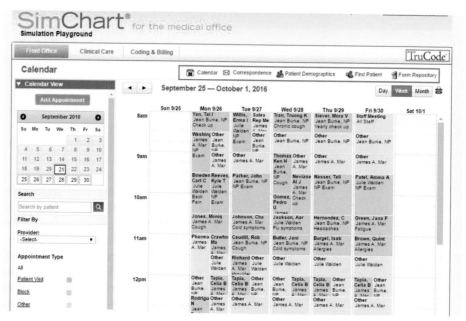

FIG. 2.4 Front Office menus.

bottom left corner of the Case section. If your instructor requires the completion of the Post-Case Quiz, you can click on Post-Case Quiz in the Info Panel. The questions in the Post-Case Quiz refer to simulation activity in some cases, but most questions address general best practices. After you have completed the questions in the Post-Case Quiz, you can then click on the Submit Assignment button to submit both your simulation work and the answers to quiz questions. Instructors manually evaluate student activity within the simulation portion of an assignment, but the system automatically grades answers to quiz questions and generates a preliminary score for the assignment. You can view your preliminary score within the Graded Assignments tab of the Info Panel. Once your instructor reviews your simulation work and approves this automatically generated score, the grade will become bold. If you click on the assignment title in the Graded Assignments tab, you will be able to see any comments your instructor has provided and also be able to reenter the simulation to review the work that you completed there.

MODULES

SCMO is organized into three modules established to simulate the medical office workflow, following a patient visit from start to finish. Just think of the patient's experience in the medical office. Typically, a patient enters the medical office, fills out paperwork, and is escorted into the examination room. After the initial intake procedures, the patient is examined by the physician, has procedures performed, and is billed for services. With this workflow in mind, SCMO is organized into Front Office, Clinical Care, and Coding & Billing.

Front Office

As mentioned, the Front Office calendar is the default landing page of the simulation (Fig. 2.4). The office staff views the calendar more frequently than most pages in order to effectively

manage patient visits. Users can create, edit, and delete new or established patient appointments. An appointment matrix can be established by adding block or other appointment slots such as staff meetings, lunch hours, or sales meetings. Other administrative functions within the Front Office module include composing patient letters, phone messages, and emails with the use of the Correspondence menu. The Patient Demographics tool is used to establish and manage patient and payer information. The Form Repository provides a comprehensive set of office forms. All of the documents and data created in the Front Office module can be viewed, saved to patient records, and printed. We will use the Front Office module in Chapter 4.

Clinical Care

View and document all patient care within the Clinical Care module, accessed by clicking the Clinical Care tab or the Find Patient icon. Once a patient is selected, SCMO will display a summary of all patient record entries known as the Patient Dashboard (Fig. 2.5). In addition to viewing the contents of the patient's record, you can add a new encounter or enter an existing encounter. All clinical documentation is performed within a patient encounter. Users must be in a patient encounter before documenting any clinical care. This reminds us that clinical documentation is performed within a visit between a patient and healthcare provider. There are several clinical records for data entry:

- Allergies
- Chief Complaint
- Health History
- Immunizations
- Medications
- Order Entry
- Patient Education
- Preventive Services

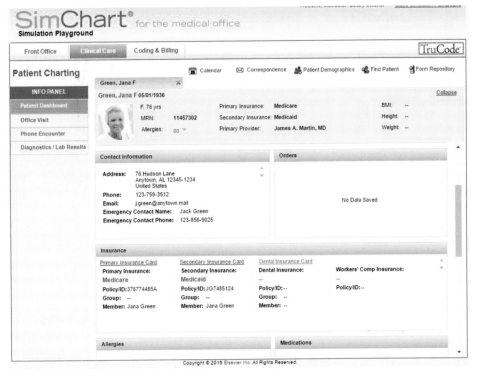

FIG. 2.5 Patient Dashboard.

- Problem List
- Progress Note
- Vitals Signs

In addition to carrying out these clinical functions, the user can upload diagnostic imaging and laboratory requests with the help of the Form Repository. All of these forms, such as the Laboratory Requisition, Neurologic Status Examination, and School Physical, are used in real medical offices. We will learn more about clinical documentation in Chapter 5. The Superbill function can also be accessed from the Clinical Care module by clicking on the Superbill link on the Patient Dashboard. This is found here because a Superbill cannot be created without an encounter.

Coding & Billing

In order for a medical office to function, services rendered must be reimbursed. Managing the monies going in and out of the office is the primary responsibility of the billing and coding department and the focus of the last SCMO module. The main features of the Coding & Billing module include:

- Superbill
- Ledger
- Claim Processing
- Day Sheet
- Reporting
- Auditing

Just like the Front Office and Clinical Care functions, the Form Repository feature plays a large role in this module as well. Insurance specialists regularly use forms such as the Insurance Claim Tracer, Patient Statement, and Bank Deposit Slip. The user can practice coding skills and understand the importance of good documentation when reviewing the progress notes by completing the Superbill and claim. We look at the Coding & Billing module in greater detail in Chapter 6.

RECURRING FEATURES IN SCMO

As you move from screen to screen through SCMO, you will notice certain visual cues that indicate functionality. Many similar cues occur in other applications, so you may already be familiar with some of them. For instance, anyone who has ever made a purchase on eBay knows that a field marked in red on the billing and shipping form must be filled out before proceeding to the next screen. SCMO uses the same functionality.

Keyboard shortcuts, icons, dialog boxes, back buttons, forward arrows, drop-down menus, scroll bars, **check boxes**, and **radio buttons** are covered in the glossary at the end of the chapter. Many SCMO functions are content-specific, meaning that the tools and buttons available are specific to the task being performed. Let's look at a few elements and functions you will use repeatedly as you navigate through SCMO.

Buttons

The **buttons** in SCMO appear on nearly every module and screen. Some have graphics (for example, the green plus sign in immunizations) on them, and others have text labels (for example, the orange Add Appointment button in the Calendar). Most are activated by a single mouse click rather than a double click. When they appear in full color, they are active, or clickable. When the color of the button is faded or "grayed" out, it is a visual cue that it is inactive and can't be selected.

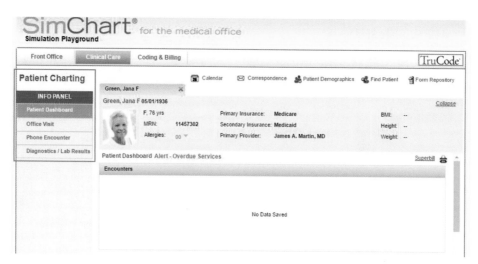

FIG. 2.6 Clinical Care Info panel.

Default Settings

Many students first learn about default settings when working with word processing software. When you open a new document in the word processing software, things like the margins, font type, and font size have already been determined but can be changed by the user. Likewise, when you open a dialog box or screen in SCMO, the options you are most likely to select have already been chosen for you. These are called default options.

Info Panel

The SCMO Info Panel is located on the left side of the screen and changes depending on the module. The Info Panel in the Clinical Care setting is used to create an encounter or to enter laboratory and diagnostic test results (Fig. 2.6). The Coding & Billing module uses the Info Panel to toggle between the various responsibilities of a reimbursement specialist. Info Panels are also used in the Form Repository and Correspondence menus to indicate which templates are available in each tool.

Structured and Unstructured Data Entry Options

There are a number of ways to enter data into electronic health record systems. The best thing you can do is get as much experience as possible in as many ways as possible. Some EHR systems allow the user to use voice dictation or enter free-text data into text fields. This type of narrative is called unstructured data entry, and it allows flexibility in the physician's communications, observations, orders, and patient cases. For many providers just starting to use an EHR system, this type of documentation is the most similar to that of paper records. It allows for a complete narrative picture of the provider's thoughts and easily illustrates a complete picture of the patient's case. Structured data entry uses coded data in several databases. The user identifies preexisting data from drop-down menus, default settings, templates, and check boxes to document individual patient information. Structured data are easier to collect and share among other computer systems,

which will aid system-wide interoperability. It also provides consistent documentation among users. At first it seems to be a quicker method of documentation because the data are already "typed" in for the user, but many providers complain that this type of data entry takes longer when searching specific content. In addition, no one database can possibly contain all of the options a patient will present with, leading to significant limitations and loss of important data. SCMO gives the user experience in both types of data entry to best prepare medical assistants for the vast number of EHR systems they might encounter during an externship/practicum and on the job. For example, patient medications can be entered using a database of drugs or in a free-text data field.

Find Patient Tool

You can imagine how time consuming and overwhelming it would be to scroll through lists and patient names to locate a particular patient. The Find Patient tool makes this task painless. When you type the first few letters of a patient's last name into the Last Name field and click the Go button, the EHR automatically displays matching items at the top of the list (Fig. 2.7).

ESTABLISHING AND MAINTAINING A PATIENT REGISTRY

Active patients are established patients who have seen a physician or any healthcare provider in the group within the past 3 years. Inactive patients are those patients who have not been seen in the past 3 years. Closed patient records are the records of those patients who will not be returning to the practice (that is, they are deceased) or have not been seen in at least 10 years (or as long as required by federal, state, or local regulations). Only registered, active patients can be scheduled for appointments. This group of active patients is called the *patient registry* or *master patient index*. Active patient health records are maintained, and closed patient records are purged from the EHR as soon as it is

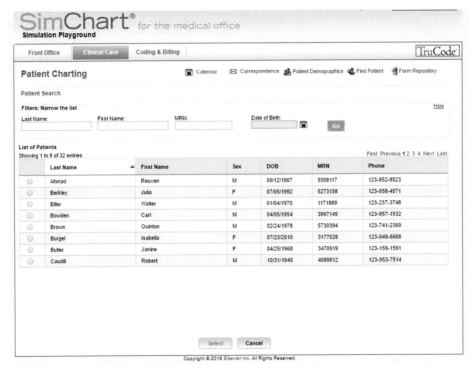

FIG. 2.7 Find Patient tool.

legally advisable to do so. Closed patient records are placed into electronic storage, where they must be kept for liabil-ity reasons in the event of a medical malpractice suit. The **retention period** is the amount of time records must be kept (retained) in storage by a medical office. Table 2.1 shows the recommended retention time for paper files. Retention time for EHR systems is specified by law and varies from state to state. SCMO has about 30 preloaded active patients in the master patient index, but you can use the Add Patient button anytime to create more patients. Next let's show you how!

CRITICAL THINKING EXERCISE 2.3

Give some other examples of technologic skills that are transferable from one version or model of an EHR product to another.

CRITICAL THINKING EXERCISE 2.4

Donna is new to your physician's office. During her training on the office EHR, she asks why inactive patient records have to be retained. What qualifies as an inactive record, and why must the record be placed in storage?

Enter a New Patient in SCMO

Just as a reminder, you need to log in to Evolve and click on Sim-Chart for the Medical Office. You will be working in the Simu-lation Playground for this activity. From the Open Assignments screen you click on the Simulation Playground button on the right side of the screen. Let's start by registering a new patient. As you follow along, register yourself as a "mock" patient.

1. From the Assignment page, click the Simulation Play-ground button located in the top right corner.
2. Select the top radio button to enter the Playground with all of the saved information from your previous session (Fig. 2.8).
3. Click the Patient Demographics icon (Fig. 2.9).
4. Attempt a patient search by entering the first couple of let-ters of the patient's last name in the Last Name field. Click the Search Existing Patients button (Fig. 2.10).
5. If no patient record exists, the Add Patient button will appear under the search field. Click on the Add Patient but-ton to create a new record (Fig. 2.11).
6. The Patient Demographics–Add Patient window appears, organized using Patient, Guarantor, and Insur-ance tabs (Fig. 2.12). Start by entering the Patient infor-mation, including name (as it appears on the insurance card or ID). The medical record number is automatically generated for the account, so there is no need to create one.
7. Complete the required fields within the Patient, Guarantor, and Insurance tabs. Red asterisks indicate required fields. New data entry is always required when a new billing account is created.
8. If a patient is legally responsible for his or her own bills, the user can select the Self radio button in the Guarantor tab, and the patient information will auto-feed from the Patient tab. If the user selects an existing guarantor, that person's data will auto-populate into the fields.
9. The Insurance tab records Primary and Secondary Insur-ance Carriers. A scanned image of the insurance card can be attached to the account using the Upload Insurance Card link.

TABLE 2.1 Records Retention Schedule

Temporary Record	Retention Period (Years)	Permanent Record (Retained Indefinitely)
Accounts receivable (patient ledger)	7	
Appointment sheets	3	Accounts payable records
Bank deposit slips (duplicate)	1	Bills of sale for important purchases (or until you no longer own them)
		Canceled checks and check registers
Bank statements and canceled checks	7	Capital asset records
		Cash books
Billing records (for outside service)	7	Certified financial statements
Cash receipt records	6	Contracts
		Correspondence, legal
Contracts (expired)	7	Credit history
Correspondence, general	6	Deeds, mortgages, contracts, leases, and property records
Day sheets (balance sheets and journals)	5	Equipment guarantees and records (or until you no longer own them)
Employee contracts	6	Income tax returns and documents
Employee time records	5	Insurance policies and records
Employment applications	4	Journals (financial)
Insurance claim forms (paid)	3	
Inventory records	3	
Invoices	6	Health records (active patients)
Health records (expired patients)	5	Health records (inactive patients)
Medicare financial records	7	
Remittance advice documents	8	Mortgages
Payroll records	7	Property appraisals and records
Petty cash vouchers	3	Telephone records
Postal and meter records	1	x-ray films
Tax worksheets and supporting documents	7	Year-end balance sheets and general ledgers

From Fordney, M. T. (2016). *Insurance handbook for the medical office* (14th ed.). St. Louis: Saunders.

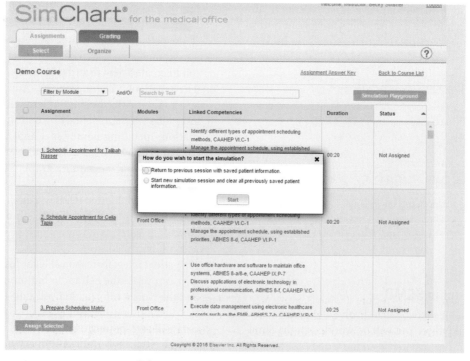

FIG. 2.8 Playground confirmation box.

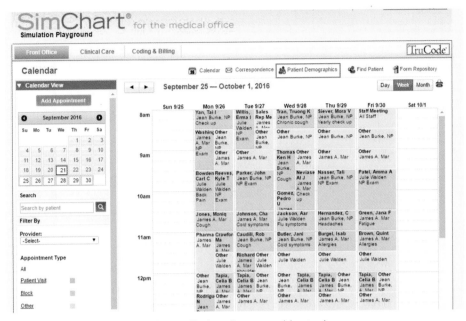

FIG. 2.9 Patient Demographics tool.

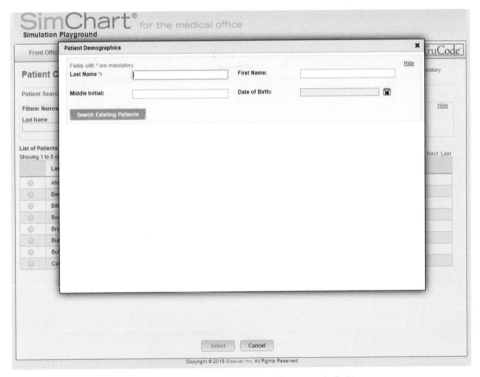

FIG. 2.10 Patient Demographics search field.

10. Scroll to the bottom of the Patient Demographics window and click the Save Patient button to create your new patient record. Your new patient is now part of the patient registry.

As patient information changes, the Patient Demographics data can be updated as well. To update information, click on the Patient Demographics icon, search for the patient by clicking on the Search Existing Patient button, verify that you have the correct patient by checking the date of birth (DOB), click on the patient's name (in blue). This will open up the Patient Demographics–Edit Patient screen. After making the changes, click on the Save Patient button.

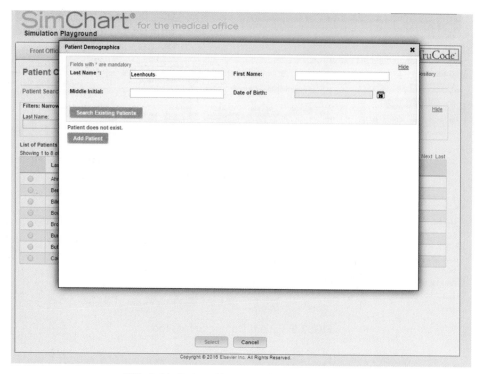

FIG. 2.11 Patient Demographics data screen.

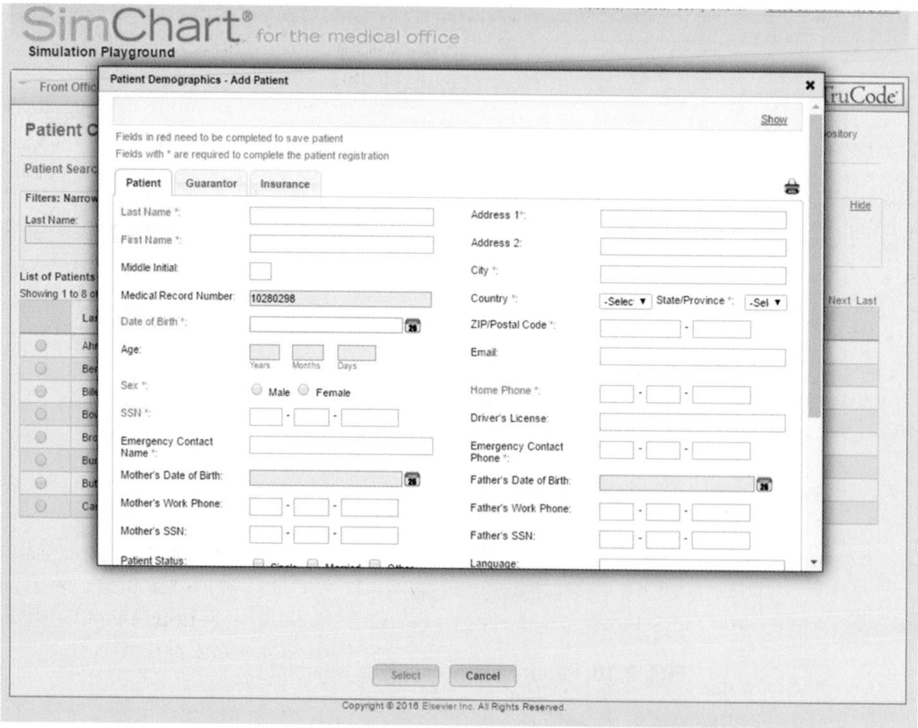

FIG. 2.12 Patient Demographics–Add Patient button.

EHR EXERCISE 2.1 Create a New Patient Record

Using the previous steps as a guide, complete the following exercise in the EHR Exercises assignment found in Open Assignments.

Now that we have walked through how to register a new patient, let's see if you can establish a new patient record for Susannah Ling. Susannah is a new patient of Dr. Martin. Use the completed Patient Information form (located at the end of this chapter) to abstract and enter her data.

EHR EXERCISE 2.2 Edit Patient Demographics

Using the previous steps as a guide, complete the following exercise in the EHR Exercises assignment found in Open Assignments.

Monique Jones, an established patient of Dr. Martin, stopped in the office this morning because the group number of her insurance has changed. Her Blue Cross/Blue Shield group number is now 78452K. Update Monique's demographics.

EHR EXERCISE 2.3 Create a New Patient Record

Using the previous steps as a guide, complete the following exercise in the EHR Exercises assignment found in Open Assignments.

Two new patients, Chase Murray and Miles Green, are establishing with Dr. Walden today. Use the completed Patient Information forms (located at the end of the chapter) to create the new patient records.

INTERNET USE IN THE MEDICAL OFFICE

Professional Use

The Internet is a great resource for the medical office. For SCMO, it is a necessary tool for access. In addition, members of the healthcare team may use it to locate testing centers for patients, identify appropriate clinical trials, find links to community support groups, and print patient education material. However, you should surf with caution. Although many reliable sites exist, many more offer bogus advice, usually in an effort to sell a useless or even harmful product or service. Patients and staff should be sure to determine what the agenda of the site is and whether the information at the URL is reliable. (See the Glossary for Computer Novices for an explanation of the terms *link* or *hyperlink*, *website* or *web page*, and *URL*.)

Personal Use

Of course, the Internet also has infinite personal uses—reading a favorite blog (or writing one), checking out friends' Facebook or Twitter status, swapping photos on Instagram, and maybe shopping for a fierce pair of Italian leather pumps from Zappos. There are more mundane uses for the Internet, too. In a spare moment you may find yourself trying to obtain the new level of Candy Crush, wandering over to see whether your check has cleared, paying your cell phone bill, or looking for a new apartment before your lease is up. It should go without saying that none of these activities is acceptable in the medical office. It may be tempting, but you should confine personal web browsing and mobile device usage to your own time, using computers unconnected with your place of employment. (See the Glossary for Computer Novices at the end of the chapter for a discussion of the term *browser*.)

Here are some sensible guidelines for Internet use in the medical office:

- Internet use should be limited to sites related to your job duties. Your Internet usage may be monitored by your employer.
- Do not use the computer to send or receive personal email messages.
- Do not open email messages, especially attachments, from unfamiliar senders.
- Perform a virus check daily. Many software programs do this for you automatically, but the programs must be kept up to date, usually by purchasing periodic upgrades.
- Be careful not to copy documents or images in violation of copyright laws.
- Do not download any software or apps to an office PC without permission.

CHAPTER SUMMARY

- A rapidly increasing rate of EHR adoption combined with up-to-date curriculum for medical assistants has made medical assisting one of the fastest-growing professions in the United States.
- There are a number of resources available for students to help with navigating SCMO. There are user guides to explain the basics of SCMO, to assist with locating and submitting assignments, and to understand the grading process.
- The Simulation Playground provides an environment for students to practice and get familiar with the modules found in SCMO. The modules reflect a patient's progress through the medical office starting with the Front Office module, moving into the Clinical Care module, and finally the Coding & Billing module.

- The functionality and navigational features in SCMO overlap with those of similar EHR products. Some common elements of SCMO include buttons, default settings, info panels, structured data entry, and patient search.
- Active patient records, inactive patient records, and closed patient records all must be handled appropriately within the medical office.
- A new patient record can be created by clicking the Patient Demographics icon and searching by last name. Once you have confirmed that the patient does not already exist in the system, click the Add Patient button at the bottom of the search field and complete the Patient, Guarantor, and Insurance tabs.

- In the medical office, the Internet should be used only for tasks related to one's job. A member of the medical office staff might use the Internet to locate testing centers for patients, find information about support groups in the community, or print patient education materials. Caution must be taken to ensure that reliable, professional sites are consulted.

CHAPTER REVIEW ACTIVITIES

Key Terms Review
Match the following key terms with their definitions.

1.	Radio button	a. The amount of time records must be kept in storage by a medical office
2.	Field	b. A secondary, related set of options displayed by holding the cursor over an entry on the main menu or by clicking to expand a list
3.	Drop-down menu	c. A specialized graphic element that toggles on and off and is used when only one response is appropriate because two of these buttons can't be depressed at the same time
4.	Retention period	d. Space allocated on a form for specific numeric or text data
5.	Active patient	e. Used to describe an established patient who currently sees the physician
6.	Check box	f. A specialized graphic element that toggles on and off. Often used when more than one answer could used.

SCMO Scavenger Hunt
Log in to Evolve and find the answers to the following questions.
1. The website to log in to Evolve is:
2. According to the Quick Tips resource, the landing page for the student is called:
3. How many ways can the calendar be displayed?
4. SCMO has multiple providers. What is the first name of the nurse practitioner?
5. What is Norma Washington's DOB?
6. Name two insurance and billing documents found in the Form Repository.
7. Name the three types of correspondence generated by SCMO.
8. List the History of Present Illness elements identified in a chief complaint.
9. Where is the patient's insurance coverage entered?
10. Who is the guarantor for patient Celia Tapia?

True/False
Indicate whether the statement is true or false.
1. _____ Most medical assistants are employed in inpatient settings.

2. _____ SCMO does not include the ability to create patient letters because it is easier to store these documents outside of the patient record.
3. _____ Unfortunately no two systems are the same, so knowing how to use one EHR will be little help in learning to use another.
4. _____ SCMO is used to document clinical data and does not function as a practice management software system.
5. _____ The user must first perform a patient search before entering a new patient record.
6. _____ When creating a new patient account, the user must randomly select a number to be the medical record number.
7. _____ SCMO allows the user to enter up to three insurance carriers.
8. _____ To submit an assignment the user should perform the EHR activity and answer quiz questions.
9. _____ Another name for a Patient Registry is a *master patient index*.
10. _____ Closed patient records are the records of patients who have not been seen in the past 6 months.
11. _____ The Add Patient screen contains a patient's contact information and demographics.
12. _____ Information from the Internet is not reliable enough to use for patient education.

Workplace Applications
Using the knowledge you obtained from this chapter, provide answers to the following cases.
1. You notice that the employees in your office have been spending company time using the Internet for personal use—primarily reading blogs, exchanging emails with friends, downloading music, and watching YouTube videos. Create an office policy for the employee handbook that prohibits the misuse of the Internet and describes in what situations it may be used.
2. Kara is new to your office and is slowly becoming familiar with the EHR. She has asked you to review some of the common elements and features in SCMO. Explore and then describe some uses to her.

PATIENT INFORMATION (Please use full legal name.)

Last Name:	Ling	Address 1:	234 Capeside Dr
First Name:	Susannah	Address 2:	--
Middle Initial:	--	City:	Anytown
Medical Record Number:	--	State:	AL
Date of Birth:	01/02/1973	Zip:	12345
Age:	43	Email:	susannah.ling@scmo.edu
Sex:	Female	Home Phone:	445-555-7897
SSN:	111-22-3333	Driver's License:	CA54841
Emergency Contact Name:	Yolanda Arnold	Emergency Contact Phone:	445-555-8525

GUARANTOR INFORMATION (Please use full legal name.)

Relationship of Guarantor to Patient:	Self		
Guarantor/Account #:	Ling, Susannah / 94556		
Account Number:	--		
Last Name:	Ling	Address 1:	234 Capeside Dr
First Name:	Susannah	Address 2:	--
Middle Initial:	--	City:	Anytown
Date of Birth:	01/02/1973	State:	AL
Age:	43	Zip:	12345
Sex:	Female	Email:	susannah.ling@scmo.edu
SSN:	111-22-3333	Home Phone:	445-555-7897
Employer Name:	Seaside Florist	Cell Phone:	--------

PROVIDER INFORMATION

Primary Provider:	James A. Martin, MD	Provider's Address 1:	1234 Anystreet
Referring Provider:	--	Provider's Address 2:	--
Date of Last Visit:	01/25/2014	City:	Anytown
Phone:	123-123-1234	State:	AL
		Zip:	12345

INSURANCE INFORMATION (If the patient is not the Insured party, please include date of birth for claims.)

Insurance:	Aetna	Claims Address 1:	1234 Insurance Way
Name of Policy Holder:	Susannah Ling	City:	Anytown
SSN:	111-22-3333	State:	AL
Policy/ID Number:	YYT5782251	Zip:	12345
Group Number:	AT12005	Claims Phone:	800-123-2222

PATIENT INFORMATION (Please use full legal name.)

Last Name:	Murray JR	Address 1:	115 Cartwright Dr
First Name:	Chase	Address 2:	--
Middle Initial:	B	City:	Anytown
Medical Record Number:	--	State:	AL
Date of Birth:	04/07/1993	Zip:	12345
Age:	21	Email:	chaser@zoom.edu
Sex:	Male	Home Phone:	970-840-1199
SSN:	630-58-4125	Driver's License:	87954285
Emergency Contact Name:	Roberta Murray	Emergency Contact Phone:	970-840-1199
Mother's Date of Birth:	04/18/1967	Mother's SSN:	654-78-9321
Mother's Work Phone:	852-788-9852		

GUARANTOR INFORMATION (Please use full legal name.)

Relationship of Guarantor to Patient:	Parent	Guarantor/Account #:	Murray, Roberta / 76320
		Account Number:	76320
Last Name:	Murray	Address 1:	115 Cartwright Dr
First Name:	Roberta	Address 2:	--
Middle Initial:	--	City:	Anytown
Date of Birth:	04/18/1967	State:	AL
Age:	46	Zip:	89754
Sex:	Female	Email:	--
SSN:	654-78-3210	Home Phone:	852-788-9852
Employer Name:	Hammer Heads Eatery	Cell Phone:	970-788-2250

PROVIDER INFORMATION

Primary Provider:	Julie Walden, MD	Provider's Address 1:	1234 Anystreet
Referring Provider:	--	Provider's Address 2:	--
Date of Last Visit:	08/2009	City:	Anytown
Phone:	123-123-1234	State:	AL
		Zip:	12345

INSURANCE INFORMATION (If the patient is not the Insured party, please include date of birth for claims.)

Insurance:	Aetna	Claims Address 1:	1234 Insurance Way
Name of Policy Holder:	Roberta Murray	City:	Anytown
SSN:	654-78-9321	State:	AL
Policy/ID Number:	77700142	Zip:	12345
Group Number:	UR4534	Claims Phone:	800-123-2222

PATIENT INFORMATION (Please use full legal name.)

Last Name:	Green	Address 1:	800 Liberty Court
First Name:	Miles	Address 2:	--
Middle Initial:	R	City:	Seacrest
Medical Record Number:	--	State:	AK
Date of Birth:	01/01/1957	Zip:	54600
Age:	57	Email:	--
Sex:	Male	Home Phone:	831-555-1954
SSN:	456-58-7782	Driver's License:	--
Emergency Contact Name:	Luke Hand	Emergency Contact Phone:	314-555-1200

GUARANTOR INFORMATION (Please use full legal name.)

Relationship of Guarantor to Patient:	Self		
Guarantor/Account #:	Green, Miles R		
Account Number:	--		
Last Name:	Green	Address 1:	800 Liberty Court
First Name:	Miles	Address 2:	--
Middle Initial:	R	City:	Seacrest
Date of Birth:	01/01/1957	State:	AK
Age:	57	Zip:	54600
Sex:	Male	Email:	--
SSN:	456-58-7782	Home Phone:	831-555-1954
Employer Name:	Baker Corrections	Cell Phone:	--------

PROVIDER INFORMATION

Primary Provider:	Julie Walden, MD	Provider's Address 1:	1234 Anystreet
Referring Provider:	Carrie Peach, MD	Provider's Address 2:	--
Date of Last Visit:	2010	City:	Anytown
Phone:	123-123-1234	State:	AL
		Zip:	12345

INSURANCE INFORMATION (If the patient is not the Insured party, please include date of birth for claims.)

Insurance:	Blue Cross Blue Shield	Claims Address 1:	1234 Insurance Place
Name of Policy Holder:	Miles Green	Claims Address 1:	--
SSN:	456-58-7782	City:	Anytown
Policy/ID Number:	PT1234098	State:	AL
Group Number:	HC345	Zip:	12345
		Claims Phone:	800-123-1111

Glossary for Computer Novices

Term	Definition

General Hardware and Computing Terms

Developer	A company that designs software with specific features and functionality and writes programming code to create the application
Keyboarding	Using a keyboard to enter data into the computer system—in a word, typing.
Keyboard shortcut	Most tasks within an application, such as copying and pasting, can be accomplished either with a series of mouse clicks or with an alternative series of keystrokes. These keystroke combinations often use the Ctrl or Alt key plus a letter. Some examples include Ctrl + C to copy data, Ctrl + V to paste data, and Ctrl + X to cut data; the F1 key is the Help key.
Workstation	In its broadest sense, a workstation is any place within the medical practice, including remotely connected locations, that is equipped with a PC, laptop computer, tablet computer, or other networked device. Workstations are usually furnished and stocked with office supplies. They may be located in offices, in clinical areas, or at reception desks. Even a handheld device, such as an iPhone, can be considered a workstation.

General Software Terms

File	A unit of organization for data stored on a computer and containing program files, text, graphics, or some combination of these. For example, in SCMO, each patient's chart is composed of records from many different files. The patient's visit information is stored in one file, the patient's appointments in another, the patient's history and examination data in another, the patient's orders in another, the patient's diagnoses in another, the patient's instructions in another, etc. A folder is a larger unit of organization than a file; files are kept in folders.
Icon	Like a blue highway sign with a white H indicating a nearby hospital, icons are miniature visual representations of tasks, commands, applications, functions, and other digital miscellany. They are part of programs we call *graphic user interfaces* (GUIs). Clicking on an icon is generally more efficient than executing a keyboard command (but not always—see *Keyboard shortcut*).

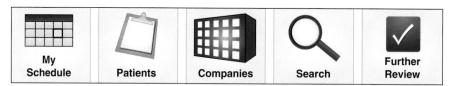

Toolbar	A collection of icons (see *Icon*) arranged in a row and used as a graphic navigational aid. Toolbars are often *context specific*. This means that the toolbar you see shows only the icons appropriate for the screen on which you're working.

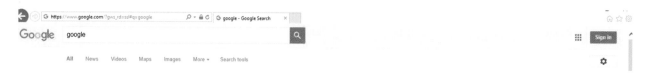

Window	In the broad sense, a window is a framed viewing area or portion of a screen that separates one part of an application from another, such as one file from another. A window can also separate one application from another. Using buttons in the upper right corner, each window can be closed (by clicking the black X), minimized—that is, made smaller (by clicking the single white line on the blue ground), or maximized—that is, resized to fill the entire computer display screen (by clicking the overlapping document icon or the large document icon). Navigational arrows (see *Back button and Forward arrow*) allow the user to move freely from window to window, minimizing and maximizing at will. Clicking the white X on the red background closes the entire program rather than just the current document. Windows can also be split, tiled, viewed side by side, and manipulated in other ways.

General Web/Internet Terms

Browser (also called Internet browser or web browser)	An application that allows you to view and download content from the Internet (the web). The four most popular browsers are Chrome, Mozilla Firefox, IE, and Safari.

Term	Definition

Term

Definition

Home page

The main page (usually the opening screen) of a website. It contains general information and navigational links, such as a search box, sidebar menus, and links to subpages. In the earlier days of the Internet, home pages used to be more like book covers, offering little information beyond the name of the site. But these "landing pages" or "splash pages" just made it harder for visitors to access the content, and few sites have them anymore. An exception is a paid advertisement that may pop up over the home page (click Close or Skip This Ad to delete it). See *website/web page.*

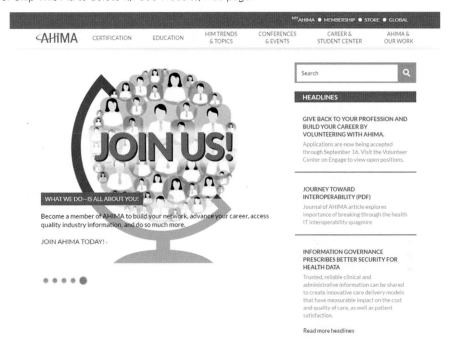

American Health Information Management Association's (AHIMA) home page.

Hyperlink (also called a link, live link, or hotlink)

An underlined web address, word, or phrase coded to jump to a new document, such as a website, or to a different part of the current document, or to select a function within SCMO. The link is activated when you click on it with your mouse (sometimes you must also press Ctrl while clicking).

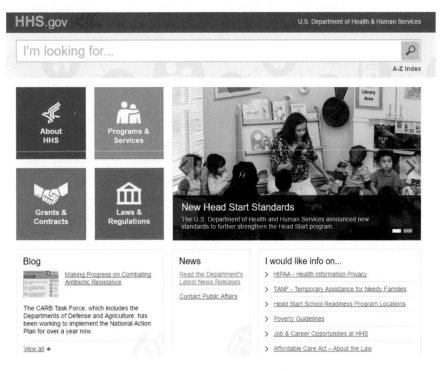

Each of the words and phrases underlined is a hyperlink. Clicking on any of the links takes you to the document described.

Continued

Term	Definition
Pop-up window	This term usually refers to the annoying ads that pop up on many commercial (.com) websites. However, within a software application such as an EHR, a pop-up screen or pop-up window is the same as a dialog box (see *Dialog box*).
URL	Uniform resource locator, or website address.
website/web page	A specific location on the web, organized under a domain name. Commercial sites are .com (dot-coms), not-for-profit organizations are .org, and government sites are .gov. Other domain-name extensions, such as .us, also exist but are not widely used. See *Home page*.

Document and Site Navigation and Manipulation Terms

Term	Definition
Back button and Forward arrow	Navigational icons, usually located in the upper left corner of a web browser or other application, used to move to the next page or screen of a document (Forward arrow) or to the previous page or screen (Back button).
Drag and drop	A function that allows you to shuffle text in a sentence or to reposition whole sentences. Just highlight the text you'd like to move (see *Highlight*), hold the mouse pointer over it, and drag it to the desired new position. To copy the text rather than move it, hold the Ctrl key as you drag. This function works for images as well.
Drop-down menu	A menu of further choices that appears (drops down) when a word on the menu bar is clicked. Many SCMO functions have a drop-down menu. In the Clinical Care module, Allergies, Medications, and Order Entry records are just a few examples of where drop-down menus are used.
Minimize/maximize/ resize	To decrease *(minimize)* or increase *(maximize)* a window so that it fills only a portion of the computer monitor screen or the entire screen, respectively. To *resize* means to manipulate the size of a window or its position on the screen by minimizing or maximizing it or by using the "grab bars" on a graphic to expand or reduce its size. See *Windows*.
Undo/redo	These buttons, found in most applications, are quick editing tools that allow you to reverse a step or series of steps (by clicking Undo) and to perform them again, if you wish, by clicking Redo.
Scroll bar	Clickable up and down arrows or left and right arrows on a vertical bar. They are the graphic equivalent of the up, down, left, and right arrows on the keyboard. Scroll bars indicate that more text is available than would fit on the screen. They're used to navigate through documents and to browse through lists.

Data Input Terms

Term	Definition
Check box	A data input choice used when there are only two possible answers. A checked box generally means "yes" or "applicable," whereas an unchecked (blank) box means "no" or "not applicable." For example, a check marked box next to Cancel means "yes." To check or uncheck a box, click it once with the mouse.
Copy and paste	An editing function that allows you to highlight text or graphics and make an exact copy to be used elsewhere in your document or in another document.
Cut and paste	An editing function that allows you to highlight text or graphics and move the selected item elsewhere in your document or to another document.
Dialog box	A pop-up box that does one of three things: (1) contains additional information (called an alert box); (2) asks you to confirm that you wish to proceed (called a confirmation box); or (3) prompts you for more information (called a prompt box). See *Pop-up window*.
Highlight	Select a word, sentence, or passage to be edited (for example, moved, reformatted, or deleted) by clicking the right mouse button, dragging it across and down, and then releasing the button. In SCMO highlighted text is shown covered in blue.

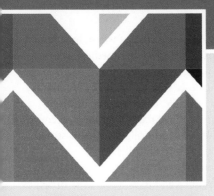

Privacy, Confidentiality, and Security

OUTLINE

CHAPTER OBJECTIVES

1. Explore the history and scope of HIPAA.
2. Discuss the legal meaning of privacy.
3. List the four implementation specifications required by the administrative safeguards outlined in the HIPAA Security Rule, and explore ways in which they might apply to a small- to medium-size medical practice.
4. Assess and complete forms related to patient privacy in the electronic health record (EHR).
5. Become familiar with patients' rights under HIPAA, and explore how they affect the EHR.
6. Identify organizations aimed at securing EHR systems.
7. Identify who is allowed access to the information in a patient's EHR and under what circumstances.
8. Describe the role of consumer reporting agencies and prescription database tools, and explain how they are regulated.
9. Discuss ways patients can protect their health information.

KEY TERMS

anonymity The patient's right to have private health data collected in a way that can never be linked or traced back to him or her.

audit trail A record that traces a user's electronic footsteps by recording activity and transactions, including unsuccessful attempts to view unauthorized screens, within the EHR system.

authentication The process of determining whether the person attempting to access a given network or EHR system is authorized to do so. User authentication can include password entry or use of biometric data (such as a digital fingerprint or voice signature) or a smart card (a data-laden microchip).

authorization A document giving a covered entity permission to use protected health information for specified purposes other than treatment, payment, or healthcare operations or to disclose protected health information to a third party specified by the patient.

business associates A person or entity that performs certain functions or activities that involve the use or disclosure of protected health information on behalf of a covered entity.

confidentiality The obligation of professionals to keep a patient's information in confidence. The patient's right and expectation that individually identifiable health information will be kept private and not disclosed without the patient's permission. Confidentiality is protected by law to varying degrees.

consent Permission given to a covered entity for uses and disclosures of protected health information for treatment, payment, and healthcare operations.

consumer reporting agency An agency regulated by the Federal Trade Commission (FTC) under the Fair Credit Reporting Act (FCRA) that sells or cooperatively exchanges consumer credit information and history.

covered entities Healthcare providers, health plans, and healthcare clearinghouses that transmit health information electronically.

disclosure Giving access to, releasing, or transferring information to a person or entity.

ethics Rules and standards of conduct that govern professional behavior and arise from our shared understanding of morality.

laws Formal enforceable rules and policies based on community standards of conduct.

minimum necessary standard A key provision of the HIPAA Privacy Rule requiring that covered entities limit unnecessary or inappropriate access to and disclosure of protected health information. Disclosures should include only the minimum necessary amount of information to accomplish a given purpose.

off-label indication A use for a prescription drug other than that for which the U.S. Food and Drug Administration (FDA) has approved it.

password A sequence of characters and sometimes spaces used to prevent unauthorized access to or disclosure of patient information contained in secure electronic files.

privacy The patient's freedom to determine when, how much, and under what circumstances his or her medical information may be disclosed.

protected health information (PHI) Individually identifiable health information (for example, demographic information, billing information, medical record numbers, account numbers, physical or mental condition, etc.) that is stored, maintained, or transmitted electronically.

safeguards Measures taken to prevent interference with computer network operations and to avert security breaches involving the unauthorized use, disclosure, modification, erasure, or destruction of protected health information; these measures are specified by the HIPAA Security Rule, which applies only to data in electronic form.

screen saver A program that displays animation or image on the screen if input (such as a keystroke) is not received for a given time period.

secondary use A use of health information that is not directly related to patient care. Such uses include statistical analysis, research, quality and safety assurance processes, public health monitoring, payment, provider certification or accreditation, and marketing and other business activities.

HEALTH INSURANCE PORTABILITY AND ACCOUNTABILITY ACT (HIPAA)

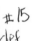

Although privacy, confidentiality, and security have always been important in the world of healthcare, it was the Health Insurance Portability and Accountability Act (HIPAA) that made it mandatory to have measures in place to protect all three. HIPAA was brought about to address the issues of protecting healthcare information in the electronic age.

The electronic age has made our lives easier, safer, and more rewarding in many ways, yet it poses problems that were inconceivable just a few years ago. Drugs that were sold on the streets are now being sold online and delivered right to the purchaser's door. Information stored in an electronic format can be hacked and identities stolen. Citizens and elected officials have struggled to sort out issues like these in every area of our lives, including healthcare and privacy. In times past, only a small number of medical personnel had access to patients' paper charts, but when electronic transmission of data became possible, more people had much easier access to health information, and this information could just as easily be shared inappropriately. In response, Congress passed the Health Insurance Portability and Accountability Act of 1996 (HIPAA). The portability section of HIPAA was designed to protect individuals from being denied insurance due to preexisting conditions and to allow employees to keep insurability when moving from one job to another. The accountability section was designed in part to protect patient information and also to standardize the process of data submission. In this chapter we are going to focus on the protection of patient information.

CONFIDENTIALITY VERSUS PRIVACY

It is important to have an understanding of some of the terms used in HIPAA. The increased use of electronic technology in the healthcare facility, including the electronic health record (EHR), has changed the way patients' confidentiality and privacy are maintained. The terms *privacy* and *confidentiality* are often used interchangeably, but in healthcare, specifically in relation to HIPAA, there is a difference. Now that everything from bank card numbers to patient test results are stored electronically, maintaining privacy has become even more difficult.

Confidentiality refers to the right of an individual to have all of his or her information, including health information, kept private. Those who work in healthcare are ethically bound to keep the patient's information confidential. Only those people directly involved in the care and treatment of the patient should be viewing or receiving this information.

Keeping patient information confidential means that you have to be diligent in what information is shared verbally in the healthcare facility. It is inappropriate to talk about a patient where other patients, family members, delivery people, pharmaceutical reps, or others could possibly overhear. When the EHR screen is being used, it should be positioned so that someone walking by cannot view the information. Daily schedules should be posted only where visitors to the healthcare facility cannot see them, or they should have a cover sheet over them. Not taking these actions can be considered a violation of HIPAA and leaves the healthcare facility open to a potential lawsuit.

Privacy refers to the patient's right to control how his or her healthcare information is used and shared with others. Before the information can be disclosed to a third party, the healthcare provider must have the patient's permission in writing. HIPAA does state that if the healthcare provider is disclosing this information for treatment, payment, or operations (TPO), the provider does not need the patient's permission to release this information. However, if a stricter state law is in place, the patient's permission must be obtained. To be safe, a patient's written permission to release that information should be obtained. HIPAA also states that a patient has the right to know who has accessed his or her health record and who has received information from his or her health record. EHR systems allow for the tracking of that information so that a report can be generated and presented to the patient if he or she requests it.

Both law and ethics require that patients be treated with respect and dignity and be offered the best care we're capable of providing, including protecting all information in the health record. **Ethics** is the set of rules and standards of conduct that grow out of our shared understanding of right and wrong and that govern our professional behavior. When we formalize (codify) these ethical principles and determine criminal or civil penalties for violating them, we call them **laws**, such as HIPAA.

Before we define a few more concepts, let's make sure we keep our discussion concrete by seeing how the laws might apply to real patients. Edmund is a 64-year-old writer of fiction and biography who has made something of a name for himself. Ed has been openly gay for many years and knows he is human immunodeficiency virus (HIV) positive. Ed's partner, a 51-year-old electrical engineer named Michael, has chosen to share his sexual orientation with the couple's wide circle of friends but not with his elderly parents. Michael would like to be tested periodically for HIV, but he is concerned about his privacy. In other words, Michael would like to decide when, how much, and with whom his medical information can be shared.

Confidential Versus Anonymous

Although the terms *confidential* and *anonymous* are often used interchangeably, a confidential test like the HIV test Michael has requested is not the same thing as an anonymous test. To adequately protect patients' privacy, it's important to know the difference. Confidentiality refers to how the recipient of the information, such as Michael's physician, handles information that a patient does not wish to have disclosed.

The notion of confidentiality presumes that the person is entitled to keep the information to himself or herself and that the provider or other person with whom the information is shared is obligated to hold it in confidence. This is often not the case. For instance, suspected child abuse must be reported to law enforcement. Sexual assault and other crimes may also be subject to reporting requirements. In some states, minors who seek family planning advice or services may be reported to parents or guardians. HIV and certain other communicable diseases, as in Michael's case, are subject to state reporting requirements so that partners can be notified and disease incidence can be tracked for public health purposes.

Confidential information may be disclosed to other parties besides public health and law enforcement officials. If Michael agrees to disclose his test results to his physician, who would then enter the information into the EHR, his test results would undoubtedly reach Michael's health insurance company. Why? Because to obtain health insurance, even for a group plan, he would have had to sign a document permitting them access to his health records.

If Michael prefers to have an anonymous test, he may be able to get one at a local public health clinic. **Anonymity** means that Michael's name will not be linked to the results. His blood sample will be submitted to the laboratory using only an identification number, and a counselor will share the results with him by phone.

Continued

TRENDS AND APPLICATIONS 3.1 Can Patients' Genetic Profiles Be Used Against Them?— cont'd

Genetic testing has the potential to help patients and providers make sound treatment decisions, aid researchers who are looking for new links between genetic mutations and disease development, lower costs for insurance companies by preventing disease (for example, in patients who undergo preventive mastectomies), and increase worker productivity for employers by reducing days off and leaves of absence for illness. Despite these obvious benefits, however, a study of patients with a family history of colorectal cancer showed that not only would many of them refuse genetic testing but also that they would not even agree to speak with a healthcare professional about their family history for fear the information would be used against them in employment and insurance coverage decisions.

According to a survey conducted by the Johns Hopkins Genetics and Public Policy Center, 93% of Americans believe that neither their insurance companies nor their employers should have access to the results of genetic tests. Yet the American public does agree that gathering genetic information is important. The same survey found that 91% of respondents said that if effective treatment were available for a particular condition, they would entrust their physicians (but not necessarily anyone else) with the genetic information necessary to diagnose and treat it.

Furthermore, new parents believe it's important to collect genetic health information about their newborns. A 2007 poll conducted by the C. S. Mott Children's Hospital at the University of Michigan found that 54% of parents approve of genetic testing even for diseases for which no effective treatment is available. In addition, 38% of parents said they would allow their child's genetic information to be linked to a nationally interoperable EHR system. Such a system would undoubtedly be an invaluable public health resource, but it would have to address the valid privacy concerns we've just discussed.

In an effort to begin addressing such concerns, in 2008 Congress passed the Genetic Information Nondiscrimination Act (GINA). Individuals who have group health insurance were already protected, but GINA extends protection to those who own individual insurance policies. Health insurers will be prohibited from raising premiums or denying coverage based on a person's genetic risk profile, and employers may not fire an employee or discriminate in hiring, promotion, or compensation on that basis.

There is also an increase in the use of the direct-to-consumer testing. With this type of testing the patient provides a sample to a laboratory, and it does the testing requested by the patient. A report is then provided to the patient. A healthcare provider neither orders this test nor receives a copy of the report. Although this type of testing provides an option for patients who do not want this information to become part of their health record, the report itself can be confusing for patients and can increase their concerns. In addition if the patient does choose to share this information with his or her provider, the provider may not have confidence in those results and order retesting to verify.

Privacy Rule

The HIPAA Privacy Rule establishes privacy standards for the use and disclosure of individually identifiable health information, promotes patients' understanding of their privacy rights, and helps patients control the ways in which their health information is used and disclosed. The rule aims to balance the necessity of making important health disclosures to authorized persons or entities against the patient's right to privacy in the healthcare arena.

Unlike other provisions of HIPAA, the HIPAA Privacy Rule applies to health information in any form: in conversation, on paper, or in electronic format. **Protected health information (PHI)**, on the other hand, refers to any individually identifiable health information stored, maintained, or transmitted electronically.

The Privacy Rule specifies that each time PHI is released for a purpose other than treatment, payment, or other healthcare operations, the disclosure must be documented and a record of it maintained for 6 years. Patients are permitted to request a log of such disclosures, which must include the following for each disclosure:

- The date of the disclosure
- The name and address, if known, of the entity or person who received the PHI
- A description of the PHI disclosed
- An explanation of the purpose of the disclosure or a copy of the patient's written **authorization**
- A copy of a written request for a disclosure, if any

The rule also requires any provider or other entity subject to the rule to do the following:

- Distribute notices informing patients of the provider's privacy practices, including its policies for handling information contained in the patient's EHR

- Designate a privacy official as well as a security officer (this may be the same person, depending on the size of the healthcare facility) to oversee adoption of privacy policies and procedures and to ensure compliance with them. In a small office this might be a staff member with other duties as well, such as an office manager. Fig. 3.1 is a detailed job description of a privacy official in a healthcare facility.
- Offer authorization forms for release of PHI
- Implement policies to protect patients' records and to give patients access to their records
- Develop procedures for amending records when they are found to be in error
- Certify that staff members or employees have been trained in HIPAA Privacy Rule standards and in the provider's privacy practices. Training may consist of simply handing out the office privacy policy and documenting that all staff members have reviewed it and understand it, or it may involve staff members completing a self-paced online HIPAA course.

There are situations where a patient's health information may be requested to help with research and various studies. EHRs can facilitate the collection of data needed for these beneficial projects. HIPAA recognizes that there is a need for this type of data collection but also recognizes the need to protect patient information. In order to allow for the collection of the data and to protect patient confidentiality, HIPAA has stated that the data can be used as long as it is de-identified. The two ways for the data to be collected and used would be:

1. Formal determination by a qualified expert
2. Removal of specified individual identifiers
   a. Names

JOB DESCRIPTION
HIPAA SECURITY OFFICER
Complete Health Care Associates

Reports to: The security officer reports to Complete Health Care Associates.

Summary: The HIPAA security officer is responsible for overseeing the development and implementation of Complete Health Care Associate's security policies and practices. The security officer is responsible for coordinating all of the practice's activities that have security implications. In addition, the security officer is responsible for monitoring the practice's services and systems to ensure it has meaningful practices with regard to security. The security officer is also responsible for advocating and protecting the security of electronic protected health information related to the practice's patients.

Essential duties and responsibilities

- Reports to Complete Health Care Associates on current and emerging federal and state legislation and regulations impacting security. Makes recommendations as to how the practice should comply with these regulations.

- Keeps Complete Health Care Associates apprised as to the status of the practice's implementation of security procedures.

- Documents the practice's security procedures.

- Monitors compliance with the practice's security policies. Responsible for documenting and responding to any problems that occur.

- Conducts security risk assessments and audits for the practice.

- Monitors internal controls to ensure that information access levels and security clearances are maintained.

- Prepares the practice's disaster recovery and emergency mode operation plans for information systems.

- Develops an employee training program regarding security requirements. Ensures that all new employees are trained within 30 days of their employment with the practice.

- Ensures that the practice appropriately protects and maintains patient information.

- Keeps abreast of new developments regarding HIPAA security and monitors any changes in the regulations.

- Maintains employees' security awareness through reminders and updates.

Qualifications

Must have strong technical skills (operating systems, hardware, security measures, firewalls, etc.).

Must have detailed knowledge of the practice's information systems and flow of electronic protected health information.

Must have good communication skills and leadership ability.

Must possess high level of integrity and trust.

Must possess excellent follow-up and documentation skills.

Must have conflict resolution skills.

Must possess ability to assess business risks and enforce appropriate security measures.

Must possess in-depth knowledge of the HIPAA Security Rule.

FIG. 3.1 A sample job description of a privacy official in a healthcare facility.

b. All geographic subdivisions smaller than a state

c. All elements of dates (except year) that are directly related to an individual

d. Telephone numbers

e. Vehicle identifiers and serial numbers

f. Fax numbers

g. Device identifiers and serial numbers

h. Email addresses

i. Web Universal Resource Locators (URL)

j. Social Security numbers

k. Internet Protocol (IP) addresses

l. Medical record numbers

m. Biometric identifiers, including fingerprints and voiceprints

n. Health plan beneficiary numbers

o. Full-face photographs and any comparable images

p. Account numbers

q. Any other unique identifying number, characteristic, or code

r. Certificate/license numbers

By de-identifying the information the patient confidentiality has been maintained, and the data can be used to help further medical knowledge.

EHR EXERCISE 3.1   Disclosure Authorization

Complete the following exercise in the EHR Exercises assignment found in Open Assignments.

Walden-Martin Family Medical Clinic has been asked to participate in a stroke prevention study conducted by the Heart Wellness and Research Group at 345 Vascula Lane, Anytown, AL 12345. Dr. Martin's patient, Erma Willis (12/09/1947), fits the patient criteria for this study. Ms. Willis has agreed to participate and understands that Walden-Martin must provide copies of any lipid panels and ECGs from the past 10 years. Use SCMO to prepare a Disclosure Authorization for Ms. Willis. The signature on file is dated as today, and this authorization will expire 1 year from today's date.

1. Click on the Form Repository icon and then select the Disclosure Authorization from the left Info Panel. Use the Patient Search button to link the document to the patient record before proceeding.

2. Fill in the blank text fields and save the completed document to the patient record using the Save to Patient Record button.

CRITICAL THINKING EXERCISE 3.2

Mr. Rogers, a letter carrier for the U.S. Postal Service, is being seen in the healthcare facility because he was bitten on the ankle by a Yorkshire terrier, and the ankle has become infected. Mr. Rogers's provider and medical assistant are discussing the patient's condition and history outside of the examination room. Mr. Edelman is heading toward the reception desk and overhears the entire conversation, including the somewhat embarrassing story of how Mr. Rogers lost a fingertip 8 years ago after offering a leftover chicken nugget to a cocker spaniel on his route. Have the provider and medical assistant violated the HIPAA Privacy Rule?

Covered Entities and Business Associates

Covered entities and **business associates** are both subject to the HIPAA Privacy Rule:

- Under the rule, the term *healthcare provider* refers broadly to any business within the healthcare industry that transmits claims electronically. Thus even medical laboratories and accounting firms that process medical bills are considered to be providers. Although it's theoretically possible for a medical practice to circumvent HIPAA by submitting claims only on paper, it would be difficult to do so because even the practice's subcontractors, such as billing agencies, would also have to submit paper claims. If the providers within the practice had any hospital affiliations, electronic transmission would be a near certainty.

- The term *health plan* is subject to a similarly open interpretation under the rule. Almost any payer of medical costs, such as Medicare or a union-sponsored health insurance plan, is considered to be a health plan. Notable exceptions, however, include law enforcement agencies (in certain circumstances), workers' compensation, and vehicle insurance policies that offer injury coverage.

- A *healthcare clearinghouse* is an information-processing company that allows healthcare services and billing companies with incompatible platforms to share data.

The covered entity is responsible for establishing a written contract with the business associate that outlines the specific requirements and responsibilities. The contract outlines the privacy and security requirements of protected health information.

Minimum Necessary Standard

The HIPAA Privacy Rule centers on a privacy standard known as the **minimum necessary standard.** According to this provision, when a covered entity makes an allowed disclosure, it should include only the minimum necessary amount of information to accomplish the task. This means that different employees in the healthcare facility may have different levels of access to patient information. The physician will have access to the complete patient record, whereas the receptionist will have access to the patient demographic information but very limited access to the clinical care information. Another application of the minimum necessary standard is the release of information in any form. Care should be taken to release only the information requested. A detailed review of the release of information form will help to ensure that you release only the information the patient has authorized for release. The standard does not apply to disclosures made to the patient, to other healthcare providers that the patient has authorized (see the following section), or to those that are required by law.

The Privacy Rule requires healthcare personnel to take reasonable precautions not to discuss patients' personal information where it might be overheard, such as in elevators and reception areas, at cashiers' windows, and so on. However, the rule does not prohibit discussion of patient information in treatment areas, at pharmacy counters, and over the phone as long as reasonable precautions, such as lowering your voice, are taken.

BOX 3.1 Components of an Authorization Form

- Complete name, date of birth, and address of the patient
- A description of the information to be disclosed (including specific dates) and for what purpose
- A description of the information that may not be disclosed
- The name of the individuals providing the information
- A list of individuals or entities to whom the information may be disclosed
- A date on which the disclosure expires
- A statement informing the patient that the authorization may be revoked if he or she changes his or her mind
- A notice advising the patient that the information disclosed could be redisclosed and therefore would no longer be protected
- The patient's signature and date signed

Authorization Versus Consent

The HIPAA Privacy Rule rests on the so-called *individual choice principle,* which states that patients should have a reasonable opportunity to make informed decisions about the collection, use, and disclosure of their individually identifiable health information. For example, Michael would like his physician to be able to discuss his test results with Ed but not with his parents. To accomplish this, Michael signs an **authorization** form, which can be used to revoke as well as to grant permission to disclose PHI. An authorization form is needed when information is to be disclosed for purposes other than treatment, payment, or operations (such as for training or for quality assurance analysis). A general authorization is usually adequate, but a specific authorization is required to disclose information considered especially sensitive, such as the results of an HIV test. An authorization form includes the components listed in Box 3.1. No authorization is required for certain kinds of disclosures, and other disclosures may be made by the patient voluntarily.

The HIPAA Privacy Rule permits but does not require covered entities to voluntarily obtain patient **consent** for uses and disclosures of protected health information for treatment, payment, and operations. Many healthcare facilities have the patient sign a form giving consent for their health information to be used for treatment, billing, research purposes, etc.

EHR EXERCISE 3.2 Authorization for the Release of Medical Records

Complete the following exercise in the EHR Exercises assignment found in Open Assignments.

Chase Murray is a new patient of Dr. Walden. Before his first visit, the provider would like to review all of Chase's records from 2010 to the present date from Dr. Marian Brown, his previous primary care physician. The medical records release will expire in 90 days or immediately after the records request is complete. Dr. Marian Brown's office is located at Medical Arts Building, Suite 3B, Anytown, AL 12345. Dr. Brown's office phone is 123-878-8989, and the fax is 123-690-2164. The records should be sent to Walden-Martin Family Medical Clinic, 1234 Anystreet, Anytown, AL 12345. Walden-Martin's phone number is 123-123-1234, and the fax number is 123-123-5678. Prepare a Medical Records Release for the patient's signature.

1. Click on the Form Respository icon and then select the Medical Records Release from the left Info Panel. Use the Patient Search button to link the document to the patient record before proceeding.
2. Fill in the blank text fields and save the completed document to the patient record using the Save to Patient Record button.

Security Rule

Given the widespread use of electronic information-sharing technologies such as EHRs and computerized provider order entry, as well as the goal of making such technologies nationally interoperable, public authorities saw a need to strengthen the security of PHI. The HIPAA Security Rule gives each covered entity four broad goals to meet:

1. Protect the integrity and confidentiality of electronic healthcare information created, received, maintained, or transmitted
2. Shield such information against security threats that can reasonably be anticipated
3. Shelter PHI against unauthorized use and disclosure, as outlined in the HIPAA Privacy Rule
4. Ensure that all employees comply with the provisions of the Security Rule

Privacy Versus Security

In plain English, the Security Rule is supposed to ensure that information is not destroyed by natural disaster or some more malicious means, and that only people who are supposed to have access to PHI can gain access to it that's in line with their job functions. As you can see from the third goal, the HIPAA Privacy and Security Rules are closely bound up with each other. So what's the difference? The HIPAA Privacy Rule governs the use and disclosure of PHI in all forms, whereas the HIPAA Security Rule outlines the administrative, physical, and technologic measures that covered entities must take in order to implement and comply with the Privacy Rule. In a nutshell, the Privacy Rule is a statement of principles, and the Security Rule is a plan for applying them.

SECURITY SAFEGUARDS IN THE MEDICAL PRACTICE

The HIPAA Security Rule, which applies only to the patient's *electronic* health information, offers safeguards designed to avert security breaches and provide contingency plans in case network operations are interrupted. Safeguards fall into three areas: administrative, physical, and technical. Instead of laying out a rigid prescription for implementation, however, the Security Rule invites a range of approaches for complying with the standards. This flexibility allows each healthcare institution, provider, or health plan to carry out the provisions of the rule in a way that makes sense given its size, organizational complexity, technologic capabilities, budget, and the kinds of risks to which it's exposed. Let's see how the EHR figures into each kind of safeguard.

Administrative Safeguards

Administrative safeguards require the medical practice or other covered entity to adopt formal processes to prevent, detect, contain, and correct security violations. These provisions are part of the Health Information Technology for Economic and Clinical Health (HITECH) Act meaningful use reporting requirements. The security management process comprises four implementation specifications:

1. **Risk analysis.** The medical office must assess threats to the confidentiality, integrity, and availability of PHI.
2. **Risk management.** The practice should put security measures in place in order to minimize risks to a level that can be managed effectively. Doing so requires strong leadership and good communication.
3. **Sanction (penalties) policy.** The practice must determine before any infraction occurs what the penalties will be for staff members who fail to comply with security measures. Penalties should increase in proportion to the severity of the offense.
4. **Information system activity review.** The office should construct a procedure to review its compliance procedures periodically. For example, after reviewing audit trails and security incident reports, it can revise policies to shore up any weaknesses in its security plan.

To carry out these implementation specifications, the practice must assign a security officer. The security officer is responsible for supervising the development and implementation of security policies, education, practices, and procedures and for coordinating all of the practice's activities that have security implications. The security officer is also responsible for advocating and protecting the security of PHI related to the practice's patients. The officer should have detailed knowledge of HIPAA requirements and EHR systems. Like the privacy officer, the security officer may be an existing employee with other job responsibilities. In a larger practice the scope of the officer's responsibilities might warrant making it a separate, full-time position.

Physical Safeguards

Covered entities, including the medical practice, must ensure the physical security of the electronic data, buildings, and equipment they maintain by guarding them against unauthorized intrusion and by shielding them from natural disasters and environmental hazards. The possibility of a national security emergency must also be considered.

Protection against unauthorized intrusion first requires securing the facility in which the EHR system is housed—for our purposes, the medical practice. This might mean using locks, security guards, employee identification and visitor badges, or video monitoring. Network security requires password protection and contingency planning for scheduled downtime, system outages, and data loss.

In addition, equipment must be protected from unauthorized access, tampering, and theft. For any workstation at which PHI can be accessed, including mobile devices, the practice must specify which security procedures limit access to patient databases. To do so, threats to desktop computers and laptops

must be assessed. The practice must specify where each laptop or desktop computer may be placed or used, and the practice must incorporate security devices that limit unauthorized access, such as screen savers. A screen saver is a program that displays moving text or images on a screen if no input, such as a keystroke, is received for a given time period (typically a few minutes). Patient information should never be left unattended on a computer screen where any passerby could view, change, or retrieve a patient's EHR. Screen savers limit unauthorized viewing of patient information while the user is away from his or her desk. When the user returns and strikes a key, the screen saver disappears and the EHR system can be accessed again. The staff must keep maintenance records indicating when screen savers and other such security devices are installed. In addition, systems will automatically log a user out of the system after a period of time with no activity.

The practice must design a plan for the receipt, removal, backup, storage, reuse, disposal, and accountability of electronic media, such as EHR systems stored on magnetic tape, disks, memory cards, and the cloud. Essentially the practice must know where its information has been, who it was with, and what it was doing there. Before any EHR is moved, an easily retrievable copy of it must be made.

Finally, the medical practice must have a plan to restore data in the event of a national emergency or natural disaster. Backing up data is a good general practice to have in place, and it should occur several times throughout the day. If the healthcare facility sees several hundred patients in a day, imagine how much information would be lost if the EHR were only backed up overnight. Backups should not be kept in the same place as the original data. If a fire or natural disaster occurs, the data must still be safe and accessible. It is also important to have a plan in place for the recovery of data in the event of a catastrophe. The recovery plan should be tested regularly, and staff should be trained in the execution of the plan.

Plans must be in place for alternative means of entering and accessing patients' records. For example, when the computer system goes down but the rest of the facility is still functioning and patient care must be continued, the documentation of patient care will be done in a paper format. It will be important to have a supply of the forms needed to continue to provide patient care and continue to document that care. When the system is up and running, paper documentation will need to be entered into the system, either by direct data entry or by scanning in the paper forms that were used.

Login Procedures

Access to files can be limited using a secure, password-based login system such as that used in the SimChart for the Medical Office (SCMO). To help practices meet physical security specifications, only physicians and staff members with an appropriate username and password are able to access the program information. The security officer will determine the level of access for the user. As mentioned earlier, the physician will have the highest level of access, and the rest of the staff will be given access to the minimum necessary information needed to do their jobs.

#17

BOX 3.2 Tips for Choosing a Strong Password

The stronger your password, the less likely it is to be guessed by another person or detected by a computer program. Here are some tips:

- Remember that the more characters you use, the stronger your password. Just think how much easier it would be to Pick 3 to win than to Pick 6 in the Lotto! A minimum of eight characters is recommended.
- Choose a combination of letters, numbers, and symbols (asterisk, exclamation point, percentage sign, etc.).
- Avoid using characters in sequence, such as ABC, 123, and 1111.
- If your password is case sensitive (that is, the computer recognizes whether a letter is capitalized), choose both uppercase and lowercase characters.
- If you have a dog named Warren, don't choose **warren1** as your password. If your new boyfriend's name is Carmine, don't use **carminerox** as your password. You get the picture—don't choose a password that can be easily guessed, including your name, Social Security number, wedding anniversary, birthday, or the birthdays of your children.
- Don't choose words that are found in a dictionary. Instead, create "words" from the first letters of phrases you can remember. Thus "Warren is the best dog in the world!" becomes "**Witbditw!**" To make the password even more impenetrable, add numbers or swap a letter for a symbol.
- Change your password often (and NEVER share it with anyone!).

Usernames and access limitations are one way to protect the EHR data. Passwords are another. Passwords used in conjunction with the username will allow access to the computer system. Passwords are character sequences chosen by the user and intended to prevent improper use or disclosure of patient information by preventing unauthorized access to records. HIPAA recommends that passwords be contain at least 8 alphanumeric characters and be changed periodically (every 30, 60, 90 days). However, a computer can verify only that the password is valid; it can't **authenticate** that the person using it is authorized to do so. Thus a strong password should be chosen (Box 3.2), should be kept in a secure place if written down at all, and should never be given to anyone else. Further steps may be required for user **authentication**, such as the entry of biometric data (fingerprint or voiceprint) or the insertion of a smart card containing encoded user data.

Technical Safeguards

The HIPAA Security Rule provides for technical safeguards that #22 protect and control access to patients' PHI. In accordance with the Privacy Rule, the covered entity, for our purposes the medical practice, must grant users the minimum necessary access to PHI they need to perform their job functions. Such a tiered system of access might give a nurse practitioner the ability to change the patient note and to refill prescriptions but might deny the receptionist those same privileges.

A description of each employee's access to the EHR should be listed in the policies and procedures manual of the healthcare facility. This information can also be given in general terms that state what kind of access each *type* of employee (medical assistant, nurse, physician, and so on) is permitted to have. The student access in SCMO is the same as the one that a physician would have. This enables the student to access all of the same functionality in the EHR that a physician can access, including

the patient's demographics, history and examination, order entry, diagnosing, patient education instructions, and billing functions. However, EHR systems allow access to specific items to be limited. For example, certain blood test results, as in Michael's HIV case, may be viewed only by the treating physician.

To create this kind of system, users must have unique usernames or numbers, and procedures for emergency access must be in place. (This part of the technical specification overlaps with the physical specification, which addresses passwords and emergency contingency plans.) Optional security measures might include automatic logoff after a period of inactivity or encryption (scrambling data into code) and decryption (translating the coded data) technology. A procedure must also be designated to terminate access by those who are no longer authorized to use the information.

CRITICAL THINKING EXERCISE 3.3

Name several situations in which it would be dangerous to the patient if a key piece of his or her health information were changed or deleted, either intentionally or inadvertently.

Assigning Employee Privileges

Fig. 3.2 shows an example of an access log for a physician's office. This log provides an explanation of employee access to the EHR. The log details the name of the employee, job title, description of physical access (full or limited), and start date of access. Once the staff member leaves the employ of the healthcare facility, the date of termination is documented as well.

CRITICAL THINKING EXERCISE 3.4

You are the practice manager for a prominent Beverly Hills plastic surgeon, and you overhear your staff talking about the rhinoplasty of a high-profile patient seen in your office. You hold an emergency staff meeting at the end of the day to address the topic of patient confidentiality. How could the discussion of the high-profile patient's rhinoplasty among the staff impact the healthcare facility?

Designing Auditing Procedures

#21 #23

Technical safeguards also include audit trails, systems tied #19 to a person's username or password that reveal the electronic bread crumb trail each of us leaves behind as we move through the EHR system. This trail helps ensure the integrity, the correctness, and completeness of the data. After all, patient records are not supposed to be like Wikipedia entries, in which anyone can add, change, or delete a patient's health information.

Periodically the security officer should examine each employee's access trail within the EHR. The audit or login function within SCMO allows the provider or practice manager (or in this case instructor) to view all modifications to a patient's record. This is typically the role of an administrator and not a general job responsibility of the usual EHR user.

EMPLOYEE ACCESS LOG

Employee Name	Description of Access (systems, building, files, etc.)	Full or Limited Access (if limited, explain)	Login/ PW	Date of Access	Date Access Removed	Deleted Login PW (√)	Retrieved Keys, Cards, etc. (√)
Jane Andrew	Medical Records Technician: Building A&B, file rooms, EHR	Limited EHR access: unable to change notes or e-prescribing	Login: Ja_files PW: XX215	01/12/XX			
Jose Martinez	Nurse: Building A&B, EHR	Full Access	Login: Jm_nurse PW: REHCC	02/04/XX			

FIG. 3.2 An example of an access log for a healthcare facility.

Limited-Access Policies for Specific Patients

Access to individual patient records can be designated as well, allowing only specified groups of staff members to view that patient's PHI. Let's say you work at a medical spa where Bobby Trendy gets Botox injections and an occasional chemical peel. Within the patient's chart, you can assign Trendy to one or more specific groups that would contain only those users who have the authority to view his chart. When this feature is set, Trendy will not show up in patient searches conducted by users outside the specified group(s). This is a customizable feature that can be set for every patient chart.

Limiting employee access to patient information is only one way of increasing patient privacy. Patients can also control who has access to their health information. The healthcare facility staff will document *disclosure information, alternative means.* An alternative means document states the patient's preference for where he or she may be contacted and whether anyone else is allowed to have access to his or her medical information (his or her spouse, for example). The medical staff can also document when a patient was given the notice of privacy practice (NPP) forms.

EHR EXERCISE 3.3   **Notice of Privacy Practice (NPP) and Patient's Bill of Rights Documents**

Complete the following exercise in the EHR Exercises assignment found in Open Assignments.

Susannah Ling (01-02-1973) has come to the office today to drop off her completed new patient paperwork before her first appointment next week. As the medical assistant, you will provide Susannah with a copy of the NPP and patient's bill of rights documents.

The office procedure is to save the documents to her patient record as acknowledgment. Use the Form Repository to link and print these documents to the patient record:

1. Click the Form Repository icon and then select the NPP from the left Info Panel (Fig. 3.3).
2. Click the Patient Search button at the bottom of the form to search for Susannah Ling's record.
3. Once you select Susannah's record, you can use the Save to Patient Record button to store the form in the patient's record. Use the Print icon to provide the patient a copy, if required by your instructor.
4. Now select the Patient Bill of Rights from the Form Repository, directly below the NPP.
5. Click on the Patient Search button at the bottom of the form to search for Susannah Ling's record.
6. Once you select Susannah's record, you can use the Save to Patient Record button to store the form in the patient's record. Use the Print icon to provide the patient a copy, if required by your instructor.

You may access these forms at any time to view or print from the Patient Dashboard in the Clinical Care module.

PATIENTS' RIGHTS UNDER HIPAA

HIPAA, originally passed in 1996, has been amended numerous times. As a result, HIPAA is often misinterpreted, not only by patients but also by healthcare personnel, resulting in misunderstanding. According to the *New York Times,* an Arizona nursing home put an end to birthday parties for residents because it was believed that revealing birth dates was a HIPAA violation. Physicians' unwarranted reluctance to release children's immunization records has stymied the creation of immunization registries nationwide. And one transplant surgeon was denied information about a donor heart because the donor's medical team did not want to violate the recently deceased patient's privacy.

It's easy to be intimidated by the law or, frankly, bored by the monotonous legalese of privacy notices, compliance data,

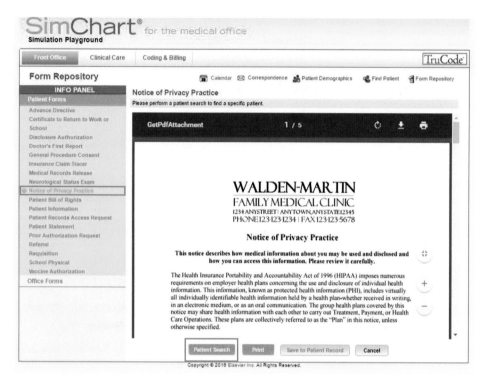

FIG. 3.3 NPP form with the form location, Patient Search button, and Print icon called out.

authorization forms, and the like. Nevertheless, as caring members of the healthcare community, we must all understand how to enforce the provisions of HIPAA without going overboard. After all, it's a real law that affects real people who make up the patient populations we serve.

Ellen, a 37-year-old with multiple sclerosis (MS), is one of them. After suffering a series of complications during a recent flare-up of her disease, Ellen decided to take a more active role in her healthcare. One of her first steps was to request copies of her records from the physicians who have been treating her—a neurologist, ophthalmologist, gastroenterologist, and general practitioner (GP). All of the practices except Ellen's GP's office sent copies of her records promptly after receiving her written request. However, Tamara, the medical assistant at the GP's office, explained (in error, as Ellen soon learned) that HIPAA prohibits releasing Ellen's own records to her. As a result, Ellen investigated HIPAA regulations and quickly determined that she, along with every other patient, has the right to the following:

- **View or receive copies of your health record.** Surprisingly, before the HIPAA Privacy Rule took effect, patients in some states could be denied access to their own health records. Now, although the insurer or medical practice may charge a reasonable fee for copying and mailing, as most of Ellen's physicians did, a patient's access to his or her own records is guaranteed by law.
- **Have inaccurate health information corrected.** If Ellen finds information that she and the provider agree is wrong, a correction (called an *amendment*) must be made within 60 days, except under special circumstances. The erroneous information need not be removed from the file, but it must

be made clear that the amended information supersedes it. And, of course, it must be obvious which is which. If the provider does not agree that the information is inaccurate, he or she is not required by HIPAA to remove or amend it. However, Ellen still has some recourse. She can file a *statement of disagreement* in her EHR to indicate which information she believes is inaccurate and why.

- **Receive a notice of privacy practices.** This notice explains how PHI can be disclosed, to whom, and under what circumstances. Typically this notice is given to patients at their first visit with the physician. It is then documented either on the paper chart or in a note in the EHR.
- **Opt out of sharing certain information with certain people.** If you want your provider to be able to discuss your medical care with your mother but not your father or with your wife but not your ex-wife, you can specify that preference, and your provider must honor any reasonable request. You can also choose, for example, to make your name and room number unavailable to the hospital switchboard or to make any other privacy request that can reasonably be carried out.
- **Have certain information withheld from certain third parties.** In addition to the option to designate certain people from whom information should be withheld, as just described, HIPAA specifies that Ellen's health information will *automatically* be kept confidential from her employer, direct marketers, and others unless she signs an authorization form to release the information to them.
- **Receive a list of disclosures of her health information.** Ellen can find out who has accessed her EHR as well as when and why.

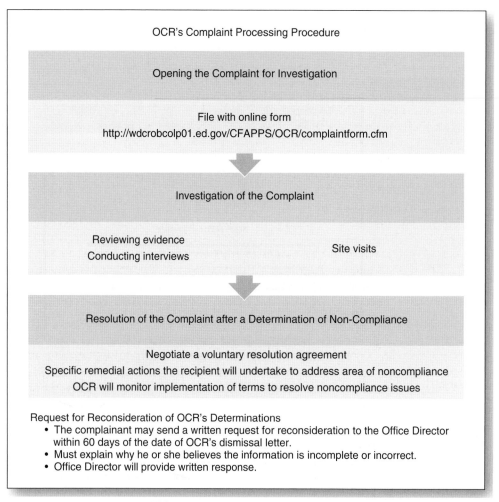

FIG. 3.4 The OCR complaint process.

- **File a complaint.** If Ellen believes that any of her providers have violated the provisions of HIPAA, she has the right to file a complaint with the Office for Civil Rights (OCR) of the U.S. Department of Health and Human Services (HHS). All HIPAA complaints made by a patient, as soon as they become known to the practice, should be documented in the patient's record and filed with the privacy official.

Ellen does not have the right to file a lawsuit against a covered entity for violating her rights under HIPAA. However, the provider is subject to civil penalties such as fines if found to be in violation. The process followed by the OCR when a patient lodges a complaint is shown in Fig. 3.4.

After Tamara was referred to the government's HIPAA website, Tamara agreed to release Ellen's records and apologized for her misunderstanding. In fact, as the privacy and security officer for the practice, Tamara has organized a lunchtime brown-bag refresher session on HIPAA for everyone on the staff.

OTHER SECURITY INITIATIVES

Along with the HIPAA regulations, other organizations and committees are trying to promote the use of secure EHR systems. The federal government's Office of the National Coordinator

for Health Information Technology, part of HHS, released its Consolidated Health Informatics initiative in 2003. The initiative is a collaborative effort involving about 20 federal agencies, including the HHS, Department of Defense, and Department of Veterans Affairs. It aims to provide consistent standards for health information interoperability, terminology, and messaging to promote the electronic exchange of clinical information within the federal government.

The HITECH Act, part of the American Recovery and Reinvestment Act of 2009, details incentive for the adoption of health information technology as a means of accelerating its meaningful implementation. In addition, HITECH details security elements that work to enforce penalties and require breach of data notifications for facilities. Meaningful use programs are discussed in more detail in Chapter 1.

ACCESS TO PROTECTED HEALTH INFORMATION

As the United States converts to using EHR systems, it's critical for Americans to have confidence that their health information will not be exploited, misused, or accessed inappropriately. However, scandals involving breaches of personal information, such as banking information, oftentimes are reported in the news and have consumers on alert. Americans are becoming increasingly uncomfortable with the idea of having external entities collect and access, sometimes even package and sell, their personal information.

When it comes to the confidentiality, privacy, and security of patient records, it seems that knowledge is power, or at least reassurance. A survey of more than 1400 patients in Massachusetts who were using an EHR with email and online patient access features found that those with more education were less likely to be concerned about security and confidentiality.

A British study by Pyper and colleagues, this one also centering on an EHR system that allowed patients to access their own files, found that patients had less apprehension after using the system. Nearly half of the study participants felt uneasy about the security of their files before viewing them, but the figure dropped to only about 40% afterward.

The idea of security rests on the notion that certain parties have permission to view private medical information, whereas others are prohibited from doing so. So who does have legal access to patients' records and in what circumstances?

Financial Institutions

In 1999 a federal law called the Financial Services Modernization Act went into effect. This law allows financial institutions—banks, securities firms, insurance companies, insurance agencies, credit unions, mortgage brokers, finance companies, check cashers, and others—to join forces and operate as a single entity.

Medical information, such as payments made to a pharmacy or medical practice, can be shared freely within these so-called financial supermarkets and can be sold to outside third parties unless the account holder objects. The law does require companies to disclose their privacy practices and to allow customers to opt out of such disclosures. However, unless a person opts out, his or her medical information could pass into the hands of a third party, such as a retailer or direct-marketing firm. Remember, only healthcare institutions are subject to HIPAA. Financial institutions, with the exception of health insurance companies and other covered entities (see following), are exempt.

SECURITY CHECKPOINT 3.1   Medical Privacy Goes Offshore

This very moment, workers in New Delhi may be transcribing court proceedings related to an obstetric malpractice case in Detroit, answering a call from a patient in Denver who wants to know whether his insurance covers smoking cessation, and entering payment information for a 90-day prescription for birth control pills given to a young woman in Dallas.

The Financial Services Modernization Act does not prohibit financial institutions from sharing medical information with service providers, such as companies with which they contract to process accounting transactions and operate customer call centers. Financial companies that operate in the United States routinely outsource these functions to low-wage foreign workers, a practice known as *offshoring*. The work is sent to nations with large English-speaking populations, such as India, Sri Lanka, the Philippines, and Hong Kong.

These offshore workers may be asked to process personal financial and medical data, such as your name, Social Security number, account numbers, and diagnosis codes. Court transcription of medical cases and general medical transcription jobs are often sent offshore as well. The data are occasionally used for fraudulent purposes, such as medical identity theft involving fraudulent claims submission. In addition, a dishonest offshore worker may sell the information to criminals operating in the United States or may share it with a subcontractor who does so.

People who are harmed, financially or otherwise, by such misuse of their personal data have little recourse because these workers are not U.S. citizens, operate outside our borders, and thus are not governed by U.S. law. Legislators are debating ways of closing this gap in HIPAA privacy protection, a loophole that wasn't anticipated when the law was passed. Companies operating in countries that are part of the European Union (EU) have solved the problem by agreeing to send private data only to so-called safe harbor countries—those that have strong, enforceable privacy protections. Because few countries have privacy policies equivalent to those of the EU nations, fewer EU companies have turned to offshoring as a way of meeting their account management needs.

Alarm over offshoring medical information may be an overreaction, however. First, companies that handle offshore transcription, accounting, call centers, and other functions have a great deal at stake and can't prosper if they handle sensitive information carelessly. Consequently, they often follow stringent internal security procedures. Second, many Americans actually feel safer having highly personal medical data handled by people on another continent than by employees who may be in the next town or city. And finally, most foreign workers, like working folks in the United States, are just doing their jobs. They're honest, hardworking people who have no intention of misusing the information—nor any interest at all in our hemorrhoids and hammertoes.

Government Agencies

The U.S. government has the right to see a patient's EHR without authorization in many circumstances. As discussed earlier when we met Michael and Ed, public health data are reported anonymously or confidentially for the purposes of tracking the incidence and spread of certain diseases. Other examples of government officials or agencies generally exempt from the HIPAA Privacy Rule include military healthcare plans, workers' compensation, correctional institutions, law enforcement officials, medical examiners, the U.S. Food and Drug Administration, and national security or intelligence officials, as required by the Patriot Act. A patient's records may even be reviewed by the HHS during the course of investigating a privacy complaint.

CRITICAL THINKING EXERCISE 3.5

Two state troopers have just burst into your healthcare facility demanding immediate help in tracking down a prisoner on the run. They believe the man may be responsible for an area carjacking, and they have a written request for a description of any distinguishing physical characteristics, such as scars and tattoos. The EHR reveals that the man has a large heart on his upper arm with the name "Pookie" written inside it. However, the officers don't have a warrant for the information. Can you give it to them? Does it matter whether the fugitive has committed a violent or a nonviolent offense?

Consumer Reporting Agencies

Most of us are aware that our credit is tracked by three major credit reporting agencies, so that when we apply for a mortgage, car loan, credit card, or another form of credit, potential lenders can check our payment history before deciding whether to approve the loan. What we may not know is that **consumer reporting agencies** exist for other purposes, such as tenant reports for landlords, homeowners' and vehicle insurance claims reports, and employment background screening reports. Life, health, disability, and long-term care insurers rely on information from consumer reporting agencies to find out about patients' health and prescription drug histories. In addition, insurers are investigating the viability of databases to collect results from patients' laboratory tests, imaging studies, and pathology reports.

These so-called downstream agencies claim to release information only with the patient's **consent,** yet the companies are not subject to HIPAA regulations. Proposed legislation would allow federal regulators to audit the companies and to impose fines for privacy violations. In addition, consumer reporting agencies are subject to the Fair Credit Reporting Act (FCRA), which is intended to protect consumer privacy and to ensure the accuracy of information supplied by consumer reporting agencies. When an insurer takes an adverse action—the denial or termination of insurance, or a rate increase—based on information obtained from a consumer reporting agency, the insurer must send a notice informing the consumer of the decision and explaining the consumer's right to request a free copy of the report in question within 60 days. However, the insurer need not explain the specific reasons for its decision.

Before obtaining medical information from an EHR, health insurers or others who wish to view it must obtain the patient's consent, which might be done in a recorded telephone statement, by email, or with a signed hard copy. Failing to do so may prompt legal action from individuals, states, or federal agencies. The Federal Trade Commission regulates compliance with the FCRA, and patients may contact the agency for information about the law or to file a complaint.

Medical Information Bureau

MIB, Inc. (MIB), known until recently as the Medical Information Bureau, is a nonprofit industry group and consumer reporting agency that maintains a database of medical information exchanged by the life, health, and disability insurers that make up its membership. You might think of it as an extensive electronic lending library where members drop by to swap information about patients' health histories. MIB saves its 470 member companies an estimated $1 billion per year by detecting and deterring fraudulent insurance claims. This savings is passed on to consumers, at least in part, in the form of lower health insurance premiums.

If a person has never been seriously injured or ill and has never made a health insurance claim, that person will not have an MIB file, just as there would be no credit report if the person has never taken out a loan or received credit of any kind. MIB reports that only about 20% of Americans have files, although this figure has not been independently confirmed.

Insurance companies are in the business of prediction, and the more information they have, the more accurate those predictions are likely to be. MIB collects any information that might have a bearing on how healthy a patient is likely to be and how long he or she is likely to live, such as the following:

- Acute and chronic illnesses
- Injuries
- Medical tests performed, the reasons the tests were ordered, and the results
- Modifiable risk factors, such as smoking, overweight, and obesity
- Lifestyle risk factors, such as gambling habits
- Substance abuse, including alcohol dependence, use of illegal drugs, and abuse of prescription drugs
- Hazardous occupations and pastimes, such as skydiving, flying private aircraft, and traveling to dangerous parts of the world
- Motor vehicle reports indicating poor driving skills and thus a likelihood of future accidents

Prescription Database Tools

Life insurance companies and other underwriters also rely on patients' prescription drug histories to make insurability decisions. About 200 million Americans' pharmacy purchases have been recorded in the files of IntelliScript or MedPoint, consumer reporting agencies that maintain databases of prescription purchasing histories. The companies sell these prescription profiles to insurance companies for about $15 each, saving insurers the time and expense of trying to retrieve the information from patients' physicians. The files are updated daily, and records stretch back 5 years.

These profiles not only tell insurers how much a patient's prescription drug costs are likely to be, but also reveal a great deal about a patient's health. A young woman receiving hydroxychloroquine (Plaquenil) and prednisone, for example, probably has lupus or a similar autoimmune disorder even if her EHR does not reveal that diagnosis directly. However, the prescription records can be misleading because so many drugs are prescribed for off-label indications. For instance, a person may be prescribed gabapentin (Neurontin) to treat neuropathic (nerve) pain. An insurance adjuster reviewing the file may presume that the person has been prescribed the drug for its primary indication, which is the treatment of epilepsy. However, when this fact is combined with information from MIB, which comes directly from the patient's EHR, a more accurate diagnostic picture tends to emerge.

Like the credit reporting bureaus, which process data from several sources in order to determine an overall credit score, the prescription database tools analyze the data in each patient's file to assign a risk score. This actual score is compared with an expected risk score to determine whether the patient is likely to be more or less expensive to insure than most patients of the same gender and age.

Employers

Group health plans that cover 50 or more employees are subject to HIPAA, but the employer still has the right to know whether an employee is enrolled in the plan, and the employer has the right to review a summary of each employee's healthcare expenses. Self-insurance plans, on-site health promotion clinics and wellness centers, and other arrangements are considered hybrid entities and are subject to special privacy rules that generally offer patients less privacy protection. In most states, employers may ask employees to authorize disclosure of information in their EHR systems. This request may be made during the hiring process, when the employee is asked to authorize a complete background check, or it might occur during an orientation session. If employees are signing multiple documents, they may not even realize they have waived their right to the privacy of their EHR. (Patients should check the HHS website for specific information.) Employers must also abide by Equal Employment Opportunity Commission regulations and by the provisions of the Americans with Disabilities Act.

Family and Friends

Disclosure to family and friends is the source of more misunderstanding than perhaps any other area of HIPAA regulations. It is not true that a healthcare professional cannot speak to a patient's family or friends about his or her condition. The HIPAA Privacy Rule says that a provider or other covered entity may discuss PHI with family members, close friends, or anyone else the patient specifies in order to inform them of the patient's general condition, location, or death, or to involve them in the patient's care, as long as the patient doesn't object.

If the patient is not available or is incapacitated and it can reasonably be inferred that the patient wouldn't object, the provider can disclose PHI directly relevant to the patient's care if he or she believes it's in the patient's best interest to do so. A covered entity is also allowed to let another person pick up prescriptions, magnetic resonance imaging films, and medical equipment, such as glucose meters and catheters.

Internet Communities

Most of us don't give a second thought to the medical information we disclose via a Facebook post or our latest tweet about going to the physician; these open web pages even link to our personal information, photographs, and physical location. Patients should review the privacy policies of every site that asks for personal information. Many sites actually capture, store, and even sell such information without patients' knowledge. Third parties have even more financial incentive to collect, sell, and swap such information, which may make its way back to the EHR and subsequently to insurance companies, marketers, and others. Patients shouldn't necessarily refrain from posting something they do not want everyone in the world to see; they should just be aware that what they say may—and probably will—leave the page, especially if they offer identifying details about themselves.

Researchers

The American Medical Informatics Association lists research as an important **secondary use** of healthcare information—an application that is not directly related to patient care—that will be facilitated by a nationally interoperable system of records. Researchers are permitted to access patients' EHR systems if they have approval from their own educational institutions to do so. Most patients don't mind this kind of disclosure. Many surveys find that most American adults would release their health information to researchers with the caveat that any personally identifying details be omitted.

Direct Marketing Firms

Direct marketing is simply another term for what most of us call junk mail or spam. The ACLU and others worry that information in EHR systems may be disclosed for the purpose of what it calls "invasive direct marketing to patients by competitors." Earlier in this chapter you met Ellen, who has MS and has decided to take a more active role in her healthcare. Her EHR reveals that she's taking Avonex, known generically as interferon beta-1a. Under certain circumstances, the pharmaceutical company that makes Rebif, a competing interferon beta-1a drug, could gain access to her EHR to get this information and then market its own product directly to Ellen. The HIPAA Privacy Rule prohibits disclosure of PHI from patients' EHR systems unless the communication occurs face to face or the direct marketer offers "a gift of nominal value." This second exception constitutes a rather large loophole. However, covered entities are prohibited from selling lists of names of patients or plan participants.

> ### CRITICAL THINKING EXERCISE 3.6
>
> You work in a practice with five gynecologists and a nurse practitioner. The office has just used its new EHR system to determine which of its female patients ages 40 and older have not yet had a mammogram or have not done so within the past year, and you and your staff have been asked to contact those patients. The patient's husband answers when you reach the third name on the list. What, if anything, can you tell him without violating your patient's privacy rights under HIPAA? Would it be better just to hang up?

HOW PATIENTS CAN PROTECT THEIR HEALTH INFORMATION

Patients are right to take an interest in protecting the integrity of their health information, which may be compromised by careless disposal or handling of records, lax security policies, and other breaches. Third parties who gain authorized or unauthorized access to a patient's health information can use it against the patient to discriminate in hiring or promotion, to reject an insurance application, to prevail in a legal proceeding, or simply to cause deliberate embarrassment. The following Security Checkpoint describes some unusually careless or devious ways in which security may be compromised.

Besides guarding against such outcomes, patients should stay vigilant to make sure their records are free of

SECURITY CHECKPOINT 3.2 Top 10 Most Creative Explanations for Privacy Breaches

We've all heard of the hacker living in his parents' basement who breaks into a patient database, and we know about the occasional stolen laptop that contains thousands of patient files. But sensitive medical information has been discarded, lost, or stolen from both paper and digital files in much more imaginative ways and for much more curious or unscrupulous reasons. Our Top 10 list describes 10 privacy or security breaches that have been documented since HIPAA was enacted. The list may have a certain entertainment value, but there's a serious message just beneath the surface: Protect patients' information vigilantly because someone is likely to want to take advantage of it if you don't.

10. **Attempted blackmail.** In a payment dispute with the Veterans Administration, an offshore contractor threatened to disclose the health information of tens of thousands of veterans. In a similar dispute with the University of California–San Francisco Medical Center, a transcriptionist in Pakistan threatened to post EHR systems on the Internet. Although he was persuaded not to do so, the medical center was unable to confirm that he had destroyed the files as requested.

9. **Winning a quarrel.** In the midst of a restructuring, whistleblowers within the Washington, D.C., emergency medical services division leaked medical information about several patients in an effort to prove their contention that the delivery of care by firefighter-paramedics was substandard. The physician who served as quality assurance director was fired over the incident.

8. **Guaranteeing future insurability.** A woman in New England admitted to a *New York Times* reporter that she had stolen multiple pages from her own paper medical chart after seeing that her physician had noted repeatedly that she was at risk for Huntington's disease, a fatal genetic condition from which the woman's mother had died. The woman did not know whether she had the disease but feared that neither she nor her children would be eligible for affordable health insurance if such a grave risk became known to the insurance companies. The pilfering patient was never caught.

7. **Dumpster ditching.** An intrepid local news team in Michigan "surveyed" Dumpsters behind area medical practices and discovered that using a paper shredder was apparently just too much of a hassle for staff members. Half of the practices had tossed intact files or other documents, many containing names, Social Security numbers, and potentially embarrassing treatment information, right into the trash. In a similar exposé, CVS and Walgreen's pharmacies in Houston were found to be dumping patients' private health information into their Dumpsters.

6. **Hitting "Reply All"—Oops!** A statistician working for Florida's Palm Beach County Health Department accidentally sent an email attachment containing the names of thousands of HIV/AIDS patients to 800 other county employees.

5. **Ambulance chasing.** In Nassau County, New York, the district attorney's office revealed that certain hospital employees had been caught accepting payola from corrupt attorneys and medical clinics for disclosing the identities of accident victims. The patients were then contacted by the lawyers or clinic staff and asked to participate in schemes involving fraudulent insurance claims.

4. **Sharing a laugh at the patient's expense.** According to the *New York Daily News,* a Brooklyn, New York, EMT was suspended without pay after a colleague reported he had scanned and emailed the medical records of patients who had been injured in circumstances that the EMT considered to be humorous. The records contained identifying details about patients as well as a description of their injuries.

3. **Protecting the environment.** An environmentally conscious San Joaquin County employee placed a box of unshredded mental health records out for curbside recycling at his home in Stockton, California. He was fired after being ratted out by a neighbor.

2. **Protecting the public.** In Pennsylvania, inmates' mental health records are considered public property under the state's "Right to Know" law.

1. **Tracking the sniffles.** The ACLU contends that forcing customers to show identification and sign a log in order to purchase pseudoephedrine-containing cold medicine (such as Sudafed), which in large quantities is used to produce methamphetamine, could unfairly place under suspicion anyone who is a regular user. These products used to be available over the counter, but in at least 35 states, customers now must purchase them at a pharmacy counter, where their identities are recorded. In Oregon, a prescription is now required to purchase pseudoephedrine.

---

inaccuracies caused by simple human error. Some inaccuracies could affect a patient's health, such as incorrect dates or frequencies of disease recurrences or even incorrect sites of amputation.

Ellen plans to take the following steps recommended by medical privacy advocates to make sure her medical information stays within her control:

- **Review medical, dental, and prescription drug records for accuracy.** Ellen requested copies of her files from MIB, IntelliScript, and MedPoint. She also requested copies of her records from the local hospital at which she has had several surgeries and from her neurologist, ophthalmologist, gastroenterologist, general practitioner, and dentist. She reviewed them for accuracy and discovered a transcription error in one of them, showing her prescription for dantrolene, a muscle relaxant, as Diprolene, a skin cream prescribed to patients with psoriasis. She requested an amendment, which was made (in compliance with HIPAA) within 60 days.

- **Request a disclosure log.** Ellen wanted to know who had accessed her records, so she requested an accounting of disclosures from her physician. The HIPAA Privacy Rule requires covered entities to account for disclosures of PHI from a patient's EHR for purposes other than treatment, payment, healthcare operations, national security or intelligence, and law enforcement, and in certain other limited circumstances.

- **Request restrictions on disclosure of sensitive information.** Patients have the right to ask a covered entity to restrict the disclosure of health information for payment purposes. The covered entity is not required to approve the request, but if it does, it then has an obligation to honor the restriction. Ellen, for instance, is insured through her husband's group plan. If she wished to do so, she could ask her provider and insurance company not to disclose her PHI to her husband even in the course of answering his payment questions.

- **Ask to receive correspondence at alternative locations.** The Privacy Rule also requires covered entities to accommodate patients who wish to receive correspondence or other communications containing PHI, such as telephone messages, by alternative means or at alternative locations. This information is documented under the HIPAA folder of the electronic patient record. For example, Ellen has asked that all messages be left on her cell phone. The covered entity may ask, in return, that the patient inform it of where bills should be sent and who will take responsibility for paying them.

- **Pay out of pocket.** Ellen has decided to seek help for depression, but she and her husband believe it's best to pay cash for the visits. Some healthcare folks call this "staying off the grid," paying directly for certain services, such as addiction counseling, rather than submitting the bills for insurance reimbursement and thus having private information disclosed to an insurer or other third party.

- **Opt for online versus paper statements and read them carefully.** Most Americans believe that some of their private health information or that of a loved one has been lost or stolen from a medical practice, healthcare institution, insurance company, employer, or government agency (such as Medicare) at one time or another. Seventy percent of Americans believe that electronic records are more likely to be lost or stolen or that paper and electronic records are subject to loss or theft about equally. This is a misconception. When it comes to identity theft, most criminals still work the old-fashioned way, by swiping mail right out of your mailbox. Remember, most statements that are printed and mailed are part of a database at the insurance company or provider network. So when a patient receives paper statements, thieves have two chances to steal the personal information. But a database is more secure than an unlocked mailbox, hands down.

Ellen used to receive paper statements from most of her physicians, declining to switch to electronic statements even when urged to do so. She also used to throw away or shred the statements without looking at them if she had a zero balance. Now she's made the switch to emailed statements. When a link to a new statement arrives in her in-box, she clicks on it and reads the Explanation of Benefits section carefully, regardless of whether she owes the provider. She also plans to check her regular credit report at least once a year to look for any medical debts that she did not incur.

EHR EXERCISE 3.4 Patient Record Access Request

Complete the following exercise in the EHR Exercises assignment found in Open Assignments.

Mr. Ken Thomas (10-25-1961) of Larkin Avenue would like to view the contents of his record to confirm that no incorrect information has been documented. He has requested an appointment with the privacy officer, who has instructed him to complete a Patient Record Access Request form. Mr. Thomas is interested specifically in Progress Notes and Hospitalizations from March 2009 to December 2013. Document the expiration date as 30 days from today.

1. Click on the Form Repository icon and then select the Patient Record Access Request from the left Info Panel.
2. Use the Patient Search button to link the document to the patient record before proceeding.
3. Fill in the blank text fields (you will not be completing the Administrative Use Only section) and save the completed document to the patient record using the Save to Patient Record button.

CHAPTER SUMMARY

- The original impetus for passage of HIPAA was to protect the insurability of patients with preexisting conditions as they switched insurers. However, the law has since been greatly expanded in an effort to ensure patient privacy and protect the security of electronic health information.

- Medical privacy is the right to decide when, how much, and with whom health information can be shared. Patients may have the expectation that this right exists, but privacy is a legal concept subject to specific exceptions and limitations.

- The HIPAA Privacy Rule specifies how healthcare providers must protect individually identifiable health information, promotes patients' understanding of their privacy rights, and helps patients control the ways in which their health information is used and disclosed.

- Administrative safeguards outlined by the HIPAA Security Rule include risk analysis, risk management, sanctions (penalties), and information system activity review. A security officer must be assigned to oversee the development and implementation of security policies, education, practices, and procedures.

- The record of a user's electronic path through the EHR system is called an audit trail. The audit trail will show who has accessed the EHR and can be used to ensure the integrity of the data found in the health record.

- Under HIPAA, patients have the right to view or receive copies of their health record, request corrections, receive the NPP, opt out of sharing certain information with certain people, have certain information withheld from certain third parties, receive a list of disclosures of their health information, and file a complaint.

- Many interested parties may have access to an employee's health information, including financial companies, insurers, public health agencies, law enforcement officials, consumer reporting agencies, schools, employers, family and friends, Internet communities, researchers, and direct marketing firms.

- Consumer reporting agencies sell or cooperatively exchange consumer information and history in areas such as credit and health. They include MIB, Inc., formerly known as the Medical Information Bureau, and for-profit prescription database tools such as IntelliScript and MedPoint.

- Patients can protect the privacy and integrity of the information in their EHR systems by reviewing their records, requesting a disclosure log, placing restrictions on whom they'd like the provider to share information with, and reviewing their statements carefully even when they owe no money.

CHAPTER REVIEW ACTIVITIES

Key Terms Review
Match the following key terms with their definitions.

1. Protected health information (PHI)

2. Covered entities

3. Laws

4. Password

5. Privacy

6. Confidentiality

7. Consent

8. Anonymity

9. Disclosure

10. Authentication

11. Audit trail

12. Secondary use

13. Minimum necessary standard

14. Ethics

15. Consumer reporting agency

a. The patient's right and expectation that individually identifiable health information will be kept private

b. Giving access to, releasing, or transferring health information to another person or entity

c. Individually identifiable health information that is stored, maintained, or transmitted electronically

d. Healthcare providers, health plans, and healthcare clearinghouses that transmit claims electronically

e. An agency that sells or cooperatively exchanges consumer information and history in areas such as credit and healthcare

f. The patient's right to have private health data collected in such a way that it can never be linked to him or her

g. A sequence of characters used to prevent unauthorized access to patient information contained in secure electronic files

h. The process of determining whether the person attempting to access a given network or EHR system is authorized to do so

i. Formal, enforceable rules and policies based on community standards of conduct

j. The patient's right to determine when, how much, and under what circumstances his or her medical information may be disclosed

k. A key provision of the HIPAA Privacy Rule requiring that disclosures include no more than the amount of information necessary to accomplish a given purpose

l. Permission given to a covered entity for uses and disclosures of protected health information for treatment, payment, and healthcare operations

m. A use of health information for a business activity or other purpose that is not directly related to patient care

n. A record that traces a user's access within the EHR system

o. Rules and standards of conduct that govern professional behavior and arise from our shared understanding of morality

True/False
Indicate whether the statement is true or false.

1. _____ All healthcare providers must maintain patient information such as test results or diagnoses.

2. _____ Covered entities—healthcare providers, health plans, and healthcare clearinghouses—are subject to the HIPAA Privacy Rule.

3. _____ The HIPAA Security Rule outlines the administrative, physical, and technologic measures covered entities must take in order to implement and comply with the HIPAA Privacy Rule.

4. _____ HITECH requires that medical offices begin implementing an EHR immediately.

5. _____ A computer can verify that a password is valid but cannot authenticate that the person using the password is authorized to do so.

6. _____ A screen saver is used to limit the view of patient information on a computer screen while the user is away from his or her desk.

7. _____ If erroneous information is found in a file, it can be removed at the patient's request.

8. _____ HIPAA prohibits financial institutions from obtaining medical information.

9. _____ A healthcare professional may speak to a patient's family or friends about the patient's general condition and location as long as the patient doesn't object or, if the patient is incapacitated, it can reasonably be inferred that he or she wouldn't object.

Workplace Applications

Using the knowledge you obtained from the chapter, provide narrative answers to the following cases.

1. You are the privacy officer for your practice, and a new employee complains to you about the excessive HIPAA training she is enduring. What can you tell this employee about why such training is necessary?
2. As you're walking toward the lunchroom, you pass a computer that has a patient's health information displayed from the EHR. You are able to clearly see a list of the patient's medications. What safety measures can the office take to prevent such unintentional disclosure of PHI?
3. Juliette Zimmerman is the volunteer coach of the high school cheerleading team. The team has earned a spot at nationals, but one of her flyers is injured and will not be able to participate. Juliette has just given an interview to a local reporter in which she made mention of this, including the girl's name. Juliette's husband, a physician, tells her that she has violated HIPAA. Is he correct?
4. You work in a psychiatry practice, and many of your patients with health insurance prefer to pay cash to protect their privacy. If a patient does submit a mental health claim, in what circumstances might that information be disclosed to a third party without the patient's authorization? How might this practice of paying "off the grid" affect public mental health services?
5. You work in a urology practice, and a 51-year-old married patient, Mr. Ratner, undergoes a vasectomy because he does not wish to have any more children. He confides to the physician that he's concerned his mistress may become pregnant. He has the procedure performed while his wife is out of town, and he requests that information about the vasectomy not be disclosed to her under any circumstances. Does Mrs. Ratner have the right to know that her husband has had a vasectomy? Does Mr. Ratner's physician or his staff have a right or an obligation to tell her? If Mrs. Ratner is also a patient in the practice, does that change your answer?
6. Chase Murray (10-20-1980) is new to the Walden-Martin office. Part of the new patient procedures is to provide the patient with a copy of the NPP and patient's bill of rights. Use SCMO to print (if required by your instructor), and save a copy of these documents to Chase's record.

EHR in Review

Complete the following exercises based on content previously covered in Chapters 1 and 2.

1. Truong Tran (05-30-1991) has picked up another insurance plan. MetLife insurance will now be his secondary insurance payer; Aetna will still remain as primary. Add this new insurance carrier to Truong's record.

MetLife Insurance
Policy ID Number: XXT65667
Group Number: PA57
Claims Address: 1234 Insurance Avenue, Anytown, AL 12345
Claims Phone Number: 800-877-0909
*Truong is the Policy Holder of this secondary insurance

---

2. What are the four main goals of the Meaningful Use program?
3. Define clinical decision support tools and give one example of how they are used.

4

Administrative Use of the Electronic Health Record Patient Letter

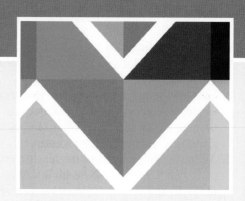

OUTLINE

CHAPTER OBJECTIVES

1. Explain the importance and typical duties of the front office assistant.
2. Discuss the necessity of respectful communication among providers, staff, and patients when answering the telephone, sending email, messaging, faxing, and scheduling appointments.
3. Create a telephone message in the SimChart for the Medical Office (SCMO).
4. Explain why a provider might send a letter to a healthcare provider or patient, and learn how to create one in an electronic health record (EHR).

5. Generate patient correspondence in SCMO.
6. Outline the procedure for the management of EHRs, including eliminating duplicate charts, the proper way of purging closed patient records, and the importance of backing up the EHR.
7. Create and manage patient appointments in the calendar.
8. Discuss the role of the front office in maintaining the waiting room.

KEY TERMS

double-booking Giving two or more patients the same appointment slot with the same provider.

encryption technology A system that keeps data secure by converting them to an unreadable code during transmission and then unencrypting the information when it reaches the recipient.

fax machine A device capable of encoding documents and sending them over a telephone line; a secure fax sends fax transmissions via secure email, eliminating many of a fax's security risks.

no-show A patient who makes an appointment and neither shows up nor calls to cancel; the term also refers to the appointment itself (a "no-show appointment").

patient flow The efficient movement of patients through the medical office as a product of accurately estimated patient volume, a consistent provider pace, and efficient scheduling practices; the term generally refers to the overall flow of patients but can refer to the path of an individual patient.

patient portal A secure website where a patient can access personal health information, schedule appointments, and refill prescriptions 24 hours a day using a username and password. Oftentimes it is part of the provider's electronic health record (EHR) system.

purging The process of separating inactive patient health records from active ones.

secure electronic messaging A component of a patient portal or personal health record that allows for secure communication between the patient and the provider.

secure email An email system capable of transmitting an encrypted message and storing it in a coded format until it is retrieved by the recipient via a secure web link.

show rate The percentage of patients in a practice who arrive for appointments as scheduled or call in advance to cancel or reschedule.

telephone etiquette A polite, helpful response and respectful manner toward callers that show patients they are cared for and valued.

~~template~~ An electronic document that has a basic format in which the required information can be entered. Templates are often created for those documents that

are needed over and over again, such as a new patient welcome letter.

views Different ways of displaying the same or similar information on a computer screen, usually with an increasing or decreasing level of detail (for example, looking at an electronic calendar in daily, weekly, and monthly views).

ROLE OF THE FRONT OFFICE ASSISTANT

When visitors arrive at a healthcare facility, the first person they encounter is usually the front office assistant. Their first impression can be created by that encounter, and we want that impression to be a positive one. The front office assistant, often a medical assistant, must have a great attitude toward patients, providers, and staff, along with the many skills to accomplish the many and varied tasks required by this position.

We have all been patients at a medical office where the staff members treat patients like unwelcome interruptions rather than valued healthcare customers. Perhaps some of us have worked in an environment where staff members pass the time by making fun of patients behind their backs rather than by figuring out ways to make an often distressing experience more pleasant. Fortunately, such offices are rare. However, it takes just one person with a poor attitude and a strong personality to taint the atmosphere for everyone else. Patients pick up on such attitudes, and many of these dissatisfied customers, so to speak, don't return.

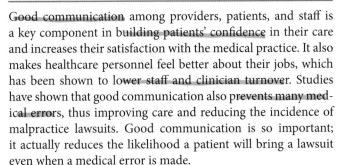

CRITICAL THINKING EXERCISE 4.1

What are the consequences for a practice if patients don't return because of what might be called customer service issues? In your answer, consider the impact on staff, providers, patient care, and practice revenue.

Staff members must be ready to help with anything the physician asks of them, within the bounds of ethics, law, and common sense. Primary front office duties usually include:

- Greeting patients on the phone and in person
- Creating the patient record and managing an electronic health record (EHR) for each patient
- Generating patient letters and other correspondence
- Maintaining the schedule
- Providing patients with registration forms and other required documents such as Notice of Privacy Practices.

COMMUNICATION IN THE MEDICAL OFFICE

~~Good communication~~ among providers, patients, and staff is a key component in ~~building patients' confidence~~ in their care and increases their satisfaction with the medical practice. It also makes healthcare personnel feel better about their jobs, which has been shown to ~~lower staff and clinician turnover~~. Studies have shown that good communication also ~~prevents many medical errors~~, thus improving care and reducing the incidence of malpractice lawsuits. Good communication is so important; it actually reduces the likelihood a patient will bring a lawsuit even when a medical error is made.

The explanation for this phenomenon is simple—patients or family members who file lawsuits tend to be upset not so much that a mistake was made but that no one ever apologized for the error and the harm it caused. As Levinson and colleagues discovered in their classic 1997 study of this topic, it's neither the error nor the poor communication alone, but the toxic combination of the two that triggers malpractice suits.

Although such studies have focused primarily on physician-patient encounters, staff interaction is important in making patients feel valued and comfortable. Levinson and colleagues found that patients appreciate being informed, for example, of what to expect. Front office assistants can play a key role in orienting patients during their visits.

When communicating patient information with other healthcare facilities, the Health Insurance Portability and Accountability Act (HIPAA) Privacy Rule allows covered entities to disclose healthcare information via email, fax, or phone without specific patient authorization, provided reasonable care is taken to avoid inappropriate disclosure or use of protected health information (PHI). If you can't tell whether the last digit of a handwritten fax number is a "7" or a "2," for instance, a reasonable safeguard might be to call the patient to verify the number before sending the fax.

Communication within the healthcare facility and between patients and healthcare professionals is continually evolving. Some medical offices now offer patient portals as a way of giving patients the option of viewing open slots on the schedule and making their own appointments online rather than having to call and ask which dates and times are available.

In the following sections we'll explore some specific means of communicating in today's healthcare setting.

CRITICAL THINKING EXERCISE 4.2

We've given an example of a reasonable safeguard you might take when sending PHI by fax. Can you think of safeguards you might need to take when calling a patient to let her know the results of a pregnancy test? What precautions might be necessary when emailing instructions to a home care nurse assigned to visit an oncology patient in your practice?

Telephone Etiquette

We have one opportunity to create a positive first impression. That opportunity can take place when the patient comes into the healthcare facility, but the initial contact between the patient and the healthcare provider's office usually occurs by phone with the medical assistant. A telephone conversation, then, gives patients their first impression of the medical office. The

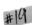

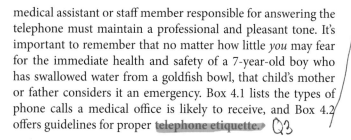

> ### BOX 4.1   Common Types of Phone Calls in the Medical Office
>
> - Appointment requests
> - Inquiries from prospective patients about the practice
> - Requests for medical advice from a physician or nurse
> - Prescription refill requests   Q5
> - Insurance and billing questions from patients
> - Information requests from insurance companies
> - Questions from pharmacists, medical supplies vendors, and other medical offices

> ### BOX 4.2   Guidelines for Proper Telephone Etiquette
>
> Following are some guidelines for telephone etiquette in the physician's office:
> - Do not use office telephone lines for personal conversations. Keep your cell phone conversations short and private, and take such calls only while on break.
> - Greet the caller by the third ring, if possible.
> - Answer the call with a professional, pleasant greeting, such as, "Good morning, Dr. Mason's office. This is Amber. How can I help you today?" The greeting should include your name so that the caller can ask for you again, if necessary, or can mention the call to another staff member (as in "I spoke to Amber yesterday about being placed on your waiting list").
> - Smile as you answer the phone. Callers will hear the cheerfulness in your voice.
> - Speak slowly and clearly, adjusting your volume if you know or suspect the caller has a hearing deficit.
> - Obtain the caller's full name, a return phone number, and the reason for the call. Verify any spelling and contact numbers for accuracy, and summarize the reason briefly and precisely.
> - If it's necessary to place the caller on hold, do so only after asking the patient's permission and awaiting a response. Few patients, if any, will refuse to be placed on hold when you make a polite request. Limit the hold time to less than a minute, if possible.
> - Document your conversation with the caller, along with the time and date and your initials.
> - To ensure that all of the caller's questions have been answered, allow her or him to end the conversation.

medical assistant or staff member responsible for answering the telephone must maintain a professional and pleasant tone. It's important to remember that no matter how little *you* may fear for the immediate health and safety of a 7-year-old boy who has swallowed water from a goldfish bowl, that child's mother or father considers it an emergency. Box 4.1 lists the types of phone calls a medical office is likely to receive, and Box 4.2 offers guidelines for proper telephone etiquette. Q3

Appointment Confirmation

Q4 A recent Medical Group Management Association study has shown that the no-show rate for healthcare facilities can be anywhere from 12% to 50%. This can mean a lot of wasted time for the healthcare facility, which can in turn mean a lot of lost revenue. This same study mentions that the longer the time between scheduling the appointment and the actual appointment date, the more likely there will be a no-show. Calling a day or two ahead to confirm appointments reduces the likelihood that patients will fail to show up, thus improving continuity of care for patients, increasing practice revenues, and helping the facility run more smoothly and productively. Automated systems are available for making confirmation calls, but in most small- and medium-size practices, front office assistants are expected to do so. Because many people have several phone numbers, leaving messages at more than one number is advisable, provided the practice has permission from the patient to do so. Text messaging and secure email can also be used to remind patients of upcoming appointments.

The Patient Dashboard in SCMO displays a record of appointment dates and times. The EHR produces a history of canceled appointments and no-shows for each patient. An excessive no-show rate will inhibit the functioning of the office. It is important for the healthcare facility to determine the most common reasons for no-shows and implement policies to help limit the number of no-shows. Patients should be encouraged to call and cancel if they can't make their appointment so that the slot can be made available to other patients. Oddly enough, healthcare facilities might be able to learn a thing or two about no-shows from the restaurant industry, for which no-shows are a perpetual problem (see Trends and Applications 4.1 and Table 4.1).

> ### TRENDS AND APPLICATIONS 4.1   What the Restaurant Industry Can Teach Us About No-Shows
>
> Anyone would be excused for thinking that the owner of Eddie's Steak and Chop has little in common with Edmund Newland Pierpont III, MD. But for restaurant owners and healthcare providers alike, no-shows are a continual annoyance and a financial drain. Both medical offices and restaurants routinely overbook in anticipation of no-shows. When the number of no-shows is overestimated, disgruntled patients and diners are subjected to long waits. When the number is underestimated, practices and kitchens are overstaffed. Because restaurants must keep perishables on hand, they also lose money by purchasing and prepping too much food.
>
>   Privately, restaurateurs have long bemoaned what they see as a scourge on the industry. According to the Operations and Information Management Department at the Wharton School, University of Pennsylvania, the industry-wide no-show rate in 2012 was estimated to be around 20% for big cities. The rate of absenteeism surges on Saturdays and can be as high as 40% on weekends and during special occasions, such as graduation day in a college town.
>
> The no-show rate among medical practices, curiously enough, falls within the same range. According to a February 2013 article in the *Pittsburgh Post-Gazette*, the average no-show rate for urban family clinics can typically be seen between 10% and 20%. However, these statistics can vary month to month or even week to week. Unfortunately, those specialty practices that are already difficult to get into can sometimes see no-show rates of as high as 50% in a single week. The no-show rate tends to be higher among practices with a large proportion of new, self-pay, or Medicare patients. The proportion is lower among practices with a large proportion of patients 46 to 64 years old and among clinics that treat more chronically ill, rather than acutely ill, patients.
>
> The restaurant industry has become remarkably aggressive and creative in combating truant diners. One restaurateur sued a would-be diner who reserved a four-top and failed to show. The court sided with the merchant, awarding him $200 in lost revenue plus the $400 that he'd paid a private eye to track down

TRENDS AND APPLICATIONS 4.1 **What the Restaurant Industry Can Teach Us About No-Shows—cont'd**

the malingerer. Another disciplinary tactic has been to embarrass deserters by listing their names on public reservations websites such as opentable.com. Perhaps a compassionate industry like healthcare can't borrow the most punitive of these strong-arm tactics, but many restaurant-industry solutions *are* adaptable to healthcare. A few clever ideas are listed in Table 4.1.

It is helpful to develop a script for making confirmation calls. With the implementation of technology, offices are using email and text messaging to confirm patient appointments. This script should become part of the office procedures manual. In addition to the date and time, the script might include the following points:

- A reminder that the physician has reserved this time especially for him or her
- A request to return the call to confirm the appointment or to reschedule if necessary
- A request to bring to the appointment a list of current medications because many patients receive prescriptions from several different specialists
- A reminder for the patient to check on his or her referral status if the patient's insurance company requires a referral
- A list of forms of payment the practice accepts (for example, "We now accept MasterCard and Visa for your copayment, or you can pay by cash or check if you prefer.")

Paper-based offices have to pull a patient's chart a day or two ahead of time to ensure that the chart can be located and that all recent correspondence received has been filed in it. An EHR eliminates that step. All test results, referral letters, and other important clinical information will already be in the patient's EHR. However, office staff should check to make sure that the provider has reviewed these items before the patient's visit. Finally, when making the confirmation call, staff should take the opportunity to check for any billing issues or insurance questions that need to be addressed.

Occasionally patients cannot be contacted via phone before their appointment because the phone was disconnected, the number was changed, or the number was entered into the EHR incorrectly. In such cases staff should ask the patient to update contact information during check-in.

Oftentimes when patients, or others who wish to speak with the provider, call with a nonurgent concern, the medical assistant in the front office will have to take a message. It is important that all of the pertinent information is obtained and documented concisely and accurately in that message. If the message is recorded in a paper format, it is best to use a product that will provide a copy of the message in case the original gets misplaced. When using an electronic system, often part of the EHR, a template is provided, and all necessary fields must be completed. The following is the basic information needed for all phone messages:

- Name of the caller
- Date and time of the call
- Who the message is for
- Who the patient is (if it is regarding a patient situation)
- Patient's date of birth (to ensure that the proper health record is referenced)
- A concise and accurate documentation of the message
- For prescription refills the medication name, pharmacy name, and number are needed

Phone contact with or about a patient needs to be documented in the health record. With an EHR this will likely happen automatically when creating the phone message. In a paper record the medical assistant should record the fact that the call has been received.

Compare the efficiency of electronic messaging systems to that of a paper-based system. Some offices use a time and date stamp to log incoming messages. Most of us recall—or perhaps are still using—those pink "While You Were Out" memo pads for transcribing phone messages. Messaging in a paper-based office might also consist of scrawling a few facts on thin little slips of perforated carbon paper no bigger than a sticky note and just as easy to misplace.

These loose message slips are then placed in a bin or a tray on the physician's desk. If the provider needs to view the patient's chart in order to respond, the chart must be pulled. The staff has little way of knowing whether the physician has read a message, reviewed a laboratory result, or returned a call. Sometimes the only clue that the physician hasn't is a third or fourth phone call from an increasingly irate patient. Once the request has been dealt with, a message is filed in the patient's paper chart. This small piece of carbon paper may be the only permanent record of the call and its content.

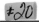

TABLE 4.1 **Reducing No-Shows**

Restaurant Industry Tactic	Adaptation for the Medical Practice
Require diners to supply their credit card number to make a deposit that's forfeited if they don't honor the reservation.	Many medical offices now notify patients that they will be charged either a percentage of the cost of a procedure or the full cost of a visit if they don't show up or cancel.
Call to remind diners of their reservation by saying, "I'm calling to confirm that you still plan to join us." Then—and here's the key—wait for an answer. Research has shown that diners who have given their word are less likely to blow off a reservation.	Medical offices can do the same—that is, call to confirm patient appointments and wait for patients to give their word that they'll either show up or call in advance to cancel.
A twist on confirming reservations is calling no-shows the following day to ask why they weren't able to come. This is a bit of a guilt trip, but it educates diners that the restaurant missed their business and was inconvenienced by their absence.	Medical offices can call patients to ask why they missed their appointments (incidentally, the most common reason is "I forgot"). Patients can be gently reminded that the physician had reserved the appointment time especially for them and can be given the option of rescheduling.
Keep callers on the phone longer. This eats up staff time, but it pays off because diners quickly develop a personal connection with the restaurant.	Scrap your recorded message and get a real person on the line chatting with college kids about their final examinations or asking after Mrs. Millikin's new grandchild. The topic doesn't matter—showing a genuine interest in the patient's life does.
Use a waiting list and walk-ins to fill tables left open by no-shows.	Johnson and colleagues found that practices with low no-show rates are more willing to take advantage of walk-in patients and to use a waiting list to fill slots left open by no-shows and last-minute cancellations.
Stop accepting reservations altogether and seat diners on a first-come, first-served basis. This idea has worked well even at high-end restaurants like celebrity chef Rick Bayless's Frontera Grill in Chicago.	Stop accepting appointments and see patients on a total or partial walk-in basis. Some practitioners use online scheduling systems to allow patients to make their own appointments, leaving as many as two-thirds of the slots open on any given day. Other practices operate in tandem a traditional appointment schedule and a fast-track room for walk-ins.

EHR EXERCISE 4.1   **Compose a Phone Message**

Complete the following exercise in the EHR Exercises assignment found in Open Assignments.

Dr. Pericardio has called at 1:15 PM today to discuss patient Noemi Rodriguez (DOB 11/04/1971). Her echocardiogram was positive for mitral valve prolapse (MVP), and Dr. Pericardio requests that Dr. Walden return his call when he is free. Dr. Pericardio can be reached after 4 PM today at 123-545-8912. Compose a phone message to communicate this information to Dr. Walden.

1. Click on the Correspondence icon and then select the Phone Message template from the left Info Panel.
2. Click the Patient Search button to perform a patient search and assign the phone message to Ms. Rodriguez.
3. Confirm the auto-populated details and enter any necessary information based on the case study.
4. Click the Save to Patient Record button.

EHR EXERCISE 4.2   **Compose a Phone Message**

Complete the following exercise in the EHR Exercises assignment found in Open Assignments.

Consumer Pharmacy called today at 10 AM to inform the Walden-Martin office that it has a shortage of Abilify. The pharmacy expects to get its shipment Saturday but will not be able to fill a prescription for Noemi Rodriguez (DOB 11/04/1971) until then. Compose a phone message to inform Dr. Martin of this shortage using the same work flow provided in EHR Exercise 4.1.

Patient Correspondence

A variety of correspondence can be created within the EHR, including physician referral letters, patient letters, and patient instructions. Providers may want to write a letter to a patient (for example, to inform the patient of test results or to summarize a plan of care), or they may want to send a letter about a patient (for instance, to provide a consultation report).

Letters in EHR systems can be prepared from standard letter templates. Templates keep providers and medical assistants from having to compose an original letter every time they send correspondence on a topic such as cholesterol results and appointment reminders.

Appointment reminder letters that are generated by the EHR system can be used to send a reminder letter about a week in advance of the appointment; it can be followed up with a confirmation call the day before. The text of the letter can provide directions for the patient to cancel or reschedule the appointment if he or she is not able to make it. A template for a letter to inform a patient of normal test results can provide information on how to have any questions answered that he or she might have.

Many EHR systems also have functionality that enables the staff members to create their own letters from the clinical documentation in the chart using macros—embedded instruction codes that automatically gather information from the patient's demographics, case information, encounter information, orders, provider's history and examination notes, healthcare professionals' documentation, prescribed medications, future appointments, referral orders to specialists, and aftercare instructions. For example, if you work for a specialist who treats burn patients and you write letters to the referring physicians to update them about a patient's progress, you can enter the term [body_surface_area] into a letter template, and the EHR will automatically use the patient's height and weight to calculate the patient's body surface area and enter it into the letter.

Physician Referral

Often a particular physician lacks the expertise or proper credentials to treat a patient with a specific condition. An example would be a family practice provider who has diagnosed a patient with diabetes and initiates treatment. Over time the patient has difficulty maintaining an appropriate blood sugar. The provider will send the patient to a board-certified physician for specialized treatment, testing, or consultation; in this case the patient would be sent to an endocrinologist. This is called a referral.

The front office assistant of the referring provider, the family practice provider in the above scenario, will complete a referral form to give the specialist a clear picture of the patient's general health, health history, and the condition for which the patient is seeking care. The front office assistant should have a basic understanding of terminology and coding systems used to complete this form. Current Procedural Terminology codes are used to designate procedures and services being requested of the specialist. *International Classification of Diseases*, 10th Revision, Clinical Modification (ICD-10) codes are used to designate the diagnosis that the patient is being referred to the specialist for. Once the specialist has seen the patient, he or she will contact the referring physician by phone or letter to outline the treatment plan. Trends and Applications 4.2 describes some benefits of copying referral letters and similar correspondence to patients.

TRENDS AND APPLICATIONS 4.2   **The Copy Letter: Should We Follow the Brits' Lead?**

In 2005 the United Kingdom's National Health Service began implementing a recommendation that patients receive copies of referrals sent to their general practitioners (GPs) after hospital consultations. Should physicians in the United States follow the United Kingdom's lead and voluntarily send referral copies to patients?

Baxter and colleagues identified four primary reasons that physicians are uncomfortable copying communication to patients. First, they worry such communication might make patients anxious about their condition. Second, they believe patients may have difficulty understanding medical terminology and don't wish to translate the information. Third, they worry that misdirected communication might violate the patient's privacy rights. Fourth, providers cite the additional workload and associated copying costs.

The first concern has not been borne out by research. Krishna and Damato interviewed patients with ocular (eye) cancer who were referred to

---

TRENDS AND APPLICATIONS 4.2   The Copy Letter: Should We Follow the Brits' Lead?—cont'd

superspecialized cancer physicians called *ocular oncologists*. The purpose of the study was to see how patients with a particularly stressful diagnosis would react to being given the additional information contained in the referral sent by the ocular oncologist to their GPs and to the referring ophthalmologist. Rather than finding the referral stressful, the patients remarked that the explanations of their condition helped them accept it. Most used the letter as a jumping off point to discuss the diagnosis with their family and friends. In fact, the researchers found that 97% of patients appreciated receiving copies of the letters.

In addition, patients have shown little difference in comprehension of letters written in medical jargon compared with those written in lay language. Among the cancer patients interviewed by Krishna and Damato, only 17% said they'd like to have the medical terms explained to them.

As to the other concerns mentioned in the study by Baxter and colleagues, HIPAA allows practitioners to communicate with patients by mail unless they specify otherwise. And finally, studies have shown that copies impose little additional burden on medical assistants and office budgets.

But why go to the extra trouble at all? Well, there are several reasons for sending copies to patients. Let's take a quick inventory:
- Promotes respect and trust between patient and provider
- Better informs patients about why they are being referred, which improves follow-up and compliance with the specialist's recommendations
- Allows patients to become more involved in their healthcare and to take responsibility for making informed choices

- Improves documentation both for the provider who copies the referrals to patients and for the specialist physician who sends patients a copy of the plan of care he or she shares with the patient's GP
- Encourages accuracy because patients have an opportunity to review the practitioner's notes, in effect, and thus correct any misinformation, such as dates of surgery and medication dosages
- Promotes a two-way exchange of information rather than an authoritative, top-down communication process
- Gives the provider an additional chance to communicate information about health promotion and healthy living

Remember, it's fairly easy to craft communication in an EHR because you can design templates that populate automatically with information from the patient's chart. Of course, providers in the United States aren't required to share their correspondence with patients. Meaningful use stage 2 requirements do require physicians to provide visit summaries, which can be helpful in improving the communication process as well.

A referral is different from a consultation. A consultation, according to the Centers for Medicare & Medicaid Services, occurs when a physician requests advice or an opinion from another physician or other qualified practitioner regarding the evaluation or management of a specific problem. Only an opinion is offered with a consultation; no treatment is provided. With a referral, treatment of the condition for which the patient was referred is transferred to the specialist physician. (Occasionally one specialist refers a patient to another specialist in a different or more highly specialized field. For example, a gynecologist might refer a patient to a gynecologic oncologist for treatment of ovarian cancer.)

EHR EXERCISE 4.3   Create a Patient Referral

Complete the following exercise in the EHR Exercise assignment found in Open Assignments.

Noemi Rodriguez (11/04/1971) is being referred to a cardiologist to perform an echocardiogram (CPT 99307) for MVP (ICD-10-CM I34.1). According to past office notes, the significant clinical information/symptoms include the fact that the patient has experienced palpitations over the past 2 months. There have been no previous treatments for the MVP. Noemi has no known allergies and takes only a multivitamin daily. The echocardiogram will be performed at Cardiology Associates, located at 445 Heart Valve Way, Anytown, AL 12345. This procedure will take one visit and will be done as an outpatient procedure. Dr. Walden is the referring provider and also the family physician. The NPI number is 8788012880, and the authorization number is NNP3234. It expires 30 days from today.

1. Click on the Form Repository icon and then select Referral from the left Info Panel. Use the Patient Search button to link the document to the patient record before proceeding.
2. Fill in the blank text fields and save the completed document to the patient record using the Save to Patient Record button.

You can access this saved form anytime by using the Patient Dashboard.

Patient Letter

Providers send letters to patients for many reasons. For example, if the medical assistant is unable to reach the patient by phone regarding normal test results, the patient may be contacted by letter. New patients are often sent a welcome letter, which outlines the office's general policies and procedures for the new patients. Appointment reminders and discharge letters are also examples of patient correspondence.

Occasionally letters are used to address unpleasant matters that must be put in writing for the legal protection of the practice. A request for payment of a delinquent balance is an example. A less common situation occurs when patients must be formally notified that the patient-provider relationship (contract) is being terminated, usually because they continually miss appointments and disregard providers' treatment plans.

EHR EXERCISE 4.4   Patient Letter

Complete the following exercise in the EHR Exercises assignment found in Open Assignments.

It is office policy to send all new patients a new patient welcome letter. Susannah Ling (01/02/1973) has recently scheduled an appointment with Walden-Martin Family Medical Clinic. Prepare a new patient welcome letter for Susannah Ling. (Susannah Ling was entered as a new patient in Chapter 2.)

1. Click on the Correspondence icon and select the New Patient Welcome template from the Letters section of the left Info Panel.
2. Click the Patient Search button at the bottom to assign the letter to Ms. Ling. The patient demographics are auto-populated.
3. Confirm the auto-populated details and include any additional information needed.
4. Click the Save to Patient Record button.

You can access this saved letter anytime by using the Patient Dashboard.

BOX 4.3 Guidelines for Sending Professional Email

Email sent from your office email account should reflect a high level of professionalism. Remember that email is a form of documentation. Accordingly, much of the email you send and receive will end up in a patient's permanent legal medical record. The following are guidelines to help you ensure that your email messages meet the highest professional standards.

- Ask yourself whether sending an email is the best way to communicate in a given situation. The tone of an email message can easily be misinterpreted, especially when addressing touchy subjects. Reread your email before sending, and consider asking a staff member for a second opinion.
- Never send an email to anyone immediately after an unpleasant incident, when you are still upset about it. If you must write it, save a draft of the message and review it when you have a cooler head. You can always send it later, but you can't take it back later.
- Triage messages as you receive them, expediting those that are urgent. You may need to refer to the patient's EHR to determine how to prioritize a message.
- Avoid the temptation to offer a diagnosis or treatment advice in response to a patient's email; leave clinical tasks to the provider.
- Use a descriptive, specific subject line (for example, Mandatory Staff Meeting, 11/15, 4:30).
- Proofread your message carefully for typographical and grammatical errors.
- Avoid using all-capital letters in the body of your message or in the subject line.
- Keep your messages brief and use a formal but conversational style.
- Never send jokes, stories, chain letters, or other inappropriate content.
- After forwarding or replying to an email, file or archive it in the correct part of the EHR. A backlog of unfiled messages creates confusion that may lead to critical errors, such as missed test results.

Secure Email

Secure email is an inexpensive, efficient system for exchanging messages through the Internet using secure encryption technology. This versatile means of communication has many different uses in the healthcare facility. The office accountant may email an insurance company to obtain an authorization. The office manager may email other staff regarding changes in office procedures. One practice may email another to request a referral for a patient office visit. Other common message topics include patient orders, notification of schedule changes, and patient education. Box 4.3 offers guidelines to ensure that email correspondence reflects professionalism.

Using the messaging system built into an EHR application ensures secure delivery of email within the practice and offers a way to communicate with staff regarding confidential patient information. Providers and staff can communicate with patients via secure email using their EHR system or any of several commercially available HIPAA-compliant secure email services. These services also offer web hosting, spam filtering, virus protection, and related accessories, such as shared calendars and address books.

Regardless of the specific use, secure email takes the place of interoffice messages—sticky notes and the like—and postal mail, which may take days to reach its destination. However, it must be used properly to prevent the unauthorized disclosure of confidential patient information. Messages must be encrypted and sent via a secure server, and a HIPAA disclosure should be attached to each message (Fig. 4.1).

SECURITY CHECKPOINT 4.1 Keeping Office Email Messages Secure

- Verify the email address of the recipient to ensure your message reaches the correct person, particularly if you have trouble reading an email address handwritten on a form.
- Inform the recipient of the sensitive nature of the email.
- If you don't receive a reply to a message in which a reply was requested, follow up by phone, mail, or fax to make sure the message was received. Don't simply resend the message to the same email address.
- Do not cc messages to others unless asked to do so, and obtain authorization when necessary.
- Develop an office policy and a related patient handout specifying what types of communication may be exchanged by email, who has access to the patients' confidential email messages, what the expected response time is, whether minors may exchange email with the office, and so on.
- Remember that your email message may end up being read by recipients other than the person for whom it was intended. A good rule of thumb is never to write anything in an email message that you wouldn't write in a letter. Fig. 4.2 shows a sample secure email agreement that can be adapted for an office and distributed to patients.

EHR EXERCISE 4.5 Patient Email Correspondence

*Complete the following exercise in the EHR Exercises assignment found in Open Assignments.

Mora Siever (01/24/1964) had a normal left ankle x-ray last Wednesday. It is Walden-Martin policy to email patients normal results. Mora's email address is m.siever@anytown.mail. Use the Correspondence menu to create a Normal Results email for Mora.

1. Click on the Correspondence icon and select the Normal Test Results template from the Emails section of the left Info Panel.
2. Click the Patient Search button at the bottom to assign the letter to Mora Siever. Confirm that the correct email address has populated the To: field.
3. Enter "x-ray Results" in the Subject field.
4. Confirm the auto-populated demographic details and document "left ankle x-ray" in the field with the Test Name watermark.
5. Document last Wednesday's date in the field with the Date of Service watermark.
6. Click the Send button.

You can access this saved email anytime by using the Patient Dashboard.

EHR EXERCISE 4.6 Compose a Patient Email Message

Complete the following exercise in the EHR Exercises assignment found in Open Assignments.

Norma Washington (DOB 08/01/1944) has been waiting for the smoking cessation program to begin at Butler Hospital, and you received word today that 6 to 8 PM classes will start this Monday in the Lawson meeting room. Compose an email message for Ms. Washington informing her of this program. Her email address is n.washington@anytown.mail.

1. Click on the Correspondence icon and select the Blank Email template from the Emails section of the left Info Panel.
2. Click the Patient Search button to assign the email message to Ms. Washington.
3. Confirm the auto-populated details and enter any necessary information based on the case study.
4. Click the Save to Patient Record button.

> *The materials in this email are private and may contain Protected Health Information (PHI). If you are not the intended recipient, be advised that any unauthorized use, disclosure, copying, distribution, or the taking of any action in reliance on the contents of this information is strictly prohibited. If you have received this email in error, please immediately notify the sender via telephone or return mail.*

FIG. 4.1 A sample HIPAA email disclosure.

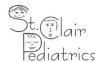 St. Clair Pediatrics

Secure E-mail Agreement

Greg T. Garrison, M.D
Jill A. Johnston, M.D
Kevin M. Ponciroli, M.D
Ginny Peter, C.P.N.P.
Kelly Harres, C.P.N.P.

Office policies regarding e-mail

Response time: E-mail will be checked only during normal office hours, 4 times per day (or more). We will make every effort to respond to e-mails within 24 hours. An e-mail sent after 12:00 PM on Friday will not receive a response until the following Monday.

E-mail access: E-mail will be managed primarily by the clinical and nursing staff. All staff members will have password-protected access to the general e-mail service. Pertinent questions and concerns will be discussed with your child's physician before the staff responds.

E-mail responses: If the question you submit can be responded to in a short and concise manner, the staff will reply via e-mail. However, for questions that require a more detailed response, the staff will contact you via telephone. Please make sure to include your phone number on all e-mails you send to us.

Office security: All desktop workstations in the office are equipped with password-protected screen savers.

E-mail security: We will not forward patient-identifiable information to a third party without your express permission. We will not use registered e-mail addresses in marketing schemes or give out your address to third parties.

Your teenager will also be allowed to use this service: Any child over the age of 13 may sign himself/herself up for the e-mail service. This allows your child to continue to communicate with his/her physician openly, honestly, and confidentially about all subject matters.

E-mail directions

E-mail must be concise: Please limit each e-mail message to one issue. This allows us to maximize message triage efficiency. Please schedule an appointment for your child if the issue is too complex or sensitive to discuss via e-mail.

All e-mails must include: The e-mail's subject line should include the reason for your e-mail followed by your child's name (i.e. "Refill Request, Joe Smith"). The body of the e-mail should include your child's date of birth and the phone number(s) where you can be reached in case the office staff needs to speak with you.

Before transmitting the e-mail: Please double-check the message and any attachments to verify that no unintended information is included.

E-mails will become a part of your child's medical record: All e-mails will be printed and/or filed in your child's medical record.

Signing up and using the service

Step 1: Read this Agreement and complete page 3. This Agreement will only be accepted in person at our office.
IMPORTANT: We will only reply to e-mails from Users that have submitted this Agreement in person.

Step 2: Log on to securesend.stclairpediatrics.com (a link can also be found on our main web page, www.stclairpediatrics.com).

Step 3: Set up your account by clicking on "Register your email address for secure sending." Enter your name, e-mail address and password. This password is the one you will use to log onto securesend.stclairpediatrics.com with your e-mail address. You then need to create a security question and password. These will be used to access a secure e-mail sent you by mydocs@stclairpediatrics.com.

To send an e-mail: Log onto securesend.stclairpediatrics.com with your e-mail address and password. You can then "Send a New Secure Message" to mydocs@stclairpediatrics.com by clicking "Compose."

To access an e-mail sent to you from mydocs@stclairpediatrics.com: The e-mail you receive will contain the line: "Click here to access your message." After clicking the link, you will be taken to a web portal, which will request two passwords. The first is the correct response to the security question you created during account registration. The second is specific to the e-mail sent to you and can be located in the body of the e-mail. You will then be taken to the actual e-mail sent to you by mydocs@stclairpediatrics.com.

IMPORTANT: Anyone can send a non-secure e-mail to mydocs@stclairpediatrics.com. The only way to ensure the information you send is secure is by logging onto securesend.stclairpediatrics.com.

Disclaimers

We are not liable for breaches of confidentiality caused by the User or any third party or for any information lost due to technical failures.

It is your responsibility to inform us of changes to your e-mail address.

This agreement describes procedures that govern an individual's use of our secure e-mail system and defines the steps that must be taken by patients or their representatives who wish to correspond via e-mail with St. Clair Pediatrics. This policy applies to the informational uses of e-mail and does not cover the ethical, legal, and regulatory issues associated with e-mail consultations.

We reserve the right to deny a User's request to communicate with him/her via e-mail.

FIG. 4.2 A sample secure email agreement. (Courtesy of St. Clair Pediatrics, Swansea, IL)

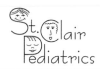

Secure E-mail Agreement

Greg T. Garrison, M.D
Jill A. Johnston, M.D
Kevin M. Ponciroli, M.D
Ginny Peter, C.P.N.P.
Kelly Harres, C.P.N.P.

E-mail us at mydocs@stclairpediatrics.com

In our continuing effort to better serve our patients and their families, we have set up an e-mail address through which you may communicate your child's protected health information with our office. It is your right to be informed about the risks of communicating via e-mail with your child's healthcare provider and about how we plan to use our secure e-mail service to maximize your child's medical management while maintaining his or her privacy as mandated by the American Health Insurance Portability and Accountability Act of 1996 (HIPAA).

Definitions for this Agreement
User: any parent/guardian or other person given access to the e-mail address listed in this Agreement.
Protected Health Information (PHI): information, including demographic information that may identify the patient, that relates to the past, present, or future physical or mental health of an individual.

What types of communication should be sent via e-mail?

Subjects appropriate for e-mail
Prescription refills
Lab results
Referral requests
Billing questions
Requests to have forms or immunization
  records completed
Non-urgent, chronic disease management
  questions

Subjects that will not be discussed through e-mail
Sensitive materials such as:
  HIV-related issues
  Other sexually transmitted diseases
  Mental health issues
  Substance abuse issues
(These topics should be discussed with your
  child's physician in person.)

What are the benefits of using e-mail?
E-mail allows quick and detailed communication with our office for non-urgent matters.
E-mail allows retention and clarification of advice provided in clinic.
E-mail is useful for information you would have to commit to writing if it were given to you orally.

What are the risks of using e-mail?
E-mail is not appropriate for urgent matters or emergency situations. E-mail, by its very nature, is a delayed communication. Our e-mail is not accessed and read continuously (see "Office policies regarding e-mail" on page 2). We cannot guarantee that any particular e-mail will be read and responded to within any particular period of time.
E-mail is sent at the touch of a button. Once sent, an e-mail message cannot be recalled or cancelled. Errors in transmission, regardless of the sender's caution, can occur.

What are the benefits of the secure e-mail service known as SecureSend used by St. Clair Pediatrics?
To comply with the guidelines regarding patient and medical records privacy set forth by HIPAA, we have engaged a third-party provider to manage our secure e-mail system: Lux Scientiae (for more information on the company, please visit www.LuxSci.com). The company uses HIPAA-compliant encrypting technology (SecureSend) to ensure security of messages sent using its system. To access these messages, the User will be required to enter two passwords. The first is a User-specific password created by each User during the on-line registration of his/her e-mail address. The second is a randomly-generated password included in each e-mail. This ensures that only the person registering a valid e-mail address has access to a child's PHI.
Everyone may use this service regardless of the type of e-mail program they have (i.e., Outlook Express, Internet Explorer, etc.). Message links embedded in the body of each e-mail direct you to a secure internet website. NOTE: You **do** need internet access to view secure e-mail messages.
In general, e-mail can be circulated, forwarded, and broadcast to unintended recipients. Using the SecureSend web portal, you con only send an email to those accounts set up through Lux Scientiae's SecureSend (which, for us, is mydocs@stclairpediatrics.com).

FIG. 4.2 cont'd

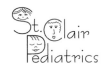

Secure E-mail Agreement

Greg T. Garrison, M.D
Jill A. Johnston, M.D
Kevin M. Ponciroli, M.D
Ginny Peter, C.P.N.P.
Kelly Harres, C.P.N.P.

Please Remember

If you have an urgent matter or an emergency situation, you should not rely on e-mail to request assistance or to describe the urgent matter or emergency situation. Instead, you should act as though provider/patient e-mail is not available to you and seek assistance by means consistent with your needs (for example, contacting the office or the on-call physician via telephone or taking your child to the emergency room).

E-mail on your computer, your laptop, and/or your PDA has inherent privacy risks – especially when your e-mail access is provided through your employer or when access to your e-mail is not continuously password protected.

In order to process and respond to your e-mail in a timely and accurate manner, individuals at St. Clair Pediatrics other than your health care provider will read your e-mail message. Your message is not a private communication between you and your child's treating physician.

Neither you nor the person reading your e-mail can see the facial expressions or gestures or hear the voice of the sender. E-mail can be misinterpreted.

Please provide the following information:

User's Name: _____

User's E-mail Address: _____

User's Mailing Address: _____

User's Phone Number: _____

For which patients do you authorize us to communicate PHI to the above e-mail address?

Patient's Name   Patient's Date of Birth   User's Relationship to Patient

_____

_____

_____

_____

_____

_____

I have read, understood, and agree to the statements in pages 1 through 3 of this Agreement. I certify the e-mail address provided on this Agreement is accurate, and that I, or my designee on my behalf, accept full responsibility for messages sent to or from this address. I understand the use of e-mail is not appropriate for urgent matters or emergency situations. I understand any e-mail sent to mydocs@stclairpediatrics.com will be read primarily by the office staff and is not a private communication between myself and my child's physician. I agree to hold harmless St. Clair Pediatrics and individuals associated with it from any and all claims and liabilities arising from or related to this Agreement.

_____   _____
Signature of Parent or Legal Guardian   Date

FIG. 4.2 cont'd

Faxing

A **fax machine** is a device that encodes documents in order to transmit them over telephone lines. The fax, like email, enables quicker message transmission than traditional mail. However, it poses several security and integrity risks:

1. Faxes can be misdirected because of human error or technical glitches.
2. The recipient of a fax cannot be verified because anyone can pick up the printed document if the machine is placed in an unsecure location.
3. It is difficult to verify that all pages were received.
4. You can mitigate these risks by following some common sense guidelines:
   a. Inform the recipient before sending any confidential patient information so that it can be retrieved immediately.
   b. Use a cover sheet when sending a fax (Fig. 4.3). The cover sheet should include the sender's contact information, a confidentiality disclaimer, and recipient information.
   c. Follow up with the intended recipient to ensure that the message was received.
   d. Document the date and time, and initial the faxed information to create a paper trail.
   e. File the completed cover sheet in the patient's chart.

An attractive alternative to faxing is to send and receive secure fax transmissions via secure email. This system for encrypting fax transmissions and sending them via email makes a fax machine obsolete, eliminating the hassles of changing toner and clearing paper jams. It also saves the practice the expense of maintaining a fax machine and paying for an additional phone line. The system works by electronically recording fax transmissions and storing them as PDF files. This then establishes the content in an electronic format, which is more compatible with EHR systems. If a hard copy is needed, these faxes can be printed, just like regular faxes.

INCIDENT REPORTS

Another responsibility for healthcare professionals is the completion of incident reports. Incident reports are used to communicate situations to the risk manager: for instance, falls, injuries, needlesticks, and medication errors. If there is a patient or employee injury, he or she would, of course, be treated for the injury and that care documented in the health record; however, an incident report would also be completed as part of risk management practices. Incident reports are used to help improve the healthcare facility. They are reviewed by the staff to see what caused the incident and what can be done to prevent it from happening again.

An incident report is completed by an employee who witnessed the accident (this may be the actual employee who was injured) and provides complete documentation of what occurred. A description of the accident and the actions taken after the accident become part of the incident report. If medical treatment is involved, it also is included in the incident report. The contributing factors and prevention measures would be documented as well. An accurate and complete incident report is an excellent tool for reducing risks for patients and employees.

MANAGING ELECTRONIC HEALTH RECORDS

The EHR is only as good as its security. It must be monitored daily to ensure the program's integrity. EHRs that are not closely

EHR EXERCISE 4.7 Complete an Incident Report

Complete the following exercise in the EHR Exercises assignment found in Open Assignments.

Carl Bowden (DOB 04/05/1954) arrived for his appointment with Dr. Walden, and as he was walking across the waiting room, he tripped on the rug. This was witnessed by the appointment coordinator, who was working at the front desk. Mr. Bowden landed facedown in front of the reception desk. The appointment coordinator, a medical assistant, called for help and went to the patient. Dr. Walden and the medical assistant assisted the patient to the examination room, where Dr. Walden concluded that Mr. Bowden had minor bruising from the fall. Complete the necessary incident report.

1. Click on the Form Repository icon, and then under Office Forms select Incident Report from the left Info Panel.
2. Document today's date, and the time was 2:30 PM.
3. Select Patient for the Incident Type and Staff as the Witness.
4. Document "Reception" in the Department field and "Waiting Room" in the Exact Location field.
5. Document "physician, medical assistant" as the Medical Team.
6. Document "scheduled appointment" as the Patient Reason for Visit.
7. Select the No radio button to indicate that this incident is not a Medication Incident.
8. Document "Patient tripped on the rug in the waiting room, landing facedown on the floor" in the Incident Description field.
9. Document "Physician and medical assistant assisted patient to examination room. Physician determined that there was minor bruising from the fall" in the Immediate Actions and Outcome field.
10. Document "Rug on floor" in the Contributing Factors field.
11. Document "Remove rug" in the Prevention field.
12. Select the No check box to indicate that the next of kin/guardian has not been notified.
13. Select the Yes check box to indicate that the medical staff has been notified.
14. Document your name in the Reported By field.
15. Document "appointment coordinator" in the Position field.
16. Document "123-123-1234" in the Contact Phone Number field.
17. Document "Dr. Walden" in the Other Persons involved field.
18. Document "physician" in the Position field.
19. Document "123-123-1234" in the Contact Phone Number field.
20. Select Julie Walden, MD from the Provider drop-down menu.
21. Document "Self-inflicted" in the Designation field.
22. Select the Signature on File check box and document the current date and time in the Date/Time field.
23. Click the Save button.

To view the completed form, click on the Saved Forms tab and select the Incident Report from the drop-down menu.

Medical Facsimile Cover Sheet

Date: _____

TO

Name	
Phone	
Fax	

FROM

Name	
Signature	
Phone	
Fax	

Patient Name	
Identifier	
Medical Record Number	

Reason for Release	

Information Released	

Total Pages_____

IMPORTANT: This facsimile transmission contains confidential information, some or all of which may be protected health information as defined by the federal Health Information Portability and Accountability Act (HIPAA) Privacy Rule. This transmission is intended for the exclusive use of the individual or entity to whom it is addressed and may contain information that is proprietary, privileged, confidential, and/or exempt from disclosure under applicable law. If you are not the intended recipient (or an employee or agent responsible for delivering this facsimile transmission to the intended recipient), you are hereby notified that any disclosure, dissemination, distribution, or copying of this information is strictly prohibited and may be subject to legal restriction or sanction. Please notify the sender by telephone (number listed above) to arrange the return or destruction of the information and all copies.

FIG. 4.3 Example of a fax cover letter.

monitored are at risk of vandalism by computer hackers and are vulnerable to destruction by natural disaster or other means. If records are damaged or destroyed, patient care could be compromised.

Maintaining the EHR is the responsibility of the entire office, and each person may have specific responsibilities. The providers, office manager, and system administrator determine which major software updates are necessary and when the changes will be made. Software updates and adding new functionality will require training sessions for all users. Planning for these updates is also important, as it may mean that the software is

unavailable for a period of time. Oftentimes the updates occur overnight, but they will require that someone be available in case of a problem with the installation and also to test the software to ensure that it is functional when the staff arrives to use it. It is important to maintain an inventory of the software and hardware assets found within the healthcare facility. The first reason is to ensure that all assets are being used to their fullest functionality, and the second is to enable replacement of equipment if needed. Staff members (medical assistants, nurses, billing staff, and receptionists) must maintain patient confidentiality, and they may be responsible for backing up the EHR. End user training sessions should be conducted not only during the process of implementing the EHR but also on an ongoing basis throughout the year. Additional training sessions will restore proficiency in forgotten applications, build competency in executing complex functions, and inform users about new EHR capabilities. In addition to ongoing end user training, technical support must also be provided. Larger organizations may have in-house technical support, especially for hardware issues. Most EHR software vendors will also offer technical support for their customers. This service may be available over the phone or in an online format.

Eliminating Duplicate Charts

The EHR should be a complete collection of a patient's health information; however, sometimes a duplicate patient chart is created in error. Perhaps the patient's last name changed due to marriage, or maybe the patient was set up as a new patient when in fact the patient had been seen before. This duplication creates a serious problem because it divides the patient information between two charts. To avoid this, the healthcare facility staff must ask pointed questions during the patient interview:

1. Ask whether the patient has ever been seen by the practice before. If so, use the already established patient EHR. Regardless of whether patients believe they are new to the office, always perform a patient search before creating a new record.
2. Ask established patients whether they have had a name change.
3. Always set up the patient EHR account using the name listed on the insurance card. Claims submitted with names that do not precisely match those on the insurance card may be denied for payment.

Purging Patient Records

Patient health records can be classified into three different groups: active, inactive, and closed. *Active records* are those of patients who have been seen within the past 3 years (see Chapter 2). These records are easily accessed and used frequently. *Inactive records* are those of patients who have not been seen by any provider in the medical office within the past 3 years. *Closed records* are those of patients who have terminated their relationship with the medical office; some have moved away, others have been asked to leave the healthcare facility because of bad debt or failure to follow the providers' advice, and some have died.

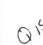

HIPAA law states that the patient health record must be kept permanently, not that it must remain in the healthcare facility. When purging, closed records are separated from active ones and stored elsewhere. Some closed records are placed on CDs or computer hard drives or maintained in inactive cloud space by the EHR vendor. Paper charts may be scanned into microfilm.

As discussed in Chapter 2, the retention period is the amount of time, by law, that patient records must be maintained by the medical office. Retention periods vary from state to state. Patient health records must be maintained for evidence of patient care in the event a lawsuit is filed.

Integrated Devices

In most healthcare facilities, the EHR system has to talk to other devices used within the organization. Scanners are used in several ways in a healthcare facility. At the front desk the insurance card is scanned in; when mail is processed, reports from other providers can be scanned, and the information is then uploaded into the health record. In the clinical area the patient may bring his or her immunization record from the previous provider to be scanned in. Faxed information needs to be documented in the EHR as well, and many machines can be integrated into the EHR so that this is a seamless process. Obtaining the patient signature electronically can be accomplished by having patients sign on a signature pad so that there is documentation of receiving the Notice of Privacy Practices (NPP), for example. Cameras are also used to help establish patient identity at check-in and to perform certain procedures within the healthcare facility.

All of these integrated devices need to be able to keep the patient information protected to remain HIPAA compliant. Being fully trained on these devices will help ensure that happens.

Backing Up the Electronic Health Record

With the use of paper-based records, protecting patient records consists of little more than storing charts in filing cabinets that are locked at the end of the day. Charts are at risk of damage from wear and tear, weather, and accidents (such as the occasional spilled cup of coffee). Paper records can be irrecoverably damaged or lost in a fire or flood, as there is no other copy of the record.

EHRs eliminate this concern if the records are backed up at a secondary, off-site location. When the software is working, the healthcare facility can run smoothly and efficiently. But no matter what precautions the medical office takes, trouble can still arise. For example, the power may be lost during severe weather, disabling computers and other electronic equipment (including the EHR). Virus attacks, hardware or software failures, and simple human error can bring a healthcare facility to a standstill.

Some medical offices store a charged portable laptop computer in the medical office. A laptop can run on battery power for a short time until the electricity is restored. Then the device should be recharged for future emergency use. Some offices may revert to written documentation while the power is off and then input the data once the software is running again. Caution should be taken, however, because rewriting documentation increases the risk of error. It's good practice to input only the data you gathered yourself and not information that a coworker gathered. This kind of backtracking can cost the practice thousands of dollars in paid overtime for office staff.

Backup takes place at a minimum of once daily to every 15 minutes or even as often as every keystroke. It's usually the job responsibility of one or two reliable workers, or the EHR vendor may conduct routine backups. Although having off-site copies of patients' charts is an advantage to patients, security must be monitored closely. Patient confidentiality and security must remain as much of a priority for the backup copies as it is for the primary EHR systems in the medical office. For this reason, backup copies should be stored in a remote location, such as a bank vault, or should be maintained by a separate entity, such as the EHR vendor. The EHR vendor may provide a data recovery package that can guarantee data backup or recovery and virus protection. An EHR vendor based as Software as a Service (SaaS) (see Chapter 2) will remotely provide backups online to minimize the risk of lost information.

The healthcare facility must, by law, have a written backup and recovery plan in place (see Chapter 3). This detailed document should be stored in the office policies and procedures manual and be easily accessible. This plan should outline what constitutes an emergency and should provide contact information for restoring the EHR (if the vendor is responsible for doing so), the location of the backup copy, instructions for managing patients while the software is down, and plans for inputting the data once the software becomes functional again.

CALENDAR

Traditionally patient appointments have been maintained using paper desk calendars or appointment books; of course, the appearance is unorganized. Scribbled names and scratched-out, overwritten, or double-booked appointments make the schedule hard to decipher. It's often difficult to reschedule appointments and find available time slots. Another disadvantage is that only one person can use the appointment book at a time.

This system has the medical assistant flipping back and forth, searching for availability within a specified time slot while perhaps one or two coworkers wait to schedule other patients. This haphazard method can cause stress for both medical assistants and patients. In addition, poor scheduling leads to longer patient wait times, a key factor in determining patient satisfaction. Patients should be seen within 5 to 10 minutes of arrival, but absolutely no more than 15 minutes of wait time should occur.

In the medical office, an electronic appointment book is the key to efficient time management. Several users can access the electronic appointment book at once. Patient appointment sheets can be printed out daily so that the physicians, medical assistants, nurses, and receptionists are all aware of the patient load for the day. Patients can be easily rescheduled, and appointment availability can be searched based on patient preferences.

When using an electronic appointment book, the medical assistant simply can search for specific appointment times, specific providers, and/or specific examination rooms (therefore ensuring the appropriate equipment is available) for the patients. At the same time, coworkers can be setting up appointments for other patients or viewing provider appointments.

Before an established patient's appointment is scheduled, his or her demographic information should be reviewed and verified. If there is change in that demographic information, it should be updated in the EHR system. When the appointment is scheduled, the demographic information is auto-populated in the schedule.

Calendar Views

In a paper system an appointment book can be viewed only two ways: open or closed. The SCMO scheduling system offers many different views, accessible from the blue tabs on the left side of the screen: Calendar View, Examination Room View, and Provider View (Fig. 4.4). Users can also view a patient's next scheduled appointment using the Search field (Fig. 4.5).

Scheduling in SCMO is done by clicking on the orange Add Appointment button from the Calendar View (Fig. 4.6) or by double-clicking within the calendar. The New Appointment box appears (Fig. 4.7). SCMO allows the user to enter three different types of appointments.

1. Patient Appointments—new and established patient visits with any of the providers in the practice
2. Block Appointments—indicates times that a provider is unavailable due to lunch, out-of-office time, office hours, or holidays
3. Other Appointments—time for staff, sales, and pharmaceutical meetings

Block an Appointment Time

Appointment slots might be blocked for a variety of reasons, such as the following:

1. To set up the appointment matrix to show when the provider is available for patient appointments
2. To account for routine days off, such as holidays
3. To schedule provider vacations, business travel, or personal time off. Some offices block out more time during the last several days before a trip and then open up the slots for urgent care patients as the need arises. During the provider's absence, the offices may also block out time on his or her partners' schedules so that they can cover urgent care visits while the physician is away.
4. To schedule provider maternity or paternity leave, family medical leave, sick leave, or other leaves of absence
5. To block out time before and after lunch or just before closing, ensuring that the staff and providers actually get to eat lunch and perhaps leave the office by quitting time

Appointment slots should be blocked out as soon as you know the time has become unavailable. Holidays and other office closings should be blocked at the beginning of the year. To block out time in the calendar, use the block appointment type.

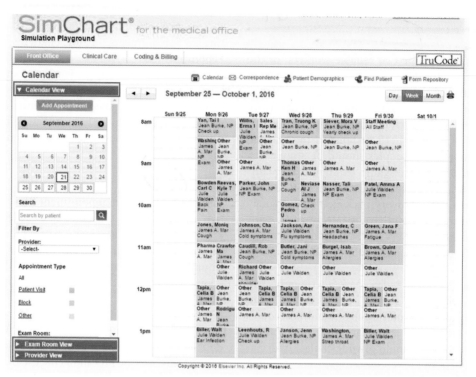

FIG. 4.4 Calendar View tabs.

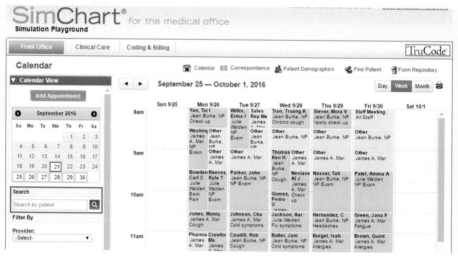

FIG. 4.5 Search field.

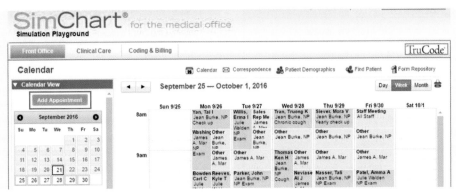

FIG. 4.6 Add Appointment button.

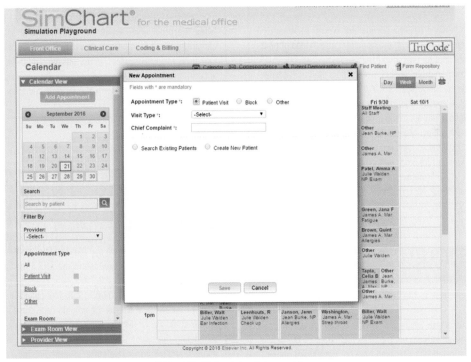

FIG. 4.7 New Appointment box.

EHR EXERCISE 4.8 Block Time for a Staff Meeting

Complete the following exercise in the EHR Exercises assignment found in Open Assignments.

The providers at Walden-Martin Family Medical Clinic want to schedule a staff meeting to discuss opening a new laboratory, new uniform requirements, and professionalism. An hour-long time slot is open this Friday at 3 PM. Coffee and water will be provided. Reserve the meeting room for this meeting.

1. Click the Add Appointment button. Select Other as the appointment type.
2. Select Staff Meeting as the Other Type.
3. Select Meeting Room as the Location.
4. Select All Staff as the Attendees.
5. Use the calendar picker to select this Friday as the meeting date.
6. Select a start time of 3 PM and an end time of 4 PM.
7. Document the agenda in the Description field as "Discussion topics: New laboratory opening, new uniforms, and professionalism. Coffee and water provided."
8. Click the Save button. A confirmation message will appear, and the meeting will be displayed on the calendar.

EHR EXERCISE 4.9 Block Out-of-Office Appointments

Complete the following exercise in the EHR Exercises assignment found in Open Assignments.

Jean Burke, NP, is attending a training seminar for wound treatment on Monday from 9 AM to 12 PM and will not be available for patient appointments during that time. Block this time for Jean Burke, NP.

1. Click the Add Appointment button. Select Block as the appointment type.
2. Select Out-of-Office as the Block type.
3. Select Jean Burke, NP, to specify who this blocked time is for.
4. Because this time will be spent out of the office, no location is needed.
5. Use the calendar picker to select Monday as the meeting date.
6. Select a start time of 9 AM and an end time of 12 PM.
7. Document "Wound treatment training" as the Description.
8. Click the Save button. A confirmation message will appear, and this time will be blocked on Jean Burke, NP's, calendar.

EHR EXERCISE 4.10 Set-Up Appointment Matrix

Complete the following exercise in the EHR Exercises assignment found in Open Assignments.

In order for everyone to know when the providers are available to see patients, you have been asked to block out the following times for the providers. This will show on the calendar as blocked time so that patient appointments will not be scheduled during that time.

a. Dr. Walden takes a 1-hour lunch break at 11:00 AM. She also likes to have a 30-minute hold on appointments from 3:00 PM until 3:30 PM for catch-up time.
b. Dr. Kahn takes a 1-hour lunch break Tuesday through Saturday at 11:30 AM. He also does rounds at the Anytown Nursing Home on Thursdays from 4:00 PM until 6:00 PM.
c. Dr. Perez is working only mornings for the next 2 months as she recovers from surgery. There should be a hold on the afternoon appointment times Monday through Friday for the next 2 months.

EHR EXERCISE 4.10 Set-Up Appointment Matrix—cont'd

1. Within the Front Office Calendar, click on the Add Appointment button.
2. Select Block as the Appointment Type, Lunch as the Block Type, and Julie Walden, MD in the For field.
3. Using the calendar picker, select today's date in the Date field.
4. For the Start Time select 11:00 AM, and for the End Time select 12:00 PM.
5. Click in the box next to Recurrence, select Daily as the Recurrence Pattern, and select End By and, using the calendar picker, select the date 6 months from today.
6. Click on the Save button, and the appointment will display on the calendar.
7. Click on the Add Appointment button.
8. Select Block as the Appointment Type, Hold as the Block Type, and Julie Walden, MD in the For field.
9. Using the calendar picker, select today's date in the Date field.
10. For the start time select 3:00 PM, and for the End Time select 3:30 PM.
11. Click in the box next to Recurrence, select Daily as the Recurrence Pattern, and select End By and, using the calendar picker, select the date 6 months from today.
12. Click on the Save button, and the appointment will display on the calendar.
13. Click on the Add Appointment button.
14. Using the steps described above, enter the Block appointments for Dr. Kahn and Dr. Perez.

After the appointment matrix has been established, it is much easier and more efficient to schedule patient appointments, as you can now clearly see when the provider is available to see patients. When scheduling patient appointments, it is important to verify the patient demographic information that is in the EHR system. If the patient's address, employment, or insurance information has changed, it is an easy process to correct it, and this will ensure that contact with the patient and that billing for services will go smoothly.

EHR EXERCISE 4.11 Edit Patient Demographic Information and Schedule an Appointment

Complete the following exercise in the EHR Exercises assignment found in Open Assignments.

Charles Johnson (DOB 03-03-1958) has called in to schedule his annual examination with Dr. Martin. He would like to come in on a Thursday morning before 10:00 AM. Dr. Martin requires 1 hour for annual examinations. Before scheduling the appointment for Mr. Johnson, you verify his address, phone number, and insurance. He states that he has moved since he was last into Walden-Martin. His new address is 1322 Flagstone Drive, Anytown, AL 12345. Update Mr. Johnson's demographic information and schedule his appointment with Dr. Martin.

1. Click on the Patient Demographics icon, enter Johnson in the Last Name field, and click on the Search Existing Patients button.
2. From the List of Patients, verify the DOB and click on Charles.
3. On the Patient tab of the Patient Demographics screen, enter Mr. Johnson's new address.
4. Scroll down and click on the Save Patient button and then close the Patient Demographics window.

EHR EXERCISE 4.11 Edit Patient Demographic Information and Schedule an Appointment—cont'd

5. Within the Front Office Calendar, click on the Add Appointment button.
6. In the New Appointment window, select Patient Visit as the Appointment Type and Annual Examination as the Visit Type.
7. Document Annual Examination as the Chief Complaint.
8. Select the Search Existing Patients button to search for Mr. Johnson's record.
9. Enter Johnson in the Last Name field of the Patient Search window, verify the DOB, and select Charles Johnson from the List of Patients.
10. Verify the Provider.
11. Use the calendar picker to select next Thursday as the appointment date.
12. Enter a Start Time of 9:00 AM and an End Time of 10:00 AM.
13. Click the Save button, and the appointment will be displayed on the calendar.

EHR EXERCISE 4.12 Schedule a Patient Appointment

Complete the following exercises in the EHR Exercises assignment found in Open Assignments.

Susannah Ling (DOB 01/02/1973) calls Walden-Martin to set up a new patient appointment with Dr. Martin next Wednesday at 10 AM. Dr. Martin requires 30 minutes for appointments with new patients. Schedule an appointment for Ms. Ling.

1. Within the Front Office, Calendar, click the Add Appointment button.
2. Within the New Appointment window, select Patient Visit as the appointment type.
3. Select New Patient Visit as the visit type.
4. Document New Patient PE as the Chief Complaint.
5. Susannah Ling was added as a Walden-Martin patient in Chapter 2, so select the Search Existing Patient radio button and click the Save button to search for Susannah's record.
6. Select James A. Martin, MD, as the provider.
7. Use the calendar picker to select next Wednesday as the appointment date.
8. Select a start time of 10:00 AM and an end time of 10:30 AM.
9. Click the Save button, and the appointment will be displayed on the calendar.

Chase Murray (added as a Walden-Martin patient in Chapter 2) called complaining of a rash on his lower extremities. The first available appointment with Dr. Martin is next Wednesday at 1 PM. Dr. Martin requires 15 minutes for urgent office visits. Schedule an appointment for Mr. Murray using examination room 4.

Prison guard Miles Green (added as a Walden-Martin patient in Chapter 2) was bitten by the drug-sniffing canine during training this morning and will need sutures. Schedule an urgent appointment with Jean Burke, NP, for 30 minutes at 4 PM.

Al Neviaser needs to schedule a follow-up appointment with Dr. Walden to check his high blood pressure. Mr. Neviaser is available next Wednesday at 11 AM. Dr. Walden requires 15 minutes for follow-up appointments and likes to perform these types of visits in examination room 6.

EHR EXERCISE 4.13 Edit an Appointment

Complete the following exercise in the EHR Exercises assignment found in Open Assignments.

Susannah Ling calls back and states that her car will not start. She would like to reschedule her appointment. Move her appointment to this Friday at 10 AM.

1. Click on Ms. Ling's existing appointment on the calendar.
2. Within the Saved Appointment window, use the calendar picker to select this Friday as the appointment date.
3. Click the Save button. A confirmation message will appear, and the appointment will be updated on the calendar.

EHR EXERCISE 4.14 Delete a Patient Appointment

Complete the following exercise in the EHR Exercises assignment found in Open Assignments.

Chase Murray calls Walden-Martin later in the day and reports that his rash turned out to be dry skin. Cancel his appointment.

1. Click on Mr. Murray's appointment on the calendar.
2. Change the status to Canceled using the Status drop-down at the bottom of the Saved Appointment window.
3. Document the reason for cancellation and click the Save button.
4. A confirmation message will appear, and the appointment will be removed from the calendar.

Double-Booking

Double-booking is a type of scheduling that may be done for any or all of the following reasons:

1. The practice expects a certain number of no-shows.
2. The practice expects certain patients to arrive early and others to arrive late, which staggers their appointment times even though the schedule shows them as being double-booked. This is an especially good scheduling strategy if patients' appointments are expected to be brief.
3. The two patients being booked in the same slot are being seen for different reasons that require different rooms and resources. For example, one patient might be scheduled for an annual physical. While the medical assistant is taking his or her vitals, another patient might be having a mole removed for evaluation by a pathologist.
4. A patient with an urgent medical problem, such as acute fever, needs to be accommodated.

You can insert a second appointment at a time you choose, or you can search for an appropriate slot by date and time, type of visit, or other criteria by following the same step for inserting a patient appointment described earlier. Keep in mind that physicians will have specific preferences as to when double-booking may occur. For example, some may allow double-booking only during the first appointment of the day, whereas others prefer double-booking slots directly before their lunch hour.

The goal of efficient scheduling is to optimize patient flow through the practice. An efficient flow requires an accurate estimation of patient volume. Scheduling must be realistic given the provider's general pace. Habitual overbooking and ineffective scheduling techniques will lengthen wait times and leave providers alternately swamped or idle.

CHAPTER SUMMARY

- The front office assistant must be well trained, versatile, and positive toward patients, providers, and other staff. Front office duties include greeting patients on the telephone and in person, taking accurate phone messages, creating and managing an EHR for each patient, scheduling appointments, and generating correspondence.
- Good communication among providers, patients, and staff improves patients' confidence in their care, increases their satisfaction with the medical practice, makes healthcare personnel feel better about their jobs, and prevents many medical errors.
- Proper telephone etiquette includes answering calls promptly, using a professional greeting, asking for the caller's full name and reason for calling, writing down a return phone number, documenting the conversation, and allowing the caller to terminate the conversation.
- Secure email is an inexpensive, efficient system for exchanging messages through the Internet using secure encryption technology.

- A fax machine is a device that encrypts and decodes documents so that they can be quickly transmitted over telephone lines. Fax transmissions can also be sent via secure email.
- Patient health records can be classified into three different groups: active, inactive, and closed. Inactive or closed medical records are purged when the retention period expires or when the patient transfers to a different practice or dies. Patients' health information stored in the EHR must be protected from destruction by computer hackers, natural disasters, terrorist attacks, and other untoward events.
- Establishing an appointment matrix is the first step in developing an efficient schedule for the healthcare facility. This clearly shows when the provider is available to see patients.
- SCMO allows the medical assistant to schedule, block, or change appointments. Using an EHR to organize appointments makes it easy to search for available slots, edit or delete appointments, keep track of patient no-shows, and double-book as needed.

CHAPTER REVIEW ACTIVITIES

Key Terms Review

Match the term in column A to the definition in column B.

1. Double-booking
2. Encryption technology
3. Secure fax
4. No-show
5. Patient flow
6. Purging
7. Secure email
8. Show rate
9. Telephone etiquette
10. Views

a. A system capable of transmitting an encrypted message and storing it in coded format until it is retrieved by the recipient via a secure web link

b. The percentage of patients in a practice who arrive for appointments as scheduled or call in advance to cancel or reschedule

c. Giving two or more patients the same appointment time with the same provider

d. The process of separating inactive patient health records from active ones

e. A polite, helpful response and respectful manner toward callers

f. A patient who makes an appointment and neither shows up nor calls to cancel

g. Different ways of displaying the same or similar information on a computer screen, usually with increasing or decreasing detail

h. A fax transmission sent via secure email

i. A system that keeps data secure by converting them into an unreadable code during transmission and then unencrypting the information when it reaches the recipient

j. A product of accurately estimated patient volume, consistent provider pace, and efficient scheduling practices

True/False

Indicate whether the statement is true or false.

1. _____ First impressions are created only when the patient enters the healthcare facility for the first time.
2. _____ The HIPAA Privacy Rule allows medical practices and other covered entities to disclose some healthcare information via email, fax, or phone without specific patient authorization, provided reasonable precautions are taken to protect privacy.
3. _____ Use of a script is a helpful way for patients to understand that the physician has reserved specific time for them.
4. _____ HIPAA-compliant secure email services may also offer web hosting services, spam filtering, virus protection, and related accessories, such as shared calendars and address books.
5. _____ Always set up the patient EHR account using the name listed on the insurance or ID card.
6. _____ Several users can access the electronic appointment book at once.
7. _____ EHR users should find the scheduling view that works best for their office and ask the administrator to program it in permanently.
8. _____ Appointment slots should be blocked out for trips, holidays, or out-of-office time using the Block Appointment type.

Workplace Applications

Using the knowledge you obtained from the chapter and SimChart for the Medical Office Simulation Playground, complete the following activities.

1. Chase Murray (DOB 04/07/1993) is having difficulty sleeping and would like to schedule an appointment with Dr. Martin next Tuesday at 9 AM. Use examination room 2 to schedule this 30-minute appointment.

2. CPR recertification training will be available for the entire staff on November 1 from noon to 4 PM in the meeting room. All staff who plan to attend must notify Marta at extension 30. Block this time on the calendar.

3. Schedule a wellness examination for Tai Yan (DOB 04/07/1956) with Dr. Walden next Monday at 9 AM. The appointment will last 30 minutes and take place in examination room 4.

4. Truong Tran (DOB 05/30/1991) needs to discuss recent episodes of depression with Jean Burke, NP. Next Monday at 1 PM will work best for him. Schedule this 30-minute office visit in examination room 7.

5. This Saturday, the Walden-Martin office will be purging health records of patients who have not been seen in the past 3 years. Use the memorandum email template in the Correspondence menu to invite available employees to assist in this process from 8:00 AM to 2:00 PM. Employees will be paid overtime, and lunch will be provided. Those interested should notify Marta at extension 30. Use the office email WMstaff@waldenmartin.com to complete this communication.

6. Maria Hernandez calls the office today for her daughter, Casey Hernandez (DOB 10/08/2000), who was exposed to poison oak while playing in the woods behind their house this weekend. She now has a red rash on her left calf that is seeping clear liquid. Casey complains that the rash is very itchy. Ms. Hernandez is working today and unable to bring Casey in. She wonders if Jean Burke, NP, could call in a prescription to help with the rash. Casey is not allergic to any medications. The Hernandez family uses Waltman's Family Pharmacy at 123-445-3200. Ms. Hernandez's work number is 123-445-5122. Compose a phone message for Jean Burke, NP, to communicate this question.

EHR in Review

This is your chance to keep past skills current. Try these activities covering previous content.

1. Interview a fellow classmate to register him or her as a new patient in SCMO. Remember to first perform a patient search within Patient Demographics to avoid creating a duplicate record. After confirming that your classmate is not registered in the system, use the Add Patient button to begin the patient registration process.

2. Noemi Rodriguez (DOB 11/04/1971) needs a copy of her electrocardiogram (ECG) from January 2014 sent to Dr. Pericardio for review before her appointment. Prepare a Medical Records Release allowing Dr. Martin to send this record. The release will expire in 30 days. Dr. Pericardio is located at 455 Heart Valve Way, Anytown, AL 45582.

3. Chris Miller, father and guarantor of patient Daniel Miller (DOB 03/21/2012), has new contact information. His cell phone number is 123-555-6363, and his work number at the auto shop is 123-540-4774. Update this contact information in the Guarantor tab of Daniel's Patient Demographics.

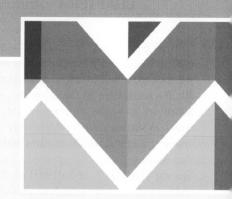

5

Clinical Use of the Electronic Health Record

CHAPTER OBJECTIVES

1. Describe the benefits of documentation in the electronic health record (EHR).
2. Explain the role of speech recognition software in medical documentation, and describe the benefits of the technology.
3. List the components of the medical, surgical, family, and social history.
4. Explain how the chief complaint and history of the present illness relate to each other.

5. Enter allergies, medications, and intolerances into an EHR.
6. Discuss what components of a patient's vaccination history should be included in the record.
7. Describe how to record vital signs and anthropometric measurements in the EHR.
8. Outline the process many physicians use for constructing a progress note.

KEY TERMS

acute condition An illness or injury that is episodic (e.g., a seizure), has a sudden onset (such as a broken bone), is of limited duration (e.g., bronchitis), and generally responds well to prompt medical attention.

anthropometric measurements Measurements of height, weight, and size used to compare the relative proportions of the human body in health and illness.

chief complaint (CC) A brief statement of the problem, condition, or symptoms that prompted the patient to seek medical care. Sometimes referred to as chief concern.

chronic condition An illness that persists for a prolonged time (typically 3 months or longer), such as diabetes mellitus, emphysema, and arthritis.

e-visit An evaluation and management service provided by a physician or other qualified health professional to an established patient using a web-based or similar electronic-based communication network for a single patient encounter that occurs over safe, secure online communication systems.

high-alert medication A medication that poses a heightened risk of injury or death when administered improperly.

history of the present illness (HPI) Details about the duration, time, location, severity, context, associated signs and symptoms, quality, and modifying factors related to the patient's illness.

medication reconciliation The process of comparing the medication list in the patient's EHR with the patient's self-report of the medications he or she has been taking.

objective Readily seen, perceived, or measured by the clinician, not only by the patient.

PFSH An abbreviation for past (medical), family, and social history.

review of systems (ROS) An organized inventory of each organ system, completed as part of the initial patient interview to pinpoint any unusual findings in the patient's history.

speech recognition A technology that converts speech into text.

subjective Perceived only by the patient and not evident to or measurable by the clinician.

DOCUMENTATION IN THE ELECTRONIC HEALTH RECORD

"If it hasn't been documented, it never happened" is the mantra drilled into the heads of medical, nursing, and medical assisting students everywhere. This is the standard for legal issues as well as for billing issues. The health record is a legal document that can be called into court as evidence to show proof of what occurred in the treatment of a patient. Health insurance companies (third-party payers) can also ask for the documentation of services provided to a patient before they make a payment on that claim. If there is no documentation of the services, the outcome of the court case can be impacted, and an insurance company will not pay for the services provided.

The electronic health record (EHR) is used to record, for instance, patient history, chief complaint, vital signs, allergies, patient education, medication lists, and orders for tests and their results. This documentation helps the provider achieve a high standard of care. Each member of the healthcare team, at various times, will need to contribute, review, or edit information in the EHR. It's important that the information added be accurate and directly reflect the actions taken during the patient encounter. Falsifying patient records is illegal and can lead to termination, civil penalties, or criminal prosecution.

Documentation is the most important responsibility of all members of the medical office. How does documentation facilitate healthcare delivery? By providing the following:

- Makes diagnosis and treatment more efficient and more likely to be effective
- Promotes patient safety and reduces medical errors by conveying critical information to other healthcare providers
- Serves as a risk management function by providing evidence of communication between the practitioner and patient and by illustrating the quality of care delivered

- Provides evidence of care delivery for third-party payer reimbursement
- In an EHR, proper documentation allows related items, such as health history, progress notes, patient letters, and patient instructions, to be linked and easily accessed.

It's not enough, though, for documentation just to be present and accounted for; it must be thorough and well organized. To ensure the best patient care, the best protection from lawsuits, and the highest level of reimbursement, an EHR should contain progress notes that are clearly written, laboratory reports and imaging studies that have been reviewed and signed, and findings and follow-up that have been neatly documented. Trends and Applications 5.1 discusses tips for ensuring proper documentation. This advice can be shared with providers and staff alike as part of a comprehensive compliance plan.

Voice Recognition

As discussed in Chapter 1, an EHR can make the problem of physicians' notoriously poor penmanship a moot point. Providers who wish to do so can document patient encounters by dictating into the medical record with the aid of speech recognition software, a technology that converts speech into text as the provider speaks into a microphone. This kind of documentation eliminates the need for a staff member to file physician documentation into a paper chart or to transcribe a tape recording into the record.

The speech recognition used in medical dictation is a different application of the same technology used in call routing (as in "Press or say 'one' now"). It's even used in the avionics systems of high-performance aircraft to allow pilots to carry out tasks such as setting radio frequencies and changing displays on cockpit gauges. It has other applications, too, ranging from computer gaming to court reporting.

TRENDS AND APPLICATIONS 5.1   Tips for Exceptional Documentation in the EHR

Composition instructors are fond of reminding students that poor writing rarely masks a brilliant insight lying just below the surface; on the contrary, jumbled sentences probably indicate muddled thinking. Clarify your ideas, and your writing will shine. Likewise, excellent documentation and high-quality care are closely related. Juries leap to conclusions about physicians whose records are sketchy, and for good reason—because it's probably true.

Good documentation prevents many errors and shows evidence of quality care. Here are some tips to improve provider and medical assistant documentation practices in your office:

1. Record all findings, both positive and negative. This includes the patient's progress since the last visit, especially if he or she is being seen for a chronic illness. Note the patient's response or lack of response to treatment, including any side effects. The documentation need not be exhaustive, but concise documentation must hit all the pertinent points.
2. Include evidence of medical decision making, unless it is clearly implied by the findings. Document treatment and follow-up, even if a wait-and-see approach is taken. Evidence of medical decision making is doubly important from a legal standpoint when the provider decides that it's wisest to do nothing.
3. Review and sign notes, reports, and letters. Leaving such documents unsigned suggests that the provider did not have a complete picture of

the patient's health status at the time he or she formulated the treatment plan.

4. Identify the patient's risk factors. Use the extensive history and relevant clinical information stored in the EHR to find the patient's greatest areas of risk. Note any conditions in the patient's family history, social history, and lifestyle or social habits that could predispose him or her toward developing certain conditions.
5. Make sure the CPT and ICD-10 codes selected are consistent with the narrative documentation. Any discrepancies could make the documentation suspect.
6. Pay special attention to prescription documentation. Refer to the list of Error-Prone Abbreviations, Symbols, and Dose Designations issued by the Institute for Safe Medication Practices (ISMP) until you know it. Use the substitutions the ISMP suggests. Avoid trailing zeros (as in "25.0"), which can make 25 mg look like 250, and avoid naked decimal points (as in .25), which can make 0.25 mg look like 25.

Does an EHR improve clinical documentation? According to a study by Rouf and colleagues, the answer is yes. They surveyed third-year medical students working in outpatient clinics, and 69% agreed that using an EHR improved their documentation. In particular, they reported that the prompts built into the system led them to ask more questions when taking a patient's history. Half of the participants said they were also more likely to review and sign patients' tests in an EHR than in a paper chart.

TRENDS AND APPLICATIONS 5.2   Use of Medical Scribes

With the push for healthcare facilities to adopt EHRs and the increase in the amount of information that must be recorded, there is a concern about the amount of time that providers are spending on these activities rather than on direct interaction with patients. This has led to the development of the medical scribe role. The Joint Commission defines a medical scribe as an unlicensed individual hired to enter information into the EHR or chart at the direction of a physician or licensed independent practitioner.

A scribe's responsibilities could include:
- Assisting the provider in navigating the EHR
- Entering information into the EHR as directed by the provider
  - HPI
  - ROS
  - Vital signs
  - Laboratory results
  - Diagnostic imaging results
  - Progress notes

- Care plans
- Medication lists
- Locating information within the EHR for provider review (laboratory and test results)
- Responding to patient requests for information as directed by the physician

A medical scribe should have an understanding of medical terminology, excellent computer skills, and a strong attention to detail. It is important that medical scribes understand that they are not obtaining the information from the patient; they are documenting the information generated by the provider and entering the information into the EHR per the provider's instructions.

Those healthcare facilities that have hired scribes have found that both the patients and providers are more satisfied with the patient encounter. The provider is establishing a better relationship with the patient because he or she is able to spend time face to face with the patient rather than interacting with a computer.

Software for the medical office incorporates a complete dictionary of medical terminology and abbreviations. The physician is able to dictate patient notes directly into the patient health record. This technology offers several advantages, including the following:
- Allows the user to work hands-free
- Eliminates the problem of misplaced or misfiled patient notes
- Decreases the rate of transcription mistakes
- Lowers the cost of transcription
- Reduces the amount of time necessary to complete documentation
- Increases the overall quality of patient care

According to a white paper by National City Corp., which finances many small medical offices, transcription costs about 11 cents per line, and an average patient encounter generates about 35 lines. That may not sound like much, but in a small clinic with two physicians, two nurse practitioners, and a load of about 14,000 visits per year, the total can swell to more than $50,000.

Speech recognition capability is available as an add-on to EHR systems. Dragon Medical, a popular speech recognition program, is compatible with many certified EHR systems.

Using Dragon Medical, you can open any of its menus. An extensive set of voice commands is used to accomplish those tasks you would normally do with the keyboard, such as "Insert a comma" and "Scratch that" to delete the last thing you said. Dragon Medical is voice recognition software that uses acoustic data to recognize your way of pronouncing things, so that the right spelling will occur if you say "tomato" and someone else in your office says "tomahto." These files also store customized terms, acronyms, and abbreviations you add to the Dragon Medical vocabulary.

Another way that documentation is occurring in EHRs is through the use of medical scribes. Many providers have found that they have been spending much of their patient contact time focusing on the computer screen rather than interacting directly with the patients. By having a scribe to enter the information into the EHR, the provider is able to focus on the patient. More information on medical scribes can be found in Trends and Applications 5.2.

CRITICAL THINKING EXERCISE 5.1

In addition to speech recognition capabilities, what advantages does electronic documentation in an EHR offer over handwritten documentation in a paper chart?

Documenting Remote Patient-Provider Encounters
Telephone Documentation

All interactions with patients, including telephone interactions, should be documented in the health record. Physicians must document all prescription refills called in or emailed to pharmacies in response to patients' phone requests. In addition medical advice offered during calls with anxious parents of feverish children, or with patients having abdominal pain or back spasms or panic attacks, must be documented.

In fact, Katz and colleagues reviewed 32 telephone-related malpractice cases and found that faulty documentation was a key factor in 88% of the errors that led to the lawsuits. These mistakes had devastating physical consequences for patients and led to an average payout of $512,000 per case for insurance companies. According to a study by Schmitt, 80% of cases are dropped if the practice is able to show, by way of excellent documentation, that a reasonable standard of care was met.

E-Visits

Advancing technology has changed not only the way patient encounters are documented but also the way patients are seen by the physician. The American Academy of Family Physicians (AAFP) defines an e-visit (also termed *web visit* or *online consultation*) as an evaluation and management service provided by a physician or other qualified health professional to an established patient using a web-based or similar electronic-based communication network for a single patient encounter that occurs over a safe, secure online communication system.

E-visits allow the patient to be "seen" by the physician without leaving his or her home or office. The patient saves travel time, decreases lost work hours, and could decrease long-term healthcare costs.

E-visits are the most successful in monitoring chronic disease. For example, diabetes, hypertension, and asthma can be monitored via e-visits on a regular basis. More and more insurance companies are beginning to pay for e-visits, reimbursing an estimated $25 to $35 per visit. Medicare, however, doesn't currently cover this service. Insurance providers who cover e-visits do require the patient to pay a regular office copayment.

The AAFP suggests the following guidelines for e-visits:
- E-visits should be offered only to established patients.
- The patient must initiate the process and agree to the terms of service. These terms include the provider's charges and privacy policy.
- Electronic communication must occur over a HIPAA-compliant online connection.
- The practitioner must appropriately document the e-visits as he or she would any other visit.
- The provider should define the time period during which the e-visit will be completed.

CRITICAL THINKING EXERCISE 5.2

In your opinion, are there any healthcare problems that should not be treated via e-visit? Why are e-visits not recommended for new patients?

CLINICAL DOCUMENTATION IN THE PATIENT RECORD

In the Who Documents in the Medical Record? section of Chapter 1, you learned that many staff members within the provider's office contribute to the medical record. After the receptionist records the basic data about the patient, the next documenter is typically the clinical medical assistant. After placing the patient in an examination room, this clinical staff member asks the patient questions related to his or her reason(s) for seeing the provider (chief complaint), the history of the chief complaint, current symptoms, previous medical history including similar injuries or illnesses, current prescriptions and over-the-counter (OTC) medications, medication

allergies, and any other nursing observations. In addition, the clinical staff member records the patient's height, weight, and vital signs, including blood pressure, temperature, pulse, and respiration rate.

Patient Encounter

Every patient visit must be documented as evidence of care. In SimChart for the Medical Office (SCMO), the patient visit is called an *encounter,* and there are eight types:
- Annual Examination
- Comprehensive Visit
- Follow-Up/Established Visit
- New Patient Visit
- Urgent Visit
- Wellness Examination
- 6-Month Visit
- Phone Encounter

The Encounters grid in the Patient Dashboard displays the encounter type, creation date, and status of existing encounters (Fig. 5.1). Users can view, edit, or create new documentation in any past encounter by clicking on the encounter in the Type column (blue underlined text).

Documenting patient care within an encounter allows the user to enter all clinical information pertaining to the date of service. To create a new patient encounter in SCMO:
1. Click the tab for the Clinical Care module or click on the Find Patient icon.
2. Perform a Patient Search. Selecting the patient will display the Patient Dashboard.
3. Click on Office Visit under Info Panel on the left side of the screen.
4. Specify the date and visit type in the Create New Encounter window. The specific provider may also be selected but is not a required field.
5. Click the Save button to add the patient encounter.
6. Clinical documentation for that encounter can begin. Users land within the Allergy record section by default but can navigate to other sections using the Record drop-down menu.

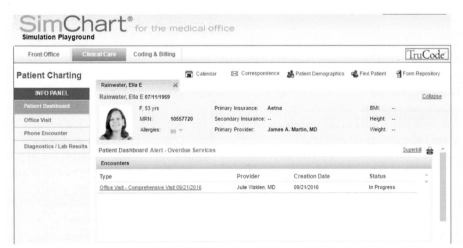

FIG. 5.1 Encounter Info panel.

ALLERGIES

One of the first requirements of Meaningful Use was that eligible providers had to maintain an active medication allergy list. This means that all patients need to be asked if they have any allergies, and the response has to be documented even if there are no known allergies (NKA). In addition to meeting the Meaningful Use criteria, knowing what the patient's allergies are is a very important factor in providing proper patient care. Patients may have many different types of allergies or intolerances, including environmental, seasonal, and contact allergies. They may also have allergies to certain medications and may have allergies to, or intolerance of, certain foods. Each patient should be asked to verify his or her allergies at the start of each visit or encounter, before medication is administered or other treatment is given, and before any medical procedures are performed. For example, before performing venipuncture, the medical assistant must ask whether the patient is allergic to latex or adhesives.

Allergies should be reviewed with the patient at every visit. If there are no allergies, this should be documented so that the patient record will show that it was reviewed but that there are no allergies at this time. If the patient indicates that he or she did have a previous allergic reaction, that reaction should also be documented in the EHR. Allergic reactions range from urticaria (hives) to pruritus (itching) to edema (swelling) to dyspnea (difficulty breathing) and chest pain. Edema of the airway may be severe enough to cause respiratory failure, so allergies must be taken seriously.

The allergies record section is the default landing page upon entering a patient encounter within SCMO. The medical assistant can verify existing allergies, document that a patient has no known allergies, and add to or edit allergies in the patient record. Most clinical records in SCMO are started by clicking the Add button, and the allergy record is no exception (Fig. 5.2). Allergies to medication, environmental factors, and food can all be documented. Allergens can be selected from a preexisting allergy database using the drop-down menu, or they can be typed directly into the field. This flexibility provides for the entry of both structured and unstructured data.

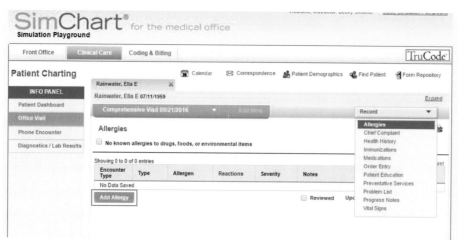

FIG. 5.2 Add Allergy button.

PATIENT HISTORY

When a new patient arrives for his or her first appointment, he or she is oftentimes asked to complete a health history form. Some healthcare facilities mail this form to the patient before the first visit for the patient to complete before arrival. In either case the form is used to collect past pertinent information about the patient, including past (medical), family, and social history (PFSH). This form could also include a comprehensive and detailed review of systems (ROS), whereas an established patient history is focused on a particular problem or condition.

All components of the history are important in treating and caring for patients and must be recorded in the EHR. The provider or other interviewer should take his or her time and consider each of the patient's responses carefully to ensure that all areas have been covered. Traditionally offices have

mailed a questionnaire to patients, asking them to complete it before their first visit. More recently, it has been possible to complete health history forms through web-based patient portals, thus reducing lost paperwork, necessary information forgotten at home, or illegible handwriting. Allowing patients to complete these forms at home gives them time to recall all important parts of their medical background in a comfortable setting. Whether the form is completed in a paper or electronic format, the content should be reviewed by the medical assistant to clarify information and ensure that no information is missed. Any positive (yes) responses to the ROS questions should prompt more specific follow-up questions.

MEDICAL AND SURGICAL HISTORY

A new patient must also be interviewed, usually by both a medical assistant and the provider, to gather as much health information as possible. This information is useful in determining a patient's risk for disease and in diagnosing, monitoring, and treating medical conditions. It includes a review of past illnesses, surgeries, hospitalizations, and treatment. During the medical history, the interviewer should also ask about drug allergies, take down a list of the patient's current medications (prescription, OTC, and supplements) and dosages, record the patient's vaccination history, and note his or her history of exposure to

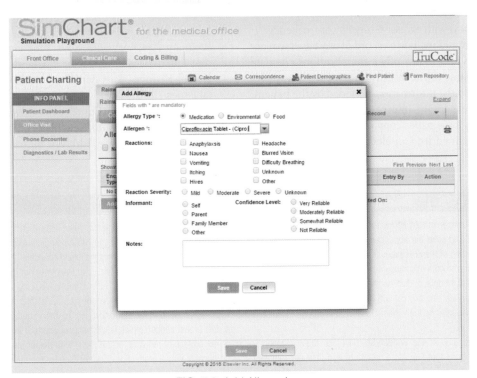

FIG. 5.3 Add Allergy box.

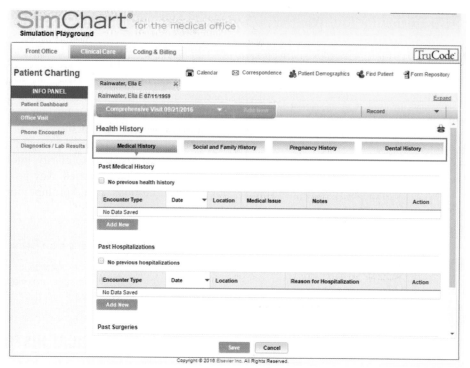

FIG. 5.4 Health History tabs.

communicable diseases, such as hepatitis and tuberculosis, if known.

Other questions asked during the medical history depend on the patient's individual needs. For example, the provider may ask an excessively thin young woman about her eating habits and about whether she has had any recent weight loss to determine whether she may have an eating or thyroid disorder. An older man may be asked whether he's experiencing any urologic problems, such as a need to urinate with excessive urgency or frequency.

Surgical history should include a record of any adverse reactions to anesthesia, a note of any other complications, the date of surgery, and the name of the institution at which it was performed. In addition to the information provided by the patient, the history may also contain information supplied by other providers. There may be a paper copy of a surgical report that would have to be scanned into an electronic format and then

uploaded to the health record. The surgery date and location would be documented in the EHR, and then the surgical report would be uploaded.

SCMO organizes health history into four tabs (Fig. 5.4):
- Medical History—Past Medical History (PMH), Past Hospitalizations, and Past Surgeries.
- Social and Family History—Safety in the Home; Paternal and Maternal Health History; marital status; employment; tobacco, drug, and alcohol use; exercise habits; and nutrition
- Pregnancy History—Previous pregnancies and significant reproductive history for female patients
- Dental History—Last dental examination, dentist, and dental issues

Once in a patient encounter, select Health History from the Record drop-down menu. New history items can be added to each tab using the orange Add New buttons.

EHR EXERCISE 5.4   Document Health History

Complete the following exercise in the EHR Exercises assignment found in Open Assignments. Download and save the appendectomy surgical report from the Additional Resources section of the EHR Exercises assignment.

If you are not already in the patient's encounter, locate the patient by clicking the tab for the Clinical Care module, or click on the Find Patient icon and perform a patient search for Susannah Ling and confirm her date of birth. Remember to enter the New Patient encounter on the Patient Dashboard in order to document in this record.

During the patient interview at the Walden-Martin office today, Susannah Ling (DOB 01/02/1973) states that she has a history of iron deficiency anemia and anxiety. Her past surgeries include an appendectomy at Butler Ambulatory

Center on November 19, 1999, and a rhinoplasty at Plastic Surgery Associates on November 1, 2013. She has a copy of the surgical report for the appendectomy with her. It was scanned when she checked in for her appointment. She has no previous hospitalizations. Ms. Ling lives with her husband, Russell, age 39, daughter Ella, age 3, and son Gunner, age 1. Ms. Ling states that she feels safe at home. She is satisfied with her job as a florist. Her father, Bert, is 64 and has hypertension and atrial fibrillation. Her mother, Shelly, is 66 and has a history of left breast cancer, which is in remission. Both of her parents are living. She drinks a glass of red wine occasionally with dinner but has never used tobacco products or illegal drugs. She does not exercise regularly or follow a special diet. She consumes two cups of coffee each day.

copy xray

EHR EXERCISE 5.4   Document Health History—cont'd

Ella was conceived naturally. Gestation was 39 weeks, and Ms. Ling was in labor for 16 hours before a vaginal delivery with no complications. Stadol was the only medication administered. Ella weighed 6 pounds, 7 ounces. Gunner was also conceived naturally. Gestation was 40 weeks, and Ms. Ling was in labor for 12 hours before a vaginal delivery with acute mastitis after delivery, which is now resolved. Ms. Ling received an epidural. Gunner weighed 8 pounds, 0 ounces. She has not had any abortions or miscarriages.

Her last dental visit was February 20, 2014, with Dr. Bonnett.

Use the Health History record to document in each of the four history tabs. Be sure to save your work when finished.

1. Within the Medical History tab, click the Add button beneath the Past Medical History grid.
2. In the Add Past Medical History window, using today's date, document "Walden-Martin Family Medical Clinic" as the location and "Iron deficiency anemia" as the medical issue. Click the Save button and repeat this work flow to document Ms. Ling's past medical history of anxiety.
3. Click the Add button beneath the Past Surgeries section.
4. In the Add Past Surgeries window, document "November 19, 1999" as the Date, "Butler Ambulatory Center" as the Location, and "Appendectomy" as the Type of Surgery. Click on the "Browse..." button in the "Upload Surgical record" section. Locate the saved appendectomy surgical report, highlight, and click the Open button. Click the Save button and repeat this work flow to document Ms. Ling's rhinoplasty (there will be no surgical report to upload).
5. Within the Social and Family History tab, click the Add New button beneath the Family History grid.
6. In the Add Family History window, document "Russell" as the name, "39" as the age, and "Husband" as the relationship. Click the Save button and repeat this work flow to add Ella and Gunner.
7. Select the Yes radio button to indicate that Ms. Ling does feel safe in her home.
8. Click the Add button beneath the Paternal section.
9. In the Add Paternal Family Member window, document "Father" as the relationship, "64" as the age, and "Hypertension and atrial fibrillation" as current medical conditions. Click the Save button and repeat this work flow for Ms. Ling's mother in the Maternal section.
10. Use the Parents Marital Status drop-down menu to indicate that Ms. Ling is married.
11. Use the Employment drop-down menu to indicate that Ms. Ling is satisfied with her job and document "Florist" in the Comments field.
12. Within the Tobacco section, select the Never radio button to indicate Ms. Ling's tobacco use.
13. Within the Alcohol/Drugs section, select the Occasionally radio button to indicate how frequently Ms. Ling drinks alcohol, and document "Red wine" in the Comments field. Select the Never radio button to indicate Ms. Ling's usage regarding illegal or addictive substances.
14. Within the Activities/Exposures/Habits section, select the No radio button to indicate that Ms. Ling does not exercise regularly.
15. Within the Nutrition section, select the No radio button to indicate that Ms. Ling does not follow a special diet but that she does consume caffeine. Document "2 cups a day" to indicate the amount of caffeine Ms. Ling consumes. Within the Pregnancy History tab, document "2" in the Gravida and Para fields to indicate the patient has had 2 pregnancies and 2 pregnancies that went to at least 20 weeks.
16. Document "0" in the Abortions and Miscarriage fields.
17. Click the Add button below the Previous Pregnancies grid to document Ella's birth history.
18. Document "3 years" to indicate that the pregnancy was 3 years ago.
19. Document "Natural" in the Conception Method field.
20. Document "39 weeks" in the Gestational Weeks field.
21. Document "16 hours" in the Duration of Labor field.
22. Document "6 pounds, 7 ounces" in the Birth Weight field.
23. Select the Female radio button to indicate the sex.
24. Document "Vaginal" in the Type of Delivery field.
25. Document "Stadol only" in the Anesthesia field.
26. Select the No radio button to indicate that this was not a preterm labor.
27. Document "None" in the Complications field and click the Save button.
28. Click the Add New button to document Gunner's birth history.
29. Document "1 year" to indicate that the pregnancy was 1 year ago.
30. Document "Natural" in the Conception Method field.
31. Document "40 weeks" in the Gestational Weeks field.
32. Document "12 hours" in the Duration of Labor field.
33. Document "8 pounds, 0 ounces" in the Birth Weight field.
34. Select the Male radio button to indicate the sex.
35. Document "Vaginal" in the Type of Delivery field.
36. Document "Epidural" in the Anesthesia field.
37. Select the No radio button to indicate that this was not a preterm labor.
38. Document "Mastitis after delivery, now resolved" in the Complications field and click the Save button.
39. Within the Dental History section, document Ms. Ling's last examination as "February 20, 2014" and dentist as "Dr. Bonnett."

CHIEF COMPLAINT

Patients come to the physician's office for many reasons. Some require medication refills. Others want to get their insurance and billing questions answered. However, the majority of patients are seeking medical care for acute or chronic problems. Acute conditions occur suddenly and are usually severe but of brief duration. Sinusitis, urinary tract infections, and fever are examples of acute conditions. Congestive heart disease, asthma, and multiple sclerosis are examples of chronic conditions. Chronic conditions are those that persist over a long time or are recurrent. Regardless of the patient's reason for seeking healthcare services, the medical assistant must determine the chief complaint.

The chief complaint (CC, or cc) is the patient's main reason for seeking medical care. Many providers now prefer to use the term *chief concern* because *complaint* has a negative connotation. Using an open-ended question such as "What brings you here today?" will prompt the patient to share the subjective information needed to accurately document the chief complaint. **The CC should be recorded using the patient's own words.**

Sometimes a patient has more than one reason for seeing the physician. It is important to know this when the patient makes the appointment to ensure that the appropriate amount of time has been set aside for the visit. In some cases, if the patient has additional, emergent issues, the physician may ask the patient to schedule another visit to accommodate the amount of time needed to address the less pressing concerns. Seeing patients for multiple problems during a brief appointment slot tends to back up appointments for the remainder of the day.

Pain Scale

Besides documenting the reason for the patient visit, the medical assistant needs to get at the progression of the current condition. This is considered the history of the present illness (HPI). As part of the HPI, the severity of the patient's condition will be assessed. The severity or intensity of the patient's pain is commonly documented on a pain scale. The patient is asked to qualify his or her pain on a scale of 1 to 10, with 10 being the worst. This, again, is based on the patient's words, just like the CC, and can be broken down to better determine how uncomfortable the patient is. For example, a value between 1 and 3 is mild pain, between 4 and 7 is moderate, and between 8 and 10 is severe pain. Other methods for determining the severity or level of discomfort for a patient include visual analog scales, in which the patient marks a spot on a 10-cm line, and the Wong-Baker FACES Pain Rating Scale used by young children. The pain scale reported by the patient is an important indicator to determine whether the patient's reported pain is consistent with the provider's physical examination findings for level of pain and to determine whether the pain is getting better or worse over time.

EHR EXERCISE 5.5   Document Chief Complaint

Complete the following exercise in the EHR Exercises assignment found in Open Assignments.

A dog bit Miles Green (DOB 08/30/1983) (added as a new patient in Chapter 2) about 3 hours ago, and Jean Burke, NP, is examining the 5-cm laceration on his left anterior palm. Mr. Green states a severity of 5 on a scale of 1 to 10 and describes the pain as throbbing and constant. Advil has helped the pain a little bit. During the review of systems, Mr. Green denies fever, chills, sweats, and fatigue, but he admits to joint swelling and injury. He reports no other signs and symptoms. Document the chief complaint in the patient record.

1. Click the tab for the Clinical Care module, or click on the Find Patient icon.
2. Perform a patient search for Miles Green and confirm his date of birth.
3. Select Office Visit from the left Info Panel.

4. Use today's date as the default, and select Urgent Visit from the Visit Type drop-down menu.
5. Click the Save button.
6. Select Chief Complaint from the Record drop-down menu.
7. Document the reason for Mr. Green's visit in the Chief Complaint field (Fig. 5.5).
8. Document symptoms associated with the chief complaint in the History of Present Illness section.
9. Within the Review of Systems section, select the No radio buttons for fever, chills, and fatigue. Select the Yes radio buttons for joint swelling and injury.
10. Document your name in the Entry By field and click the Save button.

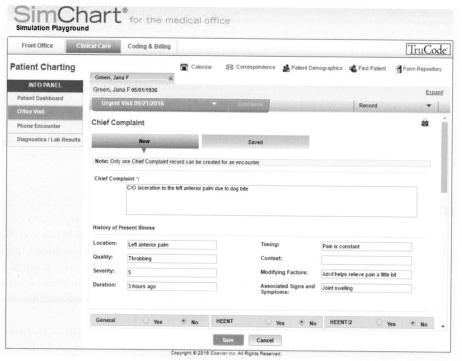

FIG. 5.5 Chief Complaint record.

MEDICATIONS

Most patients, particularly those who are elderly or chronically ill, take multiple medications that may be prescribed by several physicians and filled at more than one pharmacy. Given this complexity, it's critical to make sure the medication list in the EHR is current and complete. Any prescribed medications, OTC medications, and herbal/natural supplements the patient takes should be documented. Providers participating in Meaningful Use are required to report data on "maintaining an active medication list." Patients do not always remember their medications; after all, medications tend to look the same. Therefore, as part of the appointment confirmation, remind patients to bring to the appointment a list of their medications or even the actual medication bottles.

med reconciliation - def

EHR EXERCISE 5.6 Document Medications

Complete the following exercise in the EHR Exercises assignment found in Open Assignments.

If you are not already in the patient's encounter, locate the patient by clicking the tab for the Clinical Care module, or click on the Find Patient icon and perform a patient search for Susannah Ling and confirm her date of birth. Remember to enter the New Patient encounter on the Patient Dashboard in order to document in this record.

Susannah Ling (DOB 01/02/1973) states she is taking alprazolam XR 0.5 mg by mouth once daily, as needed for anxiety. Her daily supplements include vitamins A, D, and C by mouth with Iron OTC, an iron supplement for iron deficiency anemia. She started taking these medications 1 year ago. Document these medications in Ms. Ling's record.

1. Within the encounter, select Medications from the Record drop-down.
2. Within the Prescription Medications tab, click the Add button.
3. Within the Add Prescription Medication window (Fig. 5.6), document "Alprazolam extended-release tablet (Xanax XR)" in the Medication field, or select it from the drop-down by starting to type in "Alprazolam" in the Medication field.
4. Select 0.5 mg from the Strength drop-down.
5. Select Tablet ER from the Form drop-down.
6. Select Oral from the Route drop-down.
7. Select Daily from the Frequency drop-down.
8. Select the start date using the calendar picker.
9. Select the Active radio button to indicate the status of the medication.
10. Click the Save button to update Ms. Ling's Medication record.

Repeat this work flow within the Over-the-Counter Products tab to document the rest of Ms. Ling's medications, using the Generic Name field to either locate or type in the over-the-counter medications.

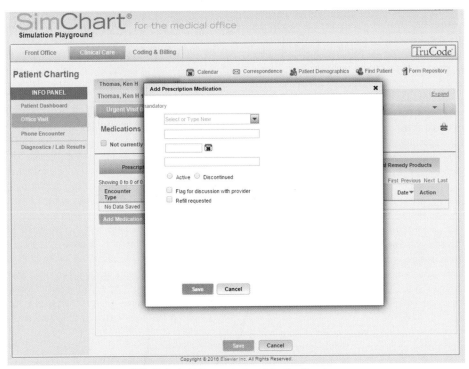

FIG. 5.6 Add Prescription Medication box.

TRENDS AND APPLICATIONS 5.3 Preventing Medication Errors in the EHR

Researchers have long known that nearly two-thirds of hospital records contain at least one medication error. An estimated 1 million medication errors occur each year, contributing to 7000 deaths. On average there is one medication error every day for every inpatient. In addition, pediatric patients have a threefold greater risk than adult patients of being seriously injured when a medication mistake is made.

Pharmacist Kathleen Orrico wanted to know whether the EHR systems of ambulatory care providers were any more likely to be accurate than hospital records. To find out she compared EHR medication lists against lists developed by nurses who conducted comprehensive telephone interviews with patients; the latter were presumably more accurate because most patients would have had access to their actual prescription bottles during phone calls taken at home. Indeed, Orrico found an average of 2.7 errors on each patient's electronic medication list.

Orrico then tried to categorize the errors by type to identify areas for quality improvement. The most common kind of discrepancy was a discontinuation (that is, about 70% of the errors represented medications listed but no longer being taken by the patient). Omission of a multivitamin was considered an error and represented 27% of the errors attributed to patients.

The errors were classified as either patient generated, such as failure to report an OTC medication, or "system" generated, which Orrico defined as the provider's failure to update the medication list. (This euphemism may spare physicians' feelings, but it's perhaps a bit misleading in an article that also refers to electronic records systems.) Eighty percent of the errors were categorized as system generated, including failure to note the date of discontinuation for medications prescribed for a limited duration, such as antibiotics.

The Institute for Healthcare Improvement and The Joint Commission recommend that physicians do **medication reconciliation** at each visit to reduce medication errors and adverse events such as allergic reactions. Medication reconciliation is also part of the stage 1 menu set measures for the Meaningful Use incentive. The objective requires eligible providers who receive a patient from another setting of care or provider of care to perform medication checks. Simply stated, the provider or a medical assistant should go over the patient's medications with him or her to make sure the list is accurate and current. Patients, too, must be accountable by bringing to each visit a list of their current medications and dosages. The list can be given not just to the patient's general practitioner but also to specialists, nurses, medical assistants, pharmacists, and other healthcare professionals who have a role in their care.

The following are some questions to ask patients when reconciling medications in the EHR:

- Inquire not only about patients' prescriptions but also about their OTC medications and about dietary supplements, such as herbal products and vitamins.
- Ask patients whether any specialist physicians or allied health practitioners, such as chiropractors, have prescribed any medications for them.
- If the patient has trouble understanding English, find out whether he or she would like an interpreter to facilitate the reconciliation process.
- Ask patients whether they ever break or cut their medication tablets; the dosage on the label is not accurate if the patient routinely breaks the tablets in half.
- Be sure to ask about oral contraceptives in female patients of childbearing age because some patients don't consider birth control pills to be medications.

- Pay special attention to verifying the dosage of high-alert medications, such as anticoagulants (blood thinners), insulin, and narcotics.

Providers, with the help of medical assistants, should document all medications, dosages, and other relevant information. The reason that a patient stops taking a specific medication should also be recorded. Perhaps the patient was taking a lipid-lowering medication that had to be discontinued because of leg cramping. Documenting such information can be used to speed insurance drug approvals, or it may remind the physician that the patient generally cannot tolerate a specific classification of drugs. As you read in the Trends and Applications 5 to 3 Preventing Medication Errors in the EHR box, it is also very important to record any OTC medications that the patient is taking, including any dietary supplements or other herbal products or vitamins. (Table 5.1 lists common prescription abbreviations.)

Immunization History

Immunizations protect people against infections caused by harmful microorganisms. Although we generally think of immunizations as being for children, some are recommended for adults as well (Table 5.2). Immunizations are required in various situations. For example, children must meet certain standards before starting school. Healthcare workers and others working in high-risk environments must have a hepatitis B immunization. A tetanus vaccine should be given every 10 years, or more frequently for those with open wound sites. The EHR can keep a running record of these vaccinations and is thus a good tool for tracking a patient's immunization history. Items documented within immunizations include:

- Name of immunization (for example, MMR [measles, mumps, rubella])
- Date given
- Name of person administering the immunization
- Date immunization is updated (if necessary)
- Route (for example, IM [intramuscular], subcut [subcutaneous], ID [intradermal])
- Site (for example, right deltoid, abdomen, left forearm)
- Manufacturer
- Type (for example, DTaP, DTP, TDap, TD)
- Expiration date
- Lot number
- Reactions (if any)

Documenting these details will assist the physician in the event of an adverse patient reaction or a recall from the manufacturer.

To maximize the physician's time with the patient, the medical assistant will want to gather some basic information about the patient's medical history. The physician will go into the patient's history in greater detail during the physician's face time with the patient. The clinical decision support functionality helps focus the medical assistant's questions to the presenting problems. In all cases, the medical assistant will want to know whether the patient has any significant medical conditions. In the case of an illness, like a cough, there should be a brief review of the patient's ears, nose, and throat. If the patient presents with a musculoskeletal issue, the medical assistant should ask about any medical history related to previous injuries or surgeries on the affected body part, and about whether the patient has any arthritis, joint problems, muscle pain or stiffness, or tendinitis.

TABLE 5.1 Common Medication Prescribing Abbreviations

Abbreviation	Spelled Out	Meaning
a.c.	ante cibum	Before meals
ATC	around the clock	Around the clock
b.i.d.	bis in die	Twice a day
gt.	gutta	A drop
m.d.u.	more dicto utendus	To be used as directed
NMT	not more than	Not more than
p.c.	post cibum	After meals
PO	per os	By mouth
p.r.n.	pro re nata	As needed
q3h	quaque 3 hora	Every 3 hours
q.i.d.	quater in die	Four times a day
S.A.	secundum artum	Use your judgment
sig.	signa	To write
SL	sublingually	Under the tongue
stat.	statim	Immediately
Tab	tabella	Tablet
t.d.s.	ter die sumendum	Three times a day
t.i.d.	ter in die	Three times a day
TPN	total parenteral nutrition	Nutrition administered via a nongastrointestinal route
troche	trochiscus	Lozenge
u.d.	ut dictum	As directed

EHR EXERCISE 5.7 Vaccine Authorization Form

Complete the following exercise in the EHR Exercises assignment found in Open Assignments.

If you are not already in the patient's encounter, locate the patient by clicking the tab for the Clinical Care module, or click on the Find Patient icon and perform a patient search for Susannah Ling and confirm her date of birth. Remember to enter the New Patient encounter on the Patient Dashboard in order to document in this record.

Dr. Martin ordered an influenza vaccine for Susannah Ling (DOB 01/02/1973) today. During the interview with the patient, Susannah denies illness or high fever. She does not have an allergy to chicken or eggs. She has not had any allergic reactions to injections before. Before Ms. Ling receives her influenza vaccine, prepare a vaccine authorization form for her to sign.

1. Click on the Form Repository icon and select the Vaccine Authorization (Fig. 5.7) from the left Info Panel.
2. Click the Patient Search button to perform a patient search for Susannah Ling and confirm her date of birth. Some of Ms. Ling's information will auto-populate.
3. Select the No radio button to indicate that Ms. Ling is not sick and does not have a fever.
4. Select the No radio button to indicate that Ms. Ling is not allergic to chicken, eggs, or egg products.
5. Select the No radio button to indicate that Ms. Ling has never had an allergic reaction to an injection.
6. Select the Unknown radio button to indicate Ms. Ling's pregnancy status.
7. Select the No radio button to indicate that Ms. Ling does not have a blood clotting disorder and is not taking a blood-thinning medication.
8. Click the Save to Patient Record button.
9. In order to print this form for Ms. Ling to sign, click the Find Patient icon to locate Ms. Ling's health record. The record will open on the Patient Dashboard.
10. Scroll down to the Forms section within the Patient Dashboard and select the Vaccine Authorization.
11. Click the Print button to print the form in order to obtain Ms. Ling's signature (if required by your instructor).

TABLE 5.2 Recommended Adult Immunization Schedule, by Vaccine and Age Group

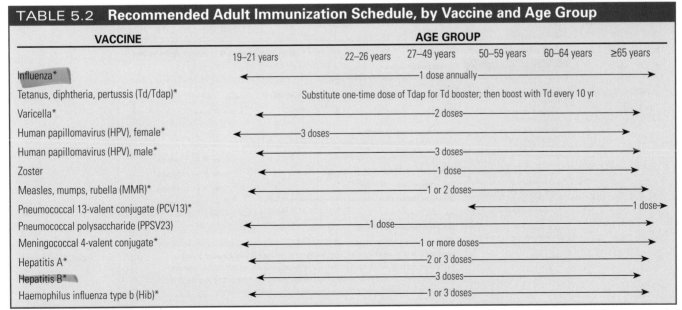

VACCINE	19–21 years	22–26 years	27–49 years	50–59 years	60–64 years	≥65 years
Influenza*	←————————————————— 1 dose annually —————————————————→
Tetanus, diphtheria, pertussis (Td/Tdap)*	Substitute one-time dose of Tdap for Td booster; then boost with Td every 10 yr
Varicella*	←————————————————— 2 doses —————————————————→
Human papillomavirus (HPV), female*	←———— 3 doses ————→
Human papillomavirus (HPV), male*	←————————————————— 3 doses —————————————————→
Zoster	←————————————————— 1 dose —————————————————→
Measles, mumps, rubella (MMR)*	←————————————————— 1 or 2 doses —————————————————→
Pneumococcal 13-valent conjugate (PCV13)*	←———————————— 1 dose ————→
Pneumococcal polysaccharide (PPSV23)	←————— 1 dose —————→
Meningococcal 4-valent conjugate*	←————————————————— 1 or more doses —————————————————→
Hepatitis A*	←————————————————— 2 or 3 doses —————————————————→
Hepatitis B*	←————————————————— 3 doses —————————————————→
Haemophilus influenza type b (Hib)*	←————————————————— 1 or 3 doses —————————————————→

For all persons in this category who meet the age requirements and who lack documentation of vaccination or have no evidence of previous infection, zoster vaccine recommended regardless of prior episode of zoster. Recommended if some other risk factor is present (e.g., on the basis of medical, occupational, lifestyle, or other indication). No recommendation.
*Covered by the Vaccine Injury Compensation Program.
Modified from Centers for Disease Control and Prevention. (2016). *Recommended adult immunization schedule, by vaccine and age group.* Available at: www.cdc.gov/vaccines/schedules/hcp/imz/adult.html. Accessed September 10, 2016.

EHR EXERCISE 5.8   Update Immunization Record

Complete the following exercise in the EHR Exercises assignment found in Open Assignments.

If you are not already in the patient's encounter, locate the patient by clicking the tab for the Clinical Care module, or click on the Find Patient icon and perform a patient search for Susannah Ling and confirm her date of birth. Remember to enter the New Patient encounter on the Patient Dashboard in order to document in this record.

Document the following immunization that Dr. Martin ordered for Susannah Ling (DOB 01/02/1973): influenza, type IIV, dose 0.5 mL, administered IM in the right deltoid. Medical Corp. manufactures this immunization, and the lot number is R5667. It expires 3 years from the current date. Ms. Ling does not have a reaction.

1. Within a patient encounter, select Immunizations from the Record drop-down menu.
2. Locate the Influenza/Flu row and click on the green plus sign to the far right of the top row. That row will become active, so you can add an immunization to Ms. Ling's record.
3. Within the Type column, select IIV.
4. Within the Dose column, document 0.5 mL.
5. Within the Date Admin column, use the calendar picker to select the date administered.
6. Within the Provider column, type "Dr. Martin" in the text box.
7. Within the Route/Site column, type "IM/right deltoid" in the text box.
8. Within the Manufacturer/Lot# column, type "Medical Corp./R5667" in the text box.
9. Document the expiration date in the Exp column.
10. Within the Reaction column, type "No reaction" in the text box.
11. Click the Save button. A confirmation message will appear, and the Immunizations table will display Ms. Ling's immunization.

Vital Signs

Every patient seen by the healthcare provider will have a set of vital signs—temperature, pulse, and respirations and blood pressure—measured by the medical assistant. Because the vital signs are measured or observed by someone other than the patient, they are considered **objective** findings. The record of these measurements must be documented in the EHR. Vital signs are an important part of the patient visit because they can indicate the presence of illness or disease. Extreme caution must be taken to ensure the accuracy of the measurements; thus, they should be taken only by trained individuals.

Anthropometric measurements (from anthropo-, meaning "human," + -metry, meaning "the process of measuring")

are not considered vital signs but are generally obtained at the same time. These measurements include height (ht), weight (wt), BMI, and head circumference (in infants).

When the weight and height are recorded, many EHR systems automatically calculate the patient's current BMI. For blood pressure readings, you can also record the patient's body position (for example, recumbent [reclining], sitting, or standing). This is important when checking for orthostatic hypotension, a form of low blood pressure that occurs when the patient changes position: lying down to sitting or standing, or sitting to standing. During a well-child examination, the EHR can plot a child's height, weight, and head circumference on age-appropriate growth charts for percentile comparisons.

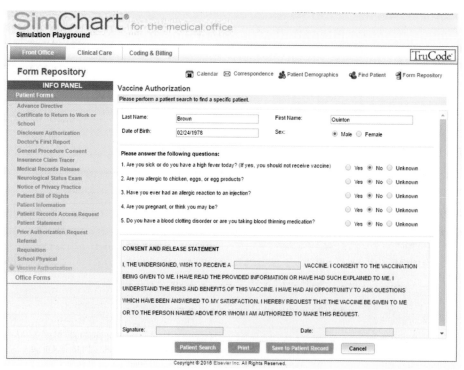

FIG. 5.7 Vaccine Authorization screen.

EHR EXERCISE 5.9 Enter Vital Signs

Complete the following exercise in the EHR Exercises assignment found in Open Assignments.

The medical assistant measures the following vital signs for Casey Hernandez (10–08–2000) during today's office visit: Ht: 4 ft, 2 in; Wt: 82 lb; T: 99.2°F, forehead; P: 78, regular (radial); R: 16, regular; BP: 120/80, sitting, left arm with manual cuff; SpO_2: 99% (obtained with digital pulse oximetry probe on the finger).

1. Click the tab for the Clinical Care module, or click on the Find Patient icon and perform a patient search for Casey Hernandez and confirm her date of birth.
2. Search and select patient record for Casey Hernandez (10/08/2000).
3. Enter the patient encounter (either select Existing Encounter from the Patient Dashboard, or create new encounter if no encounter exists).
4. Select "Vital Signs" from the Record drop-down box. The Vital Signs record is organized into a Vital Signs tab and a Height/Weight tab.
5. Within the Vital Signs tab, click Add button.
6. Document "99.2" as the temperature in the Fahrenheit field. Select Forehead from the Site drop-down menu. Notice the temperature is also displayed in Celsius after it is entered as Fahrenheit.
7. Document "78, regular" as the pulse and select Radial from the Site drop-down menu.
8. Document "16, regular" as the Respiration.
9. Document "120" as the systolic blood pressure and select Left arm from the Site drop-down menu. Document "80" as diastolic blood pressure and select Manual with cuff from the Mode drop-down menu. Select Sitting from the Position drop-down menu.
10. Document "99%" as the Oxygenation Saturation Percentage and select Digital probe, finger from the Site drop-down menu.
11. Click Save button.
12. Within the Height/Weight tab, click the Add button.
13. Document the height as "4 ft, 2 in" using the individual Height fields. Document the weight as "82" in the lb field. The BMI will auto-calculate.
14. Click the Save button.

In addition to patient information documented in preparation for the provider, there is certain information that would be documented either during the visit or after the provider has finished the visit. Those categories will be discussed below.

Order Entry

One of the best ways to decrease the number of errors and protect patients is being accomplished by adopting technology called computerized provider order entry (CPOE). The provider or licensed/credentialed healthcare professional enters orders for the patient directly into the EHR, and the system automatically checks for safety and appropriateness.

In addition to medication orders, other procedure orders and results must be documented in the EHR. Medical assistants, for example, will need to document the order and results of procedures performed in the office. For example, Snellen examinations, glucometer readings, urinalysis, electrocardiograms, and audiograms are all ordered and documented in the health record.

EHR EXERCISE 5.10 In-Office Order Entry

Complete the following exercise in the EHR Exercises assignment found in Open Assignments.

Dr. Walden ordered a peak flow measurement for Casey Hernandez (DOB 10-08-2000) using a peak flow meter (Fig. 5.8). The Patient Goal was 490, and Casey tolerated the procedure without difficulty. During the three attempts, Casey obtained 450, 480, and 480.

1. Within the Clinical Care module, perform a patient search to locate Casey Hernandez and confirm her date of birth.
2. Enter the encounter created during the previous exercise and select Order Entry from the Record drop-down menu.
3. Click the Add button located under the In-Office order grid.
4. Select Peak Flow Meter from the Order drop-down menu.
5. Document "490" in the Patient Goal field.
6. Document "450" in the First Attempt field.
7. Document "480" in the Second Attempt field.
8. Document "480" in the Third Attempt field.
9. Document your name in the Entry By field.
10. Document "Patient tolerated the procedure without difficulty" in the Notes field.
11. Click the Save button.

EHR EXERCISE 5.11 Out-of-Office Order Entry

Complete the following exercise in the EHR Exercises assignment found in Open Assignments.

Dr. Walden would like to start Casey Hernandez (DOB 10-08-2000) on Accolate 20 mg twice daily for asthma management. Prepare a 3-month prescription with one refill and document this prescription in Casey's medication record.

1. If you are no longer in the encounter for Casey, click on the Clinical Care module, perform a patient search to locate Casey Hernandez and confirm her date of birth.
2. Enter the same encounter as in the previous exercise and select Order Entry from the Record drop-down menu.
3. Click the Add button located under the Out-of-Office order grid.
4. Select Medication Prescription from the Order drop-down menu.
5. Select the check box for Julie Walden, MD.
6. Document "Asthma" in the Diagnosis field.
7. Document "Accolate" in the Drug field.
8. Document "20 mg" in the Strength field.
9. Document "Tablet" in the Form field.
10. Document "By mouth" in the Route field.
11. Document "1" in the Refills field.
12. Document "Take 1 tablet PO twice daily" in the Directions field.
13. Document "180" in the Quantity field.
14. Document "90" in the Days Supply field.
15. Document your name in the Entry By field and today's date in the Date field.
16. Click the Save button.
17. Select Medications from the Record drop-down menu.
18. Within the Prescription Medications tab, click the Add Medication button.
19. Within the Add Prescription window, select Zafirlukast tablet (Accolate) from the Medication drop-down menu.
20. Select 20 from the Strength drop-down.
21. Select Tablet from the Form drop-down.
22. Select Oral from the Route drop-down.
23. Select 2 Times/Day from the Frequency drop-down.
24. Document "40 mg per day" in the Dose field.
25. Document "Asthma" in the Indication field.
26. Select the Active radio button to indicate the Status.
27. Click Save to update Casey's medication list.

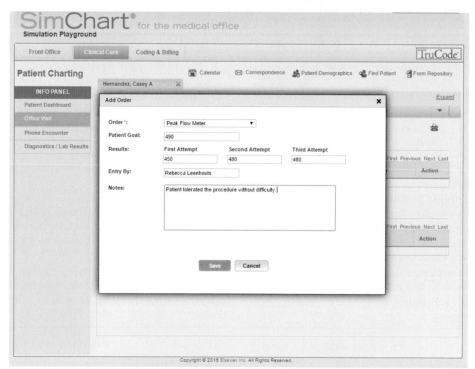

FIG. 5.8 Peak Flow Meter; Add Order box.

EHR EXERCISE 5.12 Respiratory Order Requisition

Complete the following exercise in the EHR Exercises assignment found in Open Assignments.

Dr. Walden ordered Casey Hernandez (DOB 10-08-2000) to have spirometry (with and without inhalers) on December 23 for her asthma. The authorization number is TTY7800210. The test is ordered as routine. Remember to instruct Casey to bring her inhalers from home.

1. Click on the Form Repository icon.
2. Select Requisition from the left Info Panel.
3. Select Respiratory from the Requisition Type drop-down menu.
4. Click the Patient Search button to locate Casey Hernandez's record and confirm her date of birth.

5. Use the calendar picker to document December 23 of the current year as the Service Date.
6. Document "TTY7800210" as the Authorization Number.
7. Document "Julie Walden, MD" as the Ordering Physician.
8. Document the Diagnosis as "Asthma."
9. Document the Diagnosis Code as "J44.9."
10. Select the Spirometry (with and without inhalers) check box from the Respiratory Order section.
11. Select the Routine radio button to indicate that the examination is routine.
12. Document "Patient is to bring her inhalers from home with her" in the Patient Preparation field.
13. Click Save to the Patient Record.

Problem List

Managing patient healthcare can be tedious. There are several elements and layers for managing a patient's case, and the amount of data to review can be overwhelming for even the most organized provider. EHR systems make this process manageable by providing a centralized location for a summary of a patient's acute and chronic conditions called the Problem List. Meaningful Use has recognized problem lists as one of the core objectives for improvement of patient care. According to

the American Health Information Management Association (AHIMA), the Problem Lists provide the following benefits:

- Allow customized care by identifying the most significant health concerns
- Help identify "disease-specific populations" through data analysis
- Help evaluate standard measures for specific providers and healthcare organizations
- May identify patients for possible research studies

EHR EXERCISE 5.13 Maintaining Problem List

Complete the following exercise in the EHR Exercises assignment found in Open Assignments.

Dr. Martin diagnosed Susannah Ling (DOB 01/02/1973) as having iron deficiency anemia and anxiety. Add this diagnosis to Ms. Ling's Problem List.

1. Click the tab for the Clinical Care module.
2. Perform a patient search for Susannah Ling and confirm her date of birth.
3. Select the correct encounter from Ms. Ling's Patient Dashboard.
4. Select Problem List from the Record drop-down menu and click the Add Problem button.

5. Select "Anemia, iron deficiency" as the diagnosis.
6. Select the ICD-10 Code radio button and document "D50.0" as the code.
7. Document the date identified using the calendar picker.
8. Select the Active radio button to indicate that this is a current diagnosis.
9. Click the Save button. Ms. Ling's Problem List will update to reflect her diagnosis of iron deficiency anemia (Fig. 5.9).
10. Click the Add Problem button and repeat this work flow to document Ms. Ling's anxiety, using ICD-10 code F41.1.

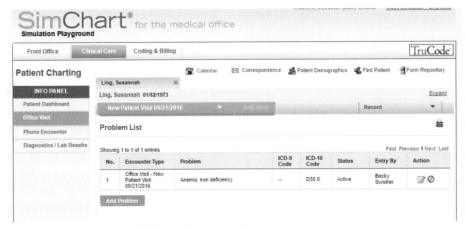

FIG. 5.9 Completed Problem List grid.

TRACKING HEALTH SCREENINGS AND IMMUNIZATIONS ~table 5.8~

Health information often reaches patients in bits and pieces. A woman may pick up a magazine at the hair salon and read about getting her daughter immunized against human papillomavirus (HPV), which causes certain types of cervical cancer. A man may hear about colon cancer screening from a colleague or neighbor who was not screened early and is now undergoing chemotherapy. A person with diabetes may be told by a friend with the condition that annual screening for diabetic retinal disease is necessary to detect vision-related complications of diabetes.

Unfortunately, patients don't always get the advice they need from those external sources. The information may be fragmented or just plain wrong. In addition, a patient's level of knowledge about healthcare often reflects disparities in income, education, age, and other variables. Tiro and colleagues studied a diverse group of American women to find out how much they knew about the role of HPV in causing cervical cancer. They found that those who knew the most were more likely to be younger, better educated, and more fully integrated into the healthcare system. The study did not measure income, but it's likely that those with better access to healthcare were in a higher tax bracket than those who did not visit a physician regularly.

In the past, relying on physicians to recommend appropriate screenings has been hit or miss. A general practitioner may be busy attending to the patient's chief concern, back pain or depression or bronchitis, or might not remember to order a screening test. Often the provider isn't aware that the patient falls into a particular risk group.

That's where the EHR comes in. Clinical decision support tools take some of the burden off physicians and patients by showing the provider which conditions the patient is at risk for and flagging the patient's chart with appropriate screening reminders. However, it's still up to the provider to act on the reminder, and it's up to the patient to make and keep the screening appointment.

Of course, patients should also strive to be health literate (that is, to stay as informed as possible about their health and to use this information to make well-considered health decisions). For example, they should learn the reason their physician is ordering a particular screening test. Depending on a patient's age and risk factors, certain testing should be done as part of a comprehensive health promotion plan. Children should be given the recommended immunizations, and adults should be vaccinated and screened for certain diseases, as indicated by their age, risk factors, or both (see Table 5.2). Screening tests might include mammograms, Pap tests, stool testing for occult blood, and laboratory tests such as a lipid (blood cholesterol) panel, complete blood count, and comprehensive metabolic panel. These tests either estimate a patient's risk for developing disease or detect its presence. A patient's insurance may or may not cover these kinds of screenings, so patients should check with their carrier before having them performed.

USING THE ELECTRONIC HEALTH RECORD FOR PATIENT EDUCATION

Healthcare providers can provide advice and treatment for the benefit of the patient. However, patients stand the best chance of living a healthy life by taking charge of their own health. The healthcare provider must create an atmosphere in which patients feel comfortable asking questions about their health status. Providers must also understand how to incorporate the resources they have within the office. These resources include written literature, videos or DVDs, educational group sessions, and even the EHR.

Although the main purpose of the EHR is to document patient-provider encounters, the EHR is also a useful tool for educating patients about their health and risk factors for disease. The EHR contains health data collected over a long time, allowing the attentive provider to identify long-term trends that indicate elevated disease risk. For example, line graphs allow weight and blood pressure trends to be monitored and compared from visit to visit. Body mass index (BMI) is a simple but powerful health promotion tool the EHR provides (Trends and Applications 5.4).

TRENDS AND APPLICATIONS 5.4 Body Mass Index as a Health Promotion Tool

When the weight and height are entered into an EHR, such as SCMO, the patient's BMI is automatically calculated. BMI is a height-weight ratio calculated by dividing the patient's weight (kilograms) by the square of his or her height (meters). The BMI is an inexpensive method of determining whether a patient is overweight or obese. It's a reliable indicator of body fatness because it has been shown to correlate strongly to the body fat percentage measured using highly accurate direct methods, such as underwater weighing. Scale weight measures pounds (or kilos, if you like) but does not indicate whether a person is overweight.

BMI is just a screening tool, though. As such, it indicates a risk for diseases related to overweight and obesity. However, taken by itself, a high BMI does not signal the presence of those diseases. The provider may choose to perform further tests or to counsel the patient about nutrition and physical activity. A person of normal weight generally has a BMI between 18.5 and 25. However, the mean BMI for an adult male in the United States is 26.6, and the average adult woman has a BMI of 26.5. Perhaps we wouldn't be wrong in suggesting that being an American has become a risk factor in itself.

EHR EXERCISE 5.14 Preventative Services Documentation

Complete the following exercise in the EHR Exercises assignment found in Open Assignments.

Susannah Ling (DOB 01/02/1973) shares her past preventative services with Dr. Martin during the patient interview. Within the past year she had a regular Pap test on March 31, a general health panel laboratory test within normal limits on February 12, and an annual general eye examination within normal limits on June 24. Document these preventative services in Ms. Ling's record.

1. Within a patient encounter, select Preventative Services from the Record drop-down menu.
2. Click the Add button below the Procedures table.
3. Within the Add Procedure window, select Pap Test from the Health Recommendation field.
4. Use the calendar picker to document the date in the Date Performed field.
5. Click the Save button.
6. Click the Add button below the Laboratory Testing table.
7. Within the Add Laboratory Testing window, select General Health Panel from the Health Recommendation field.
8. Use the calendar picker to document the date in the Date Performed field.
9. Click the Save button.
10. Click the Add button below the General Eye Examination table.
11. Within the Add General Eye Examination window, document "General eye examination" in the Health Recommendation field.
12. Use the calendar picker to document the date in the Date Performed field.
13. Click the Save button.

During an office visit patients are often given a great deal of information regarding their health status. It's helpful if patients have someone with them to help them understand and remember the details the healthcare staff provides. Written instructions help patients understand the disease process and learn to optimize quality of life while managing the symptoms of a chronic disease. The EHR stores patient information sheets on a broad range of topics that can be tailored for each patient and each visit.

As discussed in earlier chapters, the Internet is a great resource for accessing a broad range of health education and preventive medicine topics that can be tailored for each patient and every health issue. However, the medical office should establish a policy for distributing patient handouts generated from the Internet as well as a list of acceptable websites for the staff to use. Whether the education tool is maintained in the EHR system or outside on the web, the medical assistant should take time to review the printed materials with the patient. Proper communication skills are needed for the patient to fully understand the instructions. The following are a few guidelines for effective patient education:

- Speak with the patient in a quiet, well-lit area that offers as much privacy as possible.
- Use terms patients can understand, defining medical terms used.
- Provide both oral instructions and supplemental printed instructions in the patient's primary language from the EHR.
- Encourage the patient to ask questions as needed.
- Have the patient and caregiver demonstrate skills, such as insulin administration or wound dressing, before leaving the office to ensure that proper technique is used.
- Encourage patients to contact the office at any time with additional questions.

EHR EXERCISE 5.15 Patient Education

Complete the following exercise in the EHR Exercises assignment found in Open Assignments.

Maria would like to learn more about her daughter Casey Hernandez's (DOB 10/08/2000) diagnosis of asthma. The medical assistant discusses asthma with Maria and prints a patient education handout for asthma. Document Person Taught as "Parent," and Printed Handout as Teaching Methods. During the patient education, Maria states the handout is very helpful to her understanding.

1. Within the Clinical Care module, perform a patient search to locate Casey Hernandez and confirm her date of birth.
2. Create an office visit for an established patient using the encounter options in the left Info Panel.
3. Select Patient Education from the Record drop-down menu.
4. Within the New tab, select Diagnosis from the Category drop-down menu.
5. Select Respiratory System from the Subcategory drop-down menu.
6. Select the Asthma check box in the Teaching Topics section. Use the View link to review the Patient Education handouts.
7. Select the Parent check box in the Persons Taught section.
8. Select the Printed Handout Given check box in the Teaching Methods section.
9. Select the No Barriers check box in the Learning Barriers section.
10. Select the Verbalizes Understanding check box in the Outcome section.
11. Click the Save button.

THE PROGRESS NOTE

Progress notes are descriptions of the patient encounter. Accurately recording the details of a patient encounter ensures the highest level of patient care, decreases the risk of lawsuits, establishes evidence of illness, and documents the treatment plan. A patient note is created for every patient encounter. The most common method for organizing a patient encounter is called the *SOAPE note*. SOAPE is an acronym for the five components to be covered during a patient encounter: **s**ubjective data, **o**bjective data, **a**ssessment data, **p**lan of care, and **e**valuation. Let's look at each of these elements.

- **S: Subjective.** The subjective information is what the patient tells you. Generally, the problem is recorded in the patient's own words. For example, the patient might say, "Pain radiates down my left leg." Pain is a subjective (not observable or measurable to the provider) symptom because, with present technology, we have no way to measure it other than the patient's self-report. It's akin to circumstantial evidence in a court of law: Although the physician presumes the patient to be telling the truth, he or she would like some corroborating evidence, objective findings, before writing a script for Vicodin.
- **O: Objective.** Objective information is that which can be observed, measured, or collected by the healthcare provider. Vital signs, anthropometric data, imaging studies, and laboratory tests are examples of objective data. Signs are objective, whereas symptoms are subjective. Objective data, in other words, are the forensic evidence of the medical chart; it is what it is. Interpretations may differ (as to which diagnosis it points to, for instance), but no one can argue with the data. A patient with leg pain, for instance, may have a measurable elevation of pulse and a measurable loss of reflexes, both of which would corroborate a report of pain.
- **A: Assessment.** The assessment is the practitioner's summation of the diagnosis or the impression of what's wrong with the patient. For example, after a pain patient is examined, the assessment might be that he or she is suffering from sciatica, possibly caused by a herniated disk in the lumbar spine.
- **P: Plan.** The plan is just what it sounds like—the steps the provider plans to take to treat the patient. The physician may, for example, order an MRI of the lumbar spine to check for a herniated disk or may opt to order physical therapy.
- **E: Evaluation or Education.** This section of the progress note is not always used by providers, but when the information is documented, it includes advice to patients regarding treatments, advice to patients about disease, and future issues and response.

Each provider has his or her own style of documentation. Some like to dictate paragraphs based on the history and examination of the patient, which results in the data being stored in an unstructured format. Others like to use a more structured method of documentation that enables easier medical research and formats the record in an outline fashion. Providers quickly rule out many things during their examination of a patient; the structured data method of documentation provides an easy way for them to document these rule-outs.

Once the medical assistant has prepared the patient for the provider's examination or consultation, the provider sees the patient and documents the history, examination findings, plan of care, and any other observations made during the patient encounter. Providers have choices for how they want to document observations in the medical record. The most efficient way is for the provider to carry a wireless tablet (like an iPad) or touch-screen laptop into the examination room with them. Some providers are comfortable using a computer in front of patients; others are not. Providers who are not comfortable keying documentation in front of patients can use a computer in the common hallway or in their offices. The use of a scribe is also an option for those providers who are not comfortable using the computer in front of patients.

Digital Signature

Digitally signing a note is a great way to ensure a high level of security for a practice. When a note is signed electronically, the provider is representing that everything within the note is correct. A notation of when it was signed and by whom is shown below the signature line on the saved note. The digital signature process increases accountability and helps verify that the patient received the required care.

Although a batch of notes can be signed at once using the EHR, doing so may cause Medicare compliance problems. It's more prudent to sign the notes one by one as they are reviewed. The electronic signature is usually with a password given to each provider. However, a note can be saved by selecting Cancel, and the provider can sign at a later time.

CHAPTER SUMMARY

- Proper documentation makes diagnosis and treatment more efficient, promotes patient safety, and provides evidence of the quality of care delivered for both legal protection and reimbursement purposes.
- Speech recognition is a technology that converts speech into text as the provider speaks into a microphone, eliminating the need for filing or transcription.
- An encounter allows the user to document all clinical information for the patient visit.
- The EHR is used to store and record documentation gathered from the patient interview, the review of systems, the patient history, chief complaint, vital signs, allergies, medication lists, and test results.

- Allergies and medication use are important in the modification of patient treatment plans. Inaccurate documentation can lead to adverse reactions.
- The chief complaint/concern (CC or cc) is the patient's main reason for seeking medical care. A patient may have more than one chief complaint. The HPI consists of a description of the patient's symptoms, their duration, a chronology of how the symptoms have changed, and an indication of what makes the problem better or worse.
- CPOE allows the user to document medical orders and reduce the incidence of medication errors. Immunization history should be documented and monitored to ensure that a patient is up to date with necessary vaccinations. The

immunization name, date, site given, route, dose, person who administered, lot number, expiration, and manufacturer information should be documented in the EHR.

- Patient vital signs include temperature, pulse, respiration, and BP. Vital signs should be taken during every patient visit. The data collected are then entered into the EHR and can be pulled directly into the patient progress note.
- A Problem List is a central location of the patient record where a summary of patient diagnosis can be referenced and is part of Meaningful Use reporting requirements.

- Patient education can support understanding and prevention of disease process and risk factors. Progress notes are descriptions of the patient encounter and are the keystone of proper documentation. Accurately recording the details of a patient encounter ensures the highest level of patient care, decreases the risk of lawsuits, establishes evidence of medical necessity for treatment, and outlines the plan of care. The most common format for documenting a patient encounter is called the SOAPE method: **S**ubjective data, **O**bjective data, **A**ssessment, **P**lan, and **E**valuation.

CHAPTER REVIEW ACTIVITIES

Circle the Correct Term

Circle the term that correctly completes the sentence.

1. William comes to the office with bronchitis for the fourth time this year. This condition is **(acute, chronic).**
2. Kimberly is complaining of an allergic reaction to an insect bite, a(n) **(acute, chronic)** condition.
3. Beverly reports having chickenpox when she was 11 years old. This is documented in the patient's **(past medical, family, social)** history.
4. Richard reports that he has a couple of beers after work on Fridays. This is documented in the patient's **(past medical, family, social)** history.
5. Richie had called to make an appointment for a sore throat for 10 days. Upon being questioned, he also mentions difficulty swallowing and postnasal drainage. The patient's **chief complaint** is a **(sore throat, postnasal drainage, difficulty swallowing).**

Key Terms Review

Match the term in column A to the definition in column B.

1. Subjective
2. Acute condition
3. E-visit
4. Chief complaint
5. Objective
6. Review of systems
7. Anthropometric measurements
8. High-alert medication

a. An episodic illness or injury of limited duration that responds well to treatment
b. The process of comparing the medication list in the patient's EHR with the patient's self-report
c. An organized inventory of each organ system
d. Perceived only by the patient and not evident to or measurable by the provider
e. Readily seen, perceived, or measured by the provider
f. The height, weight, and size of the human body
g. A medication that poses a heightened risk of injury or death when improperly administered
h. A provider consultation with an established patient using a secure Internet service

9. History of the present illness
10. Chronic condition
11. Medication reconciliation

i. A brief statement of the problem, condition, or symptoms that prompted the patient to seek medical care
j. The duration, location, severity, context, associated signs and symptoms, quality, and modifying factors related to a patient's illness
k. A prolonged illness that requires periodic follow-up

True/False

Indicate whether the statement is true or false.

1. _____ Patient instructions should be performed in a well-lighted area with limited distractions.
2. _____ Speech recognition software can distinguish one voice from another.
3. _____ E-visits are illegal in most states.
4. _____ Physicians using the EHR must use a structured method of data entry.
5. _____ Voice recognition software does not eliminate the need to transcribe the provider's office notes.
6. _____ The chief complaint includes all of the health concerns a patient is seen for during the course of a physician's visit.
7. _____ The digital signature helps ensure the security of the patient's information.
8. _____ Immunization order and administration need not be recorded for patients ages 18 and older.
9. _____ A patient is asked for his or her allergy history only during the first visit.
10. _____ A medication list must be reconciled and updated in the EHR during each patient encounter.
11. _____ Many errors in EHR medication lists are attributable to patients' confusion about drug names and dosages.

Workplace Applications

Using the knowledge you obtained from the chapter, provide narrative answers to the following cases.

1. Paige is performing a patient interview. Determine whether the given data are part of the patient's past medical (P), family (F), or social history (S).
   - Smokes one pack of cigarettes per day

- Fixation of a broken right ankle in 1998
- Tonsillectomy 25 years ago
- Married with four children
- Socially drinks alcohol, one or two servings per month
- Mother died in 1990 of breast cancer
- Grandfather diagnosed with colon cancer

EHR in Review

1. Document the following clinical data for Truong Tran (DOB 05/30/1991). Create a patient encounter for today's Urgent Office visit.

   Chief Complaint: Pt. complains of right knee pain and swelling. Pain (4/10) started 3 weeks ago after he fell while playing tennis. Patient states pain is sharp and constant. Patient has obtained some temporary relief by taking OTC medications.

   Allergies: Patient has NKA to medications.

   Vital signs: Ht: 5′6″, Wt: 160 lb, T: 99°F, P: 66, R: 16, BP: 122/76 mm Hg

2. Al Neviaser (DOB 06/21/1968) has an appointment for a blood pressure check. Today his weight is 206 lb, his height is 67 in, and his blood pressure is 160/94 mm Hg sitting in the left arm. His pulse is 88 bpm regular. Use a follow-up visit encounter to document Mr. Neviaser's blood pressure check. Dr. Martin would like Mr. Neviaser to schedule a 30-minute appointment tomorrow at 2:00 PM to discuss his high blood pressure.

3. Casey Hernandez (DOB 10/08/2000) is recovering from the flu and needs a note to excuse her from school. She was absent Monday and Tuesday of this week. Use the Form Repository to generate an excuse for absence from school for Casey.

4. Update the Casey Hernandez (10/08/2000) problem list to include asthma.

5. Susannah Ling is ordered a glucometer. Her random blood sugar at 10:00 AM is 110 mg/dL. Document these results in In-Office Order Entry.

6. During Al Neviaser's visit, the physician requests a patient education handout for hypertension. The medical assistant prints and reviews the handout with the patient. He verbalizes understanding, and no learning barriers are present.

6

Using the Electronic Health Record for Reimbursement

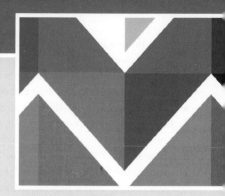

OUTLINE

CHAPTER OBJECTIVES

1. Discuss the role of the patient, the provider, and the third-party payer in the medical reimbursement process.
2. Define medical coding.
3. Discuss diagnostic coding classifications and outline the CPT coding system.
4. Evaluate the advantages and disadvantages of the pay-for-performance (P4P) incentive model.
5. List the information contained in a typical Superbill and explain how the form is used in an outpatient facility.
6. Post charges, payments, and adjustments to a patient ledger.
7. Discuss the concept of medical necessity and indicate how it affects third-party reimbursement.
8. Complete HIPAA 5010 compliant claims.
9. Define fraud and abuse, explain the difference between the two, and give examples of each.
10. Generate patient statements.
11. Explain the reporting features found within an EHR.

KEY TERMS

abstracting Collecting data from a health record. Used for determining CPT, HCPCS, or ICD-10-CM codes and for release of information.

abuse Unintentional deception in which a provider inappropriately bills for services that are not medically necessary, do not meet current standards of care, or are not medically sound.

coding variance Medical coding mistakes caused by computer error or by various kinds of human error, from simple carelessness to incorrect application of coding guidelines and procedures.

compliance plan A written set of office policies and procedures intended to ensure compliance with laws regulating billing, coding, and third-party reimbursement.

CPT (Current Procedural Terminology) A comprehensive set of medical codes that describe procedures, treatments, and services for financial reimbursement and analytical purposes.

electronic data interchange (EDI) The standardized format used to transfer data from one computer system to another.

eligibility Entitled to receive benefits from a health plan.

encounter form A form generated to reflect the services and charges for a patient visit. It includes patient information and account balance. This may also be referred to as a Superbill.

fraud Presenting claims for services that an individual or entity knows or should know to be false, resulting in a benefit to the presenting party.

guarantor The person who is legally responsible for a patient's account; the guarantor is usually the patient, but the guarantor for a minor or a person of decreased mental capacity may be a parent, trustee, or legal guardian.

HIPAA 5010 The standard electronic claim format used by a noninstitutional provider or supplier to submit a claim electronically to Medicare and most other insurance carriers for covered services.

ICD-10-CM International Classification of Diseases, Tenth Revision, with Clinical Modification. A coding system used to describe inpatient and outpatient diagnoses.

medical coding F39 The process of assigning standard numeric or alphanumeric codes to diagnoses, procedures, and treatments for research, disease tracking, and reimbursement purposes.

medical identity theft The unauthorized use of someone else's personal information to obtain medical services or to submit fraudulent medical insurance claims for reimbursement.

pay for performance (P4P) An outcomes-based payment model that offers providers financial incentives for meeting

specific standards and electronically documenting compliance with them; punitive measures may be applied to providers who fail to comply.

third-party payer An organization, other than the patient, that pays for the incurred medical expenses. This could be a federal program or a commercial insurance company (for example, Medicare, Medicaid, Blue Cross and Blue Shield, and Humana).

HEALTHCARE REIMBURSEMENT

The process of submitting insurance claims involves complete attention to detail to ensure that all of the information included is accurate. The implementation of electronic health records (EHRs) and interoperable practice management systems has made this process much easier. At first, learning the reimbursement requirements for several insurance payers can seem overwhelming, but it's more useful to think of billing and coding activities as a kind of puzzle, perhaps like deciphering a word-find puzzle, requiring attention to detail and complex pattern-recognition skills. To solve it, memory skills, critical thinking skills, and persistence are needed. Of course, having experience and using a bit of strategy can be helpful, too. All of these are needed to complete the insurance claims process correctly and efficiently.

Working with medical reimbursement means submitting claims to big insurance companies or to the federal government (Medicare or Medicaid), who are known as third-party payers. Who, then, are the first and second parties? The patient or guarantor would be the first party, and the provider would be the second party. Those third-party payers generally pay the largest share of the claim amount. To help keep down the cost, most healthcare plans (third-party payers) require that patients pay for a portion of their care. Cost sharing might include a deductible, coinsurance, and copayment. A deductible is a set dollar amount that the patient is responsible for annually before the healthcare plan starts paying for claims. In the past a deductible would be in the range of $200 to $500, but we are now seeing more and more high-deductible policies where the deductible is in the range of $2000 to $5000 annually. Once the healthcare plan has received claims for the patient totaling the deductible amount, they will start paying the claims. It is the guarantor's responsibility to pay the provider the amount that has been applied to the deductible. After the deductible amount has been met, there may be a coinsurance requirement. With coinsurance there is a percentage of the claimed amount that the healthcare plan pays, and the guarantor is responsible for the rest. Healthcare plans commonly use an 80/20 or 90/10 split. This means that after the deductible has been met, the healthcare plan will pay 80% of the claim, and the patient will be responsible for the other 20%. The last cost sharing measure is a copayment. A copayment is a set dollar amount that the patient is responsible for in the reimbursement of certain services, usually an office visit/emergency department visit. The copayment amount can range from $25 for an office visit with a primary care provider to $250 for an emergency department visit. The copayment may be higher for a specialist than it is for a

primary care provider. Many healthcare facilities require patients to pay the copayment at the time of service. This helps to reduce the outstanding accounts receivable for the healthcare facility.

TRENDS AND APPLICATIONS 6.1 Cost Sharing

There are basically three components of cost sharing when discussing healthcare plans: deductible, coinsurance, and copays. A deductible is a set dollar amount that the guarantor is responsible for annually before the healthcare plan will start paying for claims. Coinsurance is the percentage of the claim that the guarantor is responsible for once the deductible has been met. Copay refers to the set dollar amount that the guarantor has to pay for each specified type of service, such as an office visit. The copay is required whether or not the deductible has been met.

Let's look at the following example: Janine Butler was seen at Walden-Martin Family Medical Clinic by Dr. Walden for a comprehensive visit, ECG with interpretation, and a lipid panel. The total charge for this visit is $325. Ms. Butler has a $200 deductible, 20% coinsurance, and a $25 copay. Below you can see what Janine's out-of-pocket expenses would be if she had already met her deductible and if she had not met her deductible.

Deductible Has Been Met		Deductible Has Not Been Met	
Total Charge	$325.00	Total Charge	$325.00
Copay	$25.00	Copay	$25.00
Deductible	$0.00	Deductible	$200.00
Coinsurance	$60.00	Coinsurance	$20.00
Total Charge: Copay × 20%		Total Charge: Copay- Deductible × 20%	
Out-of-pocket expenses = Copay + Coinsurance	$85.00	Out-of-pocket expenses = Copay + Deductible + Coinsurance	$245.00
Healthcare Plan payment = 80% of $300.00 (total charge – copay)	$240.00	Healthcare Plan payment = 80% of $100.00 (total charge – copay – deductible)	$80.00

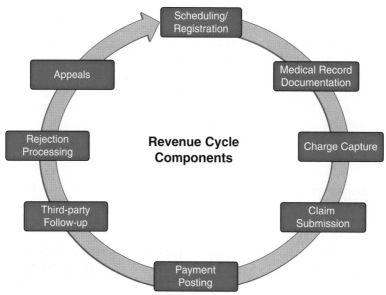

FIG. 6.1 Revenue cycle.

EHR systems have really simplified the billing process. Most EHR systems, including SimChart for the Medical Office (SCMO), have integrated practice management systems. Patient accounts are handled with practice management software, which posts the charges to the patient's ledger, creates a patient statement for provider services rendered, and generates the electronic claim for the healthcare plan.

The Health Insurance Portability and Accountability Act (HIPAA) 5010 is an electronic claim format used to submit electronic claims for reimbursement from Medicare and Medicaid and most other insurance payers. Electronic claims are not printed out; they are transmitted via a modem. Electronic data interchange (EDI) is used to transmit the information, saving money and time, as it is quicker than mailing paper claim forms. Electronic submission also decreases the amount of errors on the claim submission. Human hands enter the information once, and then the computer system collects the data needed. Payment of electronic claims is much quicker than with paper claims. Turnaround for an electronic claim is typically 14 days; it can take up to 4 to 6 weeks to receive payment for paper claims. In addition, HIPAA requires that all claims be submitted electronically for all covered entities. The law does make some exceptions for small providers' offices.

REVENUE CYCLE

The Healthcare Financial Management Association defines revenue cycle as "All administrative and clinical functions that contribute to the capture, management, and collection of patient service revenue." In other words, revenue cycle management starts with the scheduling of a patient and continues through the collection of the payment for services rendered.

When the front office person schedules a new patient for an appointment to see the provider, he or she will gather some preliminary information about who will be paying the bill. When patients arrive for their appointment, the front office person will

scan patients' picture identification cards and insurance cards to allow the billing department access to this information. This is the start of the revenue cycle. Correct identification of the patient and the patient's payers, including the appropriate payer numbers, can be the difference between a paid or denied claim. Patients' medical insurance information frequently changes. The medical staff must verify a patient's eligibility every time the patient comes into the office (Fig. 6.1).

EHR EXERCISE 6.1 Add a Secondary Insurance Plan

Complete the following exercise in the EHR exercises environment of SCMO.

Celia Tapia (DOB 05/18/1970) now has secondary medical insurance coverage effective June 24 of this year. The new payer is MetLife. The policy holder is Arnold Tapia (SSN 812-93-1341). Policy ID number is YYT1230990, and group number is TR508. Claims are submitted to 1234 Insurance Avenue, Anytown, AL 12345. The claims phone number is 800-123-4444.

1. Click the Patient Demographics icon.
2. Use the patient search fields to locate Celia Tapia's record. Click the blue "Celia" hyperlink displayed in the List of Patients table to view Ms. Tapia's demographics.
3. Within the Patient Demographics window, click the Insurance Tab to add the secondary insurance carrier.
4. Select MetLife from the drop-down menu in the Insurance field.
5. Document "Arnold Tapia" in the Name of the Policy Holder field.
6. Document "812-93-1341" in the SSN of the Policy Holder field.
7. Document "YYT1230990" in the Policy/ID Number field.
8. Document "TR508" in the Group Number field.
9. Verify the auto-populated address and phone number.
10. Click the Save Patient button.

In the previous chapter you learned that the clinical documentation serves as the basis for charges. Timely (preferably at the point of care) and accurate capture of the clinical documentation is therefore the next step in the revenue cycle. This includes ensuring that all services that were provided are accounted for on the Superbill/encounter form.

When the patient is ready to leave the healthcare facility, it is important to collect any monies due. This revenue cycle step starts the exchange of money. The patient will be asked to pay for any copayment amount due; in the case of self-pay patients, they will be asked to pay for all of the services rendered.

After the patient leaves the healthcare facility, the claim must be submitted to the third-party payer. If all goes smoothly with the claims process, the next step in the revenue cycle would be the posting of the payment received from the third-party payer and/or the guarantor. If the claim has not been paid in a timely manner, the third-party payer should be contacted to determine why. If the claim has been rejected by the third-party payer, the medical staff must determine why and submit a corrected claim. If the claim was paid but the payment was less than expected, or if the claim was denied, the appeals process must be initiated. This process could include submitting additional documentation and a cover letter from the provider explaining any special circumstances.

CODING SYSTEMS

To standardize the way claims are submitted, whether on paper or electronically, diagnostic and procedural coding systems are used. Medical coding is the process of assigning standard numeric or alphanumeric codes to diagnoses, procedures, and treatments for reimbursement and analytical purposes. Code determination is based on medical documentation in the patient health record, which serves as evidence of patient care. In addition, researchers use coding systems as a means of gathering data to monitor trends in the incidence of acute and chronic illnesses, infectious diseases, injuries, and poisoning.

Proper code assignment is not an exact science because even a single code can reflect many variables, all of which are ultimately related to the complexity of the patient's condition and thus to the amount of time, attention, and expertise required to treat the person.

As part of the standardization initiative in HIPAA, the following are the designated code sets for diagnoses, procedures, and ancillary services:
1. Diagnosis codes: International Classification of Diseases, 10th revision, with Clinical Modification (ICD-10-CM).
2. Procedure codes: Current Procedural Terminology (CPT)
3. Health Care Procedure Coding System (HCPCS)

Role of the Electronic Health Record in Medical Coding

The EHR stores complete sets of codes and links them to the appropriate diagnoses or procedures documented in the patient progress note. Coding systems are updated annually; therefore, the codes in the EHR must be updated annually as well. It's important for the medical coder to double-check the codes assigned by the software. A qualified health information technology specialist can address faulty assignment of codes, at least in part, by tweaking certain administrative options and defaults within the program. But first the problem must be recognized.

To assist with the coding process, many EHRs will have an embedded encoder, which is software that contains all of the coding information needed to correctly assign the diagnostic and procedural codes. The information contained in the encoder is the same information that is included in the coding manuals: inclusions, exclusions, and instructional notes. The encoder found in SCMO is TruCode and can be accessed with the EHR when documenting patient care or creating the necessary forms. It can also be accessed independently from the EHR.

> ### CRITICAL THINKING EXERCISE 6.1
>
> What other skills do you think would contribute to the ability to code swiftly yet accurately?

Coding and Claims Processing Errors

Coding variances, or mistakes, are caused by computer or human error of various sorts, ranging from simple carelessness to incorrect application of coding guidelines and procedures. According to the American Health Information Management Association (AHIMA), which tracks trends in coding error rates, causes can be categorized as coder, provider, or computer errors; lack of leadership (such as failure to implement an EHR effectively); and miscellaneous.

A key factor, says AHIMA, is that too few medical office staff personnel hold providers responsible for providing clear, complete documentation. If the medical biller notices incomplete documentation, whether in the health record or on the Superbill, he or she should confirm with the provider what the needed information is. There's another reason office staff must keep a close watch over claims: Errors often occur after the claim leaves the office. Reviewing the explanation of benefits is key to catching those types of errors. An error rate of 20% annually is reported among health insurers, representing millions wasted each year.

Whom you blame for this problem depends on which industry you work in, insurance or medicine. But with millions of medical claims submitted every day, mistakes are likely to happen even when people have the best of intentions. Market conditions contribute to errors as well. As insurers continue to merge and consolidate, provider networks are combined and employees are shifted to new positions, nudged into retirement, or let go. Amid changes like these, it's no surprise that claims processing can be inefficient or worse. Nevertheless, healthcare personnel can speed the reimbursement process and reduce the likelihood of claims denials by controlling coding variances on our end.

Medical practices should conduct both regular and random billing audits. During an audit the office biller or manager evaluates completed Superbills, claims, and EHR documentation for proper coding and billing procedures. An audit identifies poor coding, documentation, and billing practices so that additional training and education can occur and procedures can be adjusted. Being proactive in this area will decrease the percentage of denied or rejected claims submitted by the practice. Having a compliance plan in place is necessary as well, as explained in Trends and Applications 6.2.

Billing and collections processes are performed most often by practice management software, which is often integrated into an EHR like SCMO. Once the practice has received a payment, the payment must be posted to the correct patient's account. Part of the medical assistant's job is to ensure that patients are billed and credited properly, to see that insurance claims are submitted correctly, and to follow up on unpaid claims and delinquent patient accounts.

TRENDS AND APPLICATIONS 6.2
Designing a Compliance Plan

Coding may be a methodic, analytic process, but it's far from cut and dried. There's an awful lot of room for disagreement because the concepts involved are rather hard to pin down. Any two people, for instance, could reach different conclusions about whether the medical decision making that took place during a patient encounter was of low or moderate complexity. Opinions might also diverge over whether the history taken was brief or extended and whether the physical examination was detailed or comprehensive.

The best defense against being investigated or prosecuted for unintentional claims submission errors is to craft an effective compliance plan for the practice. A **compliance plan** is a written set of office policies and procedures intended to ensure compliance with laws regulating reimbursement. A compliance plan shows potential auditors that the practice has made a good-faith effort to comply with CMS guidelines and to conform with meaningful use requirements.

An effective compliance plan might stipulate that the practice meet the following standards:

- Undertake random and scheduled audits to identify high-risk practices.
- Keep accurate, complete patient records and immediately address any inadequacies in a provider's documentation habits.
- Conduct regular training and educational sessions for the professional development of the staff and providers.
- Enforce disciplinary standards as spelled out in the office policies and procedures manual.
- Monitor billing practices for irregularities, such as improper inducements and an excessively high rate of claims denials.
- Draw up specific plans to remedy any practices an auditor might view as disreputable. Given the legitimate differences of opinion that arise over billing and coding procedures, your practice must avoid not just impropriety but the appearance of it as well. A compliance plan documents your good intentions.

Now that we've given you a high-level view of medical billing and coding, let's zoom in on the two coding systems used most frequently in the medical office.

CRITICAL THINKING EXERCISE 6.2

Which factors do you think are most responsible for coding variances? Which ones are controllable by the medical practice, and what steps could you take to control these variances?

Current Procedural Terminology Coding (CPT)

The CPT system, introduced in 1992, is now in its fourth edition. It was devised by the American Medical Association (AMA) at the request of the federal government's Centers for Medicare & Medicaid Services (CMS). The purpose of the system was to standardize the way in which claims are submitted to the CMS, which is responsible for issuing periodic rules and guidelines for

how the codes may be applied and for conducting audits when fraud is suspected. In addition, to stay current with emerging technology, CMS publishes updated CPT codes every November.

CPT, then, is a uniform language for describing procedures and treatments performed by healthcare providers. The system consists of more than 10,000 five-digit codes that represent services rendered. Since its introduction, the code has undergone several revisions and clarifications. The CMS revision work group includes general practitioners and representatives of every medical specialty. The committee uses actual clinical cases as models to draft codes appropriate for use in general practice and in a multitude of specialty areas.

Category I

The CPT manual is separated into Category I, Category II, and Category III codes. Category I is divided into several sections, which we will explore briefly.

Evaluation and Management (99201–99499). In the print version of the CPT manual, the Evaluation and Management section is placed up front to make it easy to access because it is the most heavily used. Evaluation and management codes, usually referred to as E/M codes, are based on a trio of factors: history, physical examination, and evidence of medical decision making. Coordination and counseling, risk, and time spent with the patient are taken into account as well, but these factors are not given as much weight as the other factors. The E/M code set includes office visits, hospital visits, consultations, discharge, nursing home services, and preventive care visits. Documentation in the patient record is vital to the proper E/M code assignment. Lack of documentation during a patient visit could result in decreased reimbursement of the provider's service. For this and other reasons, it is important for the biller to have open communication with the healthcare provider so that questions may be asked and errors avoided.

CRITICAL THINKING EXERCISE 6.3

Why do you think the amount of time spent with the patient does not weigh as heavily as the other three factors in determining the proper E/M code?

An EHR can determine the proper E/M code based on the provider's documentation. A prompt will be generated if more information is required to select the right code. The EHR might, for example, ask the user to check off more morbidity and mortality risk factors from a list, or to specify which questions the patient was asked during the history taking. The system factors in other data, too, such as how long the visit lasted, the type of visit (office visit vs. consultation), and the kind of patient (new vs. established). Then the program reviews the data to generate the appropriate code. This saves the coder time by eliminating the need to manually generate a specific procedure code; however, the job responsibility now is to make sure the codes are up to date and match the services the provider performed. This is done by reviewing the progress notes and **abstracting** the information regarding the procedures that were performed and services that were provided.

Many EHR systems allow you to see the impact of your coding choices before committing to them. Of course, the actual documentation made by the provider during a visit should not be altered by anyone except the provider. In many cases, however, two virtually identical labels are available to *describe* that documentation. Ordinarily, CMS regulations allow you to choose the one that is more favorable to practice revenues.

If you like the changes you've tested and believe they accurately reflect the level of service provided during the patient's visit, you may save them. If you think a different set of codes would give you a more favorable outcome, you can scrap your changes and try a different coding scheme or return to the original CPT code (Trends and Applications 6.3). When in doubt, check with the provider because all reimbursement requests may be subject to audits by the payer.

TRENDS AND APPLICATIONS 6.3
Ensuring the Best Practice Revenues

We might like to think practice revenues are of no concern to us, but maintaining financial records and overseeing medical billing are two important aspects of the medical assistant's administrative scope of practice, as defined by the American Association of Medical Assistants. Practice revenue is what provides the money to keep the healthcare facility running. It pays the rent for the office space, pays for supplies and equipment, and pays the wages of those working there.

If the providers who own the practice believe you're looking after their financial interests and caring for their patients, you'll quickly become indispensable to them. In addition, a thriving practice is less likely to lay off staff.

Then, of course, there's the matter of raises, which tend to be commensurate with each staff member's value to the practice. You might even consider becoming a certified coder. Many providers are willing to help their medical assistants pay for such credentialing as a means of retaining qualified medical assistants. Having dual certification in medical assisting and coding is a great way to ensure your employability. If you decide to change jobs down the road, you'll be able to show potential new employers how the billing and coding practices you implemented increased practice revenues. The list below is a good place to begin.

When a claim is denied, check the simplest explanation first. Most claims are kicked back to the provider because of transposed digits, incorrect modifiers, and other elementary errors. Double-check and resubmit denied claims.

Learn as much as you can about diseases and their treatment, including common procedures. According to AHIMA, lack of knowledge in these areas is at the root of many coding variances, especially with the implementation of ICD-10-CM coding.

Take advantage of government resources, such as the Medicare Coverage Determinations website, for Medicare coding updates.

Use the coding features of your EHR to test several codes before deciding which to use. As long as your codes are accurate, CMS rules allow you to select the more profitable of two similar code selections.

Take advantage of the reporting capabilities of the EHR to track denied claims by provider and by billing code. This will help you identify trouble spots so you can work with the providers and other staff members to find targeted solutions.

Treat coding and reimbursement training as a continuous process rather than as a one-time cram session. Use the EHR's messaging capabilities to circulate information about coding modifications, newly issued codes, and coding tips.

Don't neglect to bill for your own time. The practice can bill for medical assisting services during an established patient's office visit lasting about 5 minutes for which the presence or supervision of a provider is not required (see CPT code 99211 for details). Use the EHR to track trends in the number of medical assisting visits billed.

Anesthesia (00100–01999, 99100–99150). This section is used to report the administration of anesthetic usually during surgery by an anesthesiologist, anesthetist, or other physician. Anesthesia means introducing a drug to obtain partial or complete loss of sensation in a patient. The codes used include local, regional, and general anesthesia.

Surgery (10000–69990). The surgery section makes up the bulk of the CPT manual. It categorizes surgical procedures by body system, such as the integumentary (skin), respiratory, musculoskeletal, cardiac, and reproductive systems. These codes are used to report a variety of surgical procedures performed in medical offices and in outpatient surgical centers, and to code inpatient surgeries.

Radiology (70000–79999). Radiology is the study of using radiant energy to diagnose and treat patient conditions. Codes listed in the radiology section describe radiologic imaging services, including diagnostic and therapeutic radiology, nuclear medicine, ultrasound, computed tomography, and magnetic resonance imaging.

Pathology and Laboratory (80000–89398). Pathology and laboratory codes are used to describe providers' orders for blood panel tests, such as complete blood counts, and for blood tests to check for conditions such as anemia (low blood iron content), hyperglycemia (high glucose content, which could indicate diabetes), and coagulation disorders.

Diagnostic immunology tests, which check the blood for the presence of antigens and antibodies to specific substances, fall within this category as well. Tests for conditions as diverse as pregnancy, rheumatoid arthritis, illegal drug use, and exposure to HIV are all classified as immunologic tests. Even the typing and crossmatching of blood that's done before major surgery falls into this area.

Pathology and laboratory codes are also used for anatomic pathology procedures, such as Pap tests (cell pathology), and for microscopic examination of tissue specimens (surgical pathology). For example, excised moles, intestinal polyps, or biopsied lung tissue may be examined microscopically for evidence of malignancy.

Medicine (90281–99099, 99151–99199, 99500–99607). The medicine section of the Category I CPT-4 code manual includes tests, procedures, and other services not covered in other sections of the CPT manual. These services for coding diagnostic and therapeutic services are considered to be fairly noninvasive. Examples include injections and immunizations, allergy testing, psychiatry, ophthalmology, and neurology services.

Category I Guidelines. A set of guidelines is given at the beginning of each section of the CPT Category I manual. Reading them will save you time in the long run, even if the information doesn't make for fascinating conversation at the next office picnic. The guidelines clarify terms, list procedures found within the section, and suggest codes to use for unlisted procedures. Two-digit numeric modifiers are often added to the CPT codes to specify more precisely which procedure was performed. A full list of modifiers and their descriptions is provided in Appendix A of the CPT manual.

Category II

Category II codes are supplemental codes used to help researchers collect data, track illness and disease, and measure quality of care. The use of these codes is not required, and there is no reimbursement value attached to using them.

Category III

Category III codes are temporary codes applied to emerging technology. These codes are used to minimize the number of unlisted codes being submitted to report services not otherwise described in Category I codes.

Healthcare Common Procedure Coding System (HCPCS)

In addition to CPT codes, HCPCS codes are used for nonprovider services and supplies. There are no codes in CPT for services such as ambulance services, prosthetic devices, and walkers. These services and supplies are oftentimes covered by the patient's insurance, so to submit a claim, there must be codes. Determining a correct HCPCS is very similar to the process for determining the correct CPT code. Most encoders found within EHRs have the ability to code the HCPCS services as well as CPT.

CRITICAL THINKING EXERCISE 6.4

Do you think every member of the medical office staff, including providers, should have to attend mandatory training on coding topics, or just those who code? Explain your answer.

ICD-10-CM Coding

Once the healthcare provider assesses, consults with, examines, or treats the patient and documents the encounter in a progress note, a diagnosis code is entered by the user or generated automatically by the EHR. If the diagnosis code is not indicated on the Superbill, the medical biller will need to abstract that information from the progress note. If SOAPE noting is used, the diagnosis information would be found in the assessment (A) section. It's important to remember that the code must directly reflect the provider's documentation without making assumptions. If there is any question, the healthcare provider should be consulted.

The **ICD-10-CM** codebook consists of about 70,000 codes, and the system has these characteristics:

- Codes are three to seven alphanumeric characters. The first character is a letter. The second and third characters are numbers (for example: J44.9, Bronchitis with airway obstruction).
- ICD-10 has 21 chapters without supplementary classifications.
- Coding conventions include parentheses for nonessential modifiers; see, see also, and see category for cross-references; a placeholder "X"; use of a seventh character; Excludes Notes; Code Also notes; and default codes and syndromes.

The ICD-10-CM code sets are organized into the following:

Alphabetic Index of Diseases. This volume contains diagnostic terms, in alphabetical order, to guide the location of a complete code. It contains an alphabetic index of disease and injury, Table of Neoplasms, and Table of Drugs and Chemicals.

Tabular List of Diseases. The Tabular List is organized by chapters, in alphanumeric order, based on body systems, conditions, and etiology; signs and symptoms; injuries and poisonings; factors influencing health status; and external causes of morbidity. A set of coding notes appears at the beginning of each chapter, or the subdivision of each chapter.

Official Guidelines for Coding and Reporting. The Guidelines are divided into four sections: Section I. Conventions, general coding guidelines, and chapter-specific guidelines; Section II. Selection of Principal Diagnosis; Section III. Reporting Additional Diagnoses; Section IV. Diagnostic Coding and Reporting Guidelines for Outpatient Services.

EHR EXERCISE 6.2 **Use ICD-10-CM to Document in the Problem List**

*Complete the following exercise in the EHR Exercises assignment found in Open Assignments.

Kyle Reeves (DOB 01/01/1996) is here for his follow-up appointment with Julie Walden, MD, for irritable bowel syndrome. He was first diagnosed with this problem on January 21 of this year. Update the Problem List using ICD-10-CM.

1. Click the tab for the Clinical Care module.
2. Perform a patient search for Kyle Reeves and confirm his date of birth.
3. Enter the existing encounter (if no encounter is available, create a follow-up encounter using the work flow described in Chapter 5).
4. Select Problem List from the Record drop-down menu.
5. Click the Add Problem button.
6. In the Add Problem window, enter irritable in the text box and select Irritable bowel syndrome from the Diagnosis drop-down menu.
7. Select the ICD-10 Code radio button and document "K58.9" as the diagnosis code. Refer to ICD-10-CM to confirm.
8. Using the calendar picker, document the Date Identified as 01/21 of this year.
9. Select the Active radio button.
10. Click the Save button.

Although CPT coding and ICD-10-CM coding identify different things—procedures and diagnoses, respectively—they work together to ensure that proper reimbursements occur. This will be discussed in more detail in the HIPAA 5010 Claims Processing section.

PAY FOR PERFORMANCE

Pay for performance (P4P) is an outcomes-based payment model that rewards providers for delivering evidence-based care according to specific standards and for electronically documenting compliance with those standards. This model is quickly becoming the gold standard by which most health plans (such as health maintenance organizations [HMOs] and preferred provider organizations [PPOs]) operate. These "bonus" structured payment systems are quickly turning into earned revenue as providers strive to meet specific patient targets or measures. For this reason, these value-based systems are shifting from fee-for-service systems to a combination of fee-based and performance-based payment systems.

Incentives and Penalties

To ensure that practices participate in P4P programs, private insurers and Medicare have built disincentives into the system for those who fail to meet P4P standards. For example, in 2009 providers who used a computerized provider order entry (CPOE) system to submit claims for Part D Medicare recipients were rewarded with performance pay amounting to 2% of their annual Medicare billing. This bonus has been phased out, is no longer offered. Instead, providers who choose not to use CPOE will be dinged with a penalty equal to 2% of their annual Medicare billing. The AMA has spoken out against this and other policies that reduce reimbursement based on substandard results.

CRITICAL THINKING EXERCISE 6.5

Do you believe P4P programs work to improve patient care? What other factors might motivate practitioners to improve patient care?

Use of the Electronic Health Record in P4P Compliance

Because P4P is an outcomes-based model, technology is required to measure and document the outcomes achieved. That's where the EHR system comes in. The EHR offers a way to record improvement by noting laboratory results, findings of imaging studies, and clinical progress notes. Providers who haven't adopted an EHR are at a distinct disadvantage in adhering to the program's requirements. Because hospitals and other large institutions were the first to implement electronic records systems, the P4P model has been widely used in those settings. However, large practice groups, multi-provider practices, and even solo practitioners are now being asked or even required to participate in P4P programs. The P4P model works best when applied to patients with chronic illnesses, such as diabetes, hypertension, and arthritis. Most of these patients are treated by primary care providers such as family practitioners and internists. Such practices treat nearly 70% of all ambulatory care patients in the United States.

All EHR systems have the ability to generate reports. It is these reports that can be used to demonstrate that there has been an improvement in laboratory results, that more diabetic patients are being seen on a regular basis, and that there has been an increase in mammograms in the appropriate age groups. These compilations of medical care and census data are essential for continuity of care as well as for showing that a healthcare facility's patient care plan is effective.

SUPERBILL

Practice management systems attach a Superbill (also known as an *encounter form, charge slip, route slip, fee slip,* or *checkout form*) to the patient's visit for use during an office visit. The format of the Superbill includes a list of the most commonly used CPT and ICD codes. It is important to remember that these codes are updated annually, so the Superbill should also be updated to include any new or changed codes. The provider completes this form, either on paper or electronically, and then this form is used by the medical biller to create a claim for reimbursement of services.

Patient demographics and insurance information, which are included on the Superbill, change frequently, so patient information must be verified at the beginning of every visit. Both sides of the insurance card should be scanned and the information updated right away if the policy has changed.

The patient's copy of the encounter form serves as a bill and evidence of care. This form documents charges for the office visit, any past due amounts, and a record of payment by the patient.

Of course, using an EHR vastly simplifies the process of completing a Superbill. In SCMO, the Superbill can be completed by using the Progress Note and Fee Schedule for reference. This clinical record describes the services performed during the patient visit. The Superbill serves as a summary of visit events and as a means of tracking diagnosis codes or procedure usage. The purpose of the Superbill is twofold: to collect data about the patient and to record details of the patient's visit. The form includes the following information:

- Demographic data (patient's name, address, phone number, and date of birth)
- Date of appointment
- Guarantor (the person responsible for the account)
- Insurance policy number and group ID
- Diagnosis codes
- Service codes and ranking
- Account balance including previous balance

EHR EXERCISE 6.3 Completing a Superbill

*Complete the following exercise in the EHR Exercises assignment found in Open Assignments.

Complete the Superbill for Kyle Reeves (DOB 01/01/1996) for a problem-focused, established patient visit performed today for irritable bowel syndrome. (Be sure you created the encounter from EHR Exercise 6.2 first.) The patient has a $10 copayment for office visits. Kyle's mother, Kim, has paid the copayment in cash.

1. Click the tab for the Coding and Billing module.
2. Select Superbill from the left Info Panel.
3. Perform a patient search for Kyle Reeves and confirm his date of birth.
4. Select the correct encounter in the Encounters Not Coded table (Fig. 6.2).
5. Select the ICD-10 radio button.
6. Document "Irritable bowel syndrome, K58.9" in the Rank 1 Diagnoses box.
7. Use the Fee Schedule link to determine the fee and CPT code for a problem-focused office visit for an established patient.
8. Document "1" in the Rank column for Problem focused in the Office Visit box, followed by "32.00" in the Fee column and "99212" in the Est column. Click the Fee Schedule link in the top right corner for reference.
9. Click the Save button.
10. Because this was the only service provided, click the Next button three times to progress to the fourth page of the Superbill.
11. Document "$10.00" in the Copay field (Fig. 6.3).
12. Document "$0.00" in the Previous Balance field.
13. Document "$22.00" in the Balance Due field.
14. According to Kyle's Patient Demographics, he is covered by Kim Reeves. Document "Kim Reeves" in the Insured's Name field.
15. Click the Same Address as Patient check box.
16. Select the Child radio button for the Patient Relationship to Insured field.
17. Select the Single radio button for the Patient Status field.
18. Select the No radio button to indicate that there is no other health benefit plan.

Continued

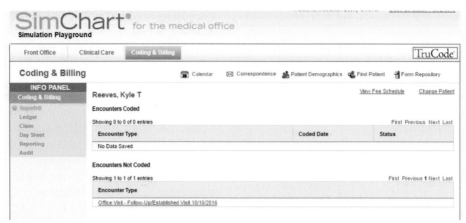

FIG. 6.2 Encounters Not Coded section.

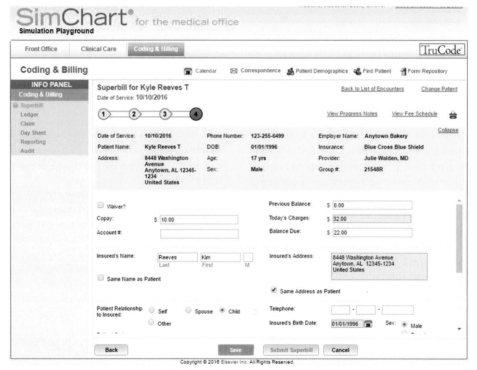

FIG. 6.3 Superbill, page 4.

EHR EXERCISE 6.3   Completing a Superbill—cont'd

19. Select the No radio buttons to indicate that the patient condition is not related to employment, an auto accident, or other accident.
20. Click the Save button.
21. Click the Next button.
22. Click the check box to indicate that you are ready to submit the Superbill.
23. Select the Yes radio button to indicate that a signature is on file.
24. Enter today's date in the Date field.
25. Click Save button.
26. Click the Submit Superbill button.

PATIENT LEDGER

There is much more to maintaining a patient record in the EHR than just clinical documentation. The billing information is also stored in a central location inside the EHR. A summary of all payments, charges, and adjustments to an account in SCMO is called the ledger. The services provided to the patient are posted to the ledger on the date of service, using the CPT or HCPCS codes for services and/or procedures. As payments are received, they are also posted to the ledger on the date that they are received. Oftentimes there is an adjustment that needs to be made when a payment is received from a third-party payer.

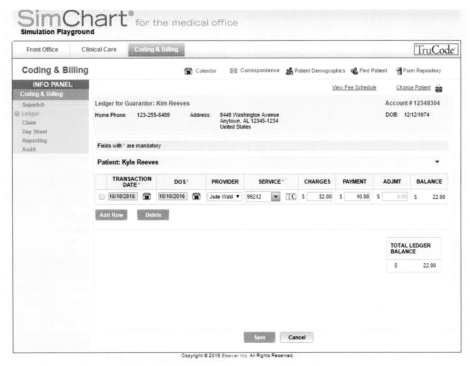

FIG. 6.4 Ledger for Guarantor page.

With managed care contracts the provider has agreed to a discount for services provided to the members of that managed care organization. The adjustments would be posted at the same time as the payment. There are no CPT codes for payments and adjustments that are posted to the ledger, so many healthcare facilities come up with their own service codes such as INSPYMT to represent a payment received from the insurance company and PTPYMT to represent a payment received from a patient.

The ledger is organized by guarantor, but the search for the account is still performed using the patient's name. Proper entry of the guarantor in the Patient Demographics screen will facilitate the creation of the correct ledger in the Coding and Billing module. The Ledger, located in the left Info Panel of the Coding and Billing module, is not linked to a patient encounter, which allows the user to document payments and charges at any time.

EHR EXERCISE 6.4   Completing a Patient Ledger

*Complete the following exercise in the EHR Exercises assignment found in Open Assignments.

Document the copayment and charge for Kyle Reeves's (DOB 01/01/1996) office visit with Dr. Walden in the Ledger of the Coding and Billing module.

1. Click the tab for the Coding and Billing module.
2. Select Ledger from the left Info Panel.
3. Perform a patient search for Kyle Reeves and confirm his date of birth.
4. The Ledger for Kyle Reeves will display "Ledger for Guarantor: Kim Reeves" because she is Kyle's mother and is responsible for his account.
5. Click on the arrow on the right side of the screen, across from Kyle's name.

---

6. Document today's date in the Transaction Date and DOS using the calendar picker.
7. Select Julie Walden, MD, from the Provider drop-down menu.
8. Document "99212" in the Service column.
9. Document "32.00" in the Charges column.
10. Document "10.00" in the Payment column.
11. The Balance of $22.00 is auto-populated based on the amounts listed in the previous columns (Fig. 6.4).
12. Click the Save button.

EHR EXERCISE 6.5   Posting Payments and Adjustments

*Complete the following exercise in the EHR Exercises assignment found in Open Assignments.

Walden-Martin Family Medical Clinic has received a payment from Aetna for services provided to Casey Hernandez (DOB 10-08-2000) on 09/27/2016. Aetna paid $147.80, and because Walden-Martin is part of the Aetna PPO, there is a 10% adjustment needed ($16.43). Document the insurance payment and adjustment received for Casey in the Ledger of the Coding and Billing module.

1. Click the tab for the Coding and Billing module.
2. Select Ledger from the left Info Panel.
3. Perform a patient search for Casey Hernandez and confirm her date of birth.
4. The Ledger for Casey Hernandez will display "Ledger for Guarantor: Sofia Hernandez" because she is Casey's mother and is responsible for her account.
5. Click on the arrow on the right side of the screen, across from Casey's name.
6. Click on the Add Row button.
7. Document the today's date in the Transaction Date and DOS using the calendar picker.

Continued

8. Document "INSPYMT" in the Service column.
9. Document "147.80" in the Payment column.
10. Document "-16.43" in the Adjustment column. Be sure to include the minus sign in front of the dollar amount so that the amount is subtracted from the balance.
11. Click the Save button.
12. The Balance and Total Ledger Balance will be auto-calculated.

HIPAA 5010 CLAIM PROCESSING

Once the Superbill is submitted and once services and payments have been entered in the ledger, it's time to request reimbursement for those services from the third-party payer. The electronic format of the claim form is HIPAA 5010. This form lists the patient information: name, address, insurance, diagnosis codes, services, and charges, along with the provider and payment information for the payer to review. The procedure codes must be linked to the diagnosis code so that the healthcare plan can see why the services were provided. It will demonstrate medical necessity, which will be discussed in the next section. Once the claim is submitted, it is paid, pending, or denied. It is important for the medical assistant to accurately complete and review the claims before submission to decrease the incidence of denials due to data entry errors. The claim data in SCMO is pulled from two sources: Patient Demographics and the Superbill. Besides the fields that are auto-populated are several fields that require manual entry. These fields pertain to charges for services, assignment of benefits, and acknowledgment that a HIPAA form is on file for the patient.

EHR EXERCISE 6.6   Prepare a Claim

*Complete the following exercise in the EHR Exercises assignment found in Open Assignments.

Using the Superbill completed in EHR Exercise 6.3 for reference, prepare a Claim for Kyle Reeves's (DOB 01/01/1996) visit.

1. Click the tab for the Coding and Billing module.
2. Select Claim from the left Info Panel.
3. Perform a patient search for Kyle Reeves and confirm his date of birth.
4. The submitted Superbill appears under the Encounter Type in the List of Superbills for Kyle Reeves.
5. Click the icon (paper and pencil) under the Action column to progress to the Claim.
6. Review the information auto-populated in the Patient Info, Provider Info, and Payer Info tabs.
7. Within the Encounter Notes tab, select the Yes radio button to indicate that the HIPAA form is on file and document the date. Note that the diagnosis entered in Superbill is in the DX1 field under Encounter Diagnosis.
8. Click the Save button.
9. Within the Claim Info tab, select the No radio buttons to indicate that Kyle's condition is not related to employment or an auto accident.
10. Select the Yes radio button in the Release of Info field.
11. Select the Yes radio button in the Assignment field.
12. Select the Yes radio button to indicate that the signature is on file.
13. Click the Save button.
14. Click the Charge Capture tab.
15. Document today's date in the DOS From and DOS To columns.

16. Document "99212" in the CPT/HCPCS column.
17. Document "11" in the POS column. Click the Place of Service link in the top right corner for reference.
18. Document 1 in the DX column to link the procedure code to the diagnosis listed in the Encounter Notes tab.
19. Document "32.00" in the Fee column. This amount will auto-populate in the Total Charges field below the table.
20. Document "1" in the Units column.
21. Document "10.00" in the Amount Paid field below the table. The balance of $22.00 will auto-populate in the Balance Due field.
22. Click the Save button.
23. Click the Submission tab.
24. Select the check box to indicate that you are ready to submit the Claim.
25. Select the Yes radio button to indicate that a signature is on file.
26. Document the date in the Date field.
27. Click the Save button.
28. Click the Submit Claim button to submit the Claim electronically.
29. If your instructor wants you to print out your work to turn in, click the printer icon in the top right corner. The work completed within the claim will display as a PDF in a separate window. (NOTE: The print functionality within the 5010 is only to submit your 5010 form to your instructor or to save in a portfolio. This does *not* generate a 1500 form.) To view or print as a 1500 claim form (paper form), click the Output Claim button.

TABLE 6.1   Medical Necessity

Primary diagnosis: sore throat J02.9
Second diagnosis: diabetes mellitus type 2 E11.9
Third diagnosis: hypertension I10

Services	Linked Diagnoses
99213 office visit	J02.9
	E11.9
	I10
87081 throat culture	J02.9
82962 blood glucose	E11.9

MEDICAL NECESSITY

Medical necessity is a legal doctrine that holds that medical services rendered must be reasonable and necessary according to generally accepted clinical standards. Claims that fail to meet such standards will be denied. An error in the billing process could create an issue with medical necessity. Let's look at a scenario where a patient was seen in the office with a chief complaint of a sore throat but also had type 2 diabetes mellitus and hypertension. After assessing the sore throat, the provider decided that a blood glucose should be done, and the patient's blood pressure was taken and discussed. Three diagnosis codes would be used for this visit: sore throat (J02.9), diabetes mellitus type 2 (E11.9), and benign hypertension (I10). The sore throat diagnosis is the primary diagnosis because it was the main reason for the patient visit. The services provided would be an office visit (99213), throat culture (87081), and a blood glucose (82962). As stated in the HIPAA 5010 section, the services provided need to be linked to a diagnosis code. Table 6.1 demonstrates that linking.

If the throat culture had been linked to the diagnosis code for diabetes mellitus type 2, there would be a medical necessity issue, as it is not generally accepted medical standards to do a throat culture for diabetes. If the blood glucose had been linked to the sore throat diagnosis code, there would be a medical necessity issue, as it is not generally accepted medical standards to do a blood glucose for a sore throat. The diagnosis can confirm that a procedure or service was truly medically necessary. Another example is a rhinoplasty (nose job). Most people think of a rhinoplasty being done for cosmetic reasons. This is not considered a medical necessity, but a rhinoplasty performed to correct a nasal deformity that affects a patient's ability to breathe would be. The CPT would be the same in both scenarios; it is the ICD-10-CM code that would make the difference.

Furthermore, if claims deemed medically unnecessary are discovered during an audit, Medicare or the insurance carrier may demand that the provider pay back the reimbursement received for such services. A pattern of such claims may indicate intentional fraud, in which case the practitioner would be likely to lose his or her Medicare provider eligibility, have his or her medical license revoked, and endure criminal prosecution.

The provider's establishment of medical necessity ensures that a patient's treatment is consistent with the diagnosis and is provided in the appropriate setting under adequate supervision. Clinical decision support systems can significantly aid providers with selecting treatments that are consistent with the diagnosis. Most EHR systems automatically line up the most likely orders for the chief complaint, thus enabling the provider to place orders based on medical necessity. By monitoring procedures and testing, insurance payers can ensure that the correct level of care is being provided.

If the provider believes a service might not be covered, preauthorization to perform the procedure should be obtained before scheduling it. The office staff may request a preauthorization over the phone, by fax, or electronically. Regardless of the method, the patient's insurance information, diagnosis, service requested, and clinical information must be provided. It's also smart to ask the patient to agree in writing to pay for the procedure if the claim is denied.

A little planning goes a long way when you're requesting a preauthorization. Make sure you have all the information you need at hand before making the call. Once the procedure has been approved, the authorization number and expiration date should be documented in the EHR. The procedure can then be scheduled. Remember that every insurance contract has its own set of guidelines regarding which services and procedures require authorization. Creation of an insurance manual can help you keep track of these requirements. In addition, the EHR's reporting capabilities can be used to identify codes that are consistently being rejected.

---

1. Click Form Repository icon in the top right corner.
2. Select Prior Authorization Request from the left Info Panel.
3. Click the Patient Search button to locate Erma Willis and confirm her date of birth.
4. Confirm all auto-populated fields.
5. Document "Julie Walden, MD" in the Ordering Physician field.
6. Document your name in the Provider Contact Name field.
7. Document "Eagle Physical Therapy, 301 Gunner Way, Anytown, AL 54622" in the Place of Service/Treatment and Address field.
8. Document "Physical Therapy" in the Service Requested field.
9. Document the date in the Starting Service Date field.
10. Document 2 weeks from the current date in the Ending Service Date field.
11. Document "3 times a week for 2 weeks" in the Frequency field.
12. Document "DDD M51.3" in the Diagnosis/ICD Code field.
13. Select the No radio buttons to indicate that this request is not injury related or workers' compensation related.
14. Document "GUN02282013" in the Authorization Number field.
15. Document today's date in the Effective Date field.
16. Document the expiration date of 30 days in the Expiration Date field.
17. Click the Save to Patient Record button.
18. Access the Forms section of the Patient Dashboard to print the form if required.

CRITICAL THINKING EXERCISE 6.6

Which other functions of the EHR can help to streamline billing and coding practices? How would you integrate them into the office routine?

When working with insurance claims, it is important to keep track of whether claims have been processed, either paid or denied. An EHR, specifically the practice management software, can generate reports that will show the medical biller which claims are still pending. Remember that electronic claims are generally processed within 14 days. If it has been longer than that, the medical biller should follow up with the third-party payer to determine what happened to the claim. One way to do that is to submit an insurance claim tracer to the third-party payer. An insurance claim tracer is a form that is submitted to the third-party payer that includes the claim information such as claim number, DOS, CPT codes, ICD-10-CM codes, and fees. The form is sent to the third-party payer asking for the status of the claim. The response from the third-party payer will help resolve the outstanding claim. You may need to resubmit the claim with additional information.

EHR EXERCISE 6.7   Documenting a Prior Authorization Request

*Complete the following exercise in the EHR Exercises assignment found in Open Assignments.

Dr. Walden ordered physical therapy for Erma Willis (DOB 12/09/1947) three times a week beginning today and lasting for the next 2 weeks for degenerative disk disease of the lumbar spine (DDD). The order is effective starting today and expires in 30 days. The service will be performed at Eagle Physical Therapy located at 301 Gunner Way in Anytown, AL 54622. This order is not related to an injury or workers' compensation. The authorization number is GUN02282013.

EHR EXERCISE 6.8   Create an Insurance Claim Tracer

*Complete the following exercise in the EHR Exercises assignment found in Open Assignments.

While reviewing claims, the medical assistant notices an outstanding claim for Mora Siever (DOB 01/24/1964) for an ECG with interpretation for mitral valve prolapse on 07/08/2011. The claim number is 1357246, and it was submitted to Aetna on 07/09/2016. The service fee is $89.

1. Click Form Repository icon in the top right corner.
2. Select Insurance Claim Tracer from the left Info Panel.
3. Click the Patient Search button to locate Mora Siever and confirm her date of birth.

Continued

FRAUD AND ABUSE

Fraud is misrepresentation of the medical services provided to deceive or mislead another person or entity, such as Medicare. Fraudulent schemes are carried out primarily for financial gain. Sometimes physical or emotional harm is inflicted on patients or others in the process. Regardless of the motive, fraud is unacceptable and is not tolerated by the government, by private insurers, or by patients. They may be able to fly under the radar for a time, but once exposed, few courts have any sympathy for those who cheat the system. Judges don't hesitate to impose stiff fines. Committing fraud can also result in being removed as a Medicare/Medicaid provider.

If you suspect that fraud is being committed by someone associated with the healthcare facility, you should report it to your supervisor. If it is your supervisor, you may need to take it to the office manager or even report it to the Insurance Commissioner in your state.

Medical identity theft is a different kind of fraud in which the patient—or someone posing as one—is the con artist. They try to use someone else's insurance information to have their medical services paid for. The victim is a current patient or any person who has healthcare coverage.

This crime harms its victims in two ways: medically and financially. The medical harm comes from having the victim's health record riddled with false information that can be traced to the imposter's medical history. That means a patient's medical history and EHR can include someone else's information. In some cases, the entire file can contain the wrong patient's medical history. This erroneous information can be life threatening, such as when the real patient has a drug allergy and the imposter doesn't, or when the patient and the imposter have different blood types.

The damage can create financial disarray that takes years to sort out. Unpaid medical bills may lead to a dismal credit score. The imposter may have expensive hospitalizations, surgeries, and other treatments that push the real policy owner's total above the insurer's lifetime caps. Extensive claims may make it impossible for the victim to purchase new medical insurance.

To make matters worse, victims may not be aware that a theft has occurred until years later, when they develop a medical condition or are tracked down by creditors seeking payment for bills racked up by the imposter. The thief seeking care or fraudulent reimbursement under someone else's name often arranges to have bills and other correspondence sent to a post office box to avoid alerting the real policy owner of the fraud. This allows the scammer to conceal the crime for a long time.

Unscrupulous office workers and employees of healthcare systems are paid as much as $15 for palming off the medical information of a single patient. That's a princely sum compared with the chump change a waiter pockets, as little as 40 cents, for swiping a diner's credit card information and selling it online. Although the interoperability of EHR systems may make it easier for thieves to steal entire databases of patient information, most security consultants agree that an electronic file is infinitely more secure than any mailbox.

To prevent medical identity theft, many healthcare facilities require that the patient present photo identification to confirm that they really are who they say they are. Other healthcare facilities take a picture of the patient and include the photo in the patient information screen of the EHR so that the office staff members who check in the patient can easily see if the person at the counter is the same person who was registered initially. This can be seen on the patient dashboard in SCMO.

Abuse is an unintentional deception in which a provider inappropriately bills for services that are not medically necessary, do not meet current standards of care, or are not medically sound. The difference between fraud and abuse is this: Fraud occurs when a provider bills for services that were never rendered or were not rendered at the level of service indicated, whereas abuse takes place when dubious or excessive tests and treatments are administered.

Once the abusive practice has been recognized, efforts must be made to retrain the employee so the abusive practice is stopped. If a healthcare worker is suspected of fraudulent practices, the situation must be reported to a supervisor immediately. You, as a healthcare professional and patient advocate, have a responsibility to your patient and your employer. Examples of fraud and abuse are given in Box 6.1. The best way to ensure that your office is not engaging in abusive practices is to create and enforce a compliance plan.

PATIENT STATEMENTS

Another aspect of reimbursement for medical services involves collecting money from the patient for his or her portion of the bill. Many times there is a coinsurance responsibility or non-covered services that the patient is responsible for. Generating a patient statement is how the healthcare facility lets the patient know what is owed and why. The statement should show which services were provided and any payments or adjustments that were made to the account. It looks very much like the information found on the patient ledger. Statements are generated on a regular schedule, usually monthly. In larger healthcare facilities, patient statement generation is spread out over the whole month. Patients from a certain section of the alphabet (by guarantor last name) would receive their statements each week of the month. This helps to keep the money flowing in on a steady basis and helps to spread out the phone calls regarding billing questions as well.

EHR Exercise 6.9   Generate a Patient Statement

*Complete the following exercise in the EHR Exercises assignment found in Open Assignments.

Using the Ledger completed in EHR Exercise 6.4 for reference, prepare a Patient Statement for Kyle Reeves's (DOB 01/01/1996) visit.

1. Click on the Form Repository icon in the top right corner.
2. Select Patient Statement from the left Info Panel.
3. Perform a patient search for Kyle Reeves and confirm his date of birth.
4. Confirm all auto-populated fields.
5. Document today's date in the Date of Service field.
6. Document Office Visit 99212 in the Description field.
7. Document 32.00 in the Amount field.
8. Document $32.00 in the Patient's Responsibility field.
9. In the second line of the Patient Statement, document today's date in the Date of Service field.
10. Document Patient Payment in the Description field.
11. Document 10.00 in the Amount field.
12. Document 22.00 in the Patient's Responsibility field.
13. Document 22.00 in the Total Amount Due field.
14. Click on the Save to Patient Record button.

BOX 6.1   Examples of Fraud and Abuse

Fraud

Falsifying a provider's note

Altering test results

Misrepresenting the person who provided the service in order to bill at a higher level

Falsifying dates of service

Inserting codes for services not documented in the patient progress note

Submitting duplicate claims for reimbursement

Changing the diagnosis to receive a higher level of reimbursement, a practice known as "upcoding"

Offering patients kickbacks, gifts, or perks of any kind to accept services that can be billed to Medicare

Failing to refund credit balances due to patients or third-party payers

Balance billing (billing the patient for the difference between the provider's fee and the Medicare allowable amount)

Abuse

Calling patients back for repeated and unnecessary visits

Charging excessively for services and supplies

Performing more diagnostic tests than necessary

Using different fee schedules for Medicare recipients and those with private insurance

Waiving fees and deductibles

REPORTING FEATURES OF AN EHR

To meet the requirements of Meaningful Use an EHR must be able to generate reports that can be used in multiple ways within the healthcare facility. Within the practice management tools should be the ability to generate various aging reports. To stay on top of accounts receivable the healthcare facility needs to know which accounts or insurance claims are not being paid. The EHR should be able to generate a report listing patient accounts and showing the balances and how old those balances are. The categories generally seen on aging reports are 0 to 30 days, 31 to 60 days, 61 to 90 days, 91 to 120 days, and older than 120 days. A useful patient account aging report will also include when the last payment was made on the account and whether it was a patient payment or a third-party payment. The aging categories are used to determine what collection steps will be taken. If an account balance is sitting in the 61- to 90-day category, it is likely that the medical biller will attempt to call the patient and send a reminder letter. If the account balance is older than 120 days, it would appear that all previous collection actions have been unsuccessful, and it may be time to turn the account over to a collection agency. Insurance claim aging reports use the same categories, but the actions taken are focused on the third-party payer rather than on the patients. It must be determined why the claim has not been paid. Oftentimes the third-party payer is looking for additional information from either the provider or the patient. If it is from the provider the medical biller can locate and send the requested information. If it is from the patient, the medical biller can contact the patient and remind him or her that the third-party payer needs information from them and that if it is not provided, the claim could be denied and the patient will be responsible for the full balance.

Accounts receivable is part of the financial picture, but other factors must be considered when judging the financial state of the healthcare facility. Provider productivity is also looked at by the office manager. An EHR can produce reports that will show how many patients a particular provider has seen as well as what services each provider has billed for. These statistical reports can be used for multiple purposes; financial analysis is just one of them. Generating a report of the most common diagnoses used within the healthcare facility can help to determine what additional services should be offered. If the report shows that many patients have been diagnosed with diabetes mellitus, the facility may decide to hire a dietitian to help with the education of those patients. Or the facility may decide to offer a support group that is facilitated by one of the providers. These statistical reports can also be used when making equipment purchase decisions. The report could show how many patients would be helped with the purchase of the new equipment, or it could show that sending the patients somewhere else to get the test done would make more sense.

The reporting function can also be used for quality assurance measures. Information can be obtained and compared with accepted standards to ensure that the healthcare facility is in compliance with those standards. A report could be run to determine whether patients over the age of 50 are getting the appropriate health screenings such as colonoscopies. The reporting function could also be used to determine whether certain services are being overused, for example if a provider is ordering Lyme disease testing on every patient seen during June, July, and August.

All of the reports discussed above can and have been generated without an EHR. It is just more efficient and accurate to use the EHR. You can give the system the parameters you are looking for, such as the specific provider during a specific time frame, and quite quickly you should have the results you are looking for.

CHAPTER SUMMARY

- In the medical reimbursement process, claims are submitted by the provider (the second party) to Medicare or a private insurance carrier (the third-party payer) on behalf of the patient (the first party). It's within the medical assistant's scope of practice to ensure that patients are billed and credited properly, to see that insurance claims are submitted correctly, and to follow up on unpaid claims and delinquent patient accounts.
- Medical coding systems are used in the provider's office as a standardized way of submitting diagnostic and procedural information from a patient encounter. Codes are used primarily for reimbursement purposes, but they're also useful to researchers in collecting data.
- The ICD-10-CM coding system translates complex medical diagnoses into a uniform language used to facilitate reimbursement and tracking of diagnoses. CPT codes are used to report services and procedures performed by the healthcare provider.
- The P4P payment model rewards providers for delivering evidence-based care according to specific standards and for electronically documenting compliance with those standards.
- The Superbill, or encounter form, is attached to every patient visit, and the provider uses it to record the procedure and diagnosis codes for the visit. In addition, the encounter form details patient demographics, insurance information, charges, payments, and any balance due.

- The ledger is used to track all of the charges for services provided to the patient as well as all payments and adjustments applied to the patient account.
- Claims submitted electronically to third-party payers are submitted using the HIPAA 5010 format. This format contains all of the patient demographic information, provider information, and encounter information needed by the third-party payer to make a payment determination.
- The concept of medical necessity holds that services rendered must be reasonable and necessary according to generally accepted clinical standards.
- Fraud is misrepresentation of the medical services provided to deceive or mislead, usually for the purpose of financial gain. Abuse occurs when a provider defrauds Medicare or insurance companies by rendering services that are inappropriate or not medically necessary.
- Patient statements are the tool used to let patients know what their financial responsibility is for the services provided at the healthcare facility. They can easily be generated by the EHR system, specifically the practice management component.
- EHRs can generate a multitude of useful reports. The reports can be used for collection practices (from both patients and third-party payers), for assessing the financial status of the healthcare facility, and for quality assurance.

CHAPTER REVIEW ACTIVITIES

Fill in the Blanks
Read the scenario and fill in the blanks.

Janelle uses the _____ filled out by the provider during the office visit to submit claims. The form includes _____ codes for procedures and services provided and _____ codes for the diagnoses to complete the _____ for submission to the healthcare plan. Once the claim has been submitted, the _____ reviews the claim and provides reimbursement for the patient visit.

Key Terms Review
Match the term in column A to the definition in column B.

1. HIPAA 5010	**a.** Presenting (or causing to be presented) claims for medical services that an individual or entity knows or should know to be false, resulting in a benefit to the presenting party
2. ICD-10-CM	**b.** A coding system used to describe inpatient and outpatient diagnoses
3. Third-party payer	**c.** Assigning standard numeric or alphanumeric codes to diagnoses, procedures, and treatments for reimbursement purposes
4. CPT	**d.** The person who bears ultimate financial responsibility for a patient's account
5. Electronic data interchange (EDI)	**e.** An outcomes-based payment model that offers providers financial incentives for meeting specific standards
6. Compliance plan	**f.** A document that lists the diagnosis and procedure codes most often used in the practice, along with other pertinent information
7. Encounter form	**g.** A coding system describing procedures, treatments, and services
8. Guarantor	**h.** The unauthorized use of someone else's personal information to obtain medical services or submit fraudulent medical insurance claims for reimbursement

9. Fraud
   i. Technology that makes possible the rapid, accurate transfer of encrypted data in a standardized format
10. Pay for performance (P4P)
   j. An organization that pays for the incurred medical expenses
11. Coding variance
   k. Standard claim format used by a noninstitutional provider or supplier to bill Medicare and most other insurance carriers for covered services
12. Copayment
   l. Unintentional deception in which a provider inappropriately bills for services that are not medically necessary, do not meet current standards of care, or are not medically sound
13. Medical identity theft
   m. A written set of office policies and procedures intended to ensure compliance with laws regulating reimbursement
14. Medical coding
   n. Medical coding mistakes
15. Abuse
   o. A set dollar amount that is the patient's responsibility for certain services

True/False

Indicate whether the statement is true or false.

1. _____ The HIPAA 5010 claim format cannot be filed electronically.
2. _____ Evaluation and management code assignment is ultimately related to the complexity of the patient's condition and thus the amount of time, attention, and expertise required to treat the person.
3. _____ Coding systems are updated annually with new, revised, and deleted codes.
4. _____ The medical assistant is permitted to correct minor errors in provider documentation.
5. _____ CPT codes were revised using actual clinical cases as models to draft codes appropriate for use in general practice and in a multitude of specialty areas.
6. _____ Evaluation and management codes are used to describe office visits for new and established patients.
7. _____ The P4P payment model has forced many providers to return to paper-based record keeping.
8. _____ The encounter form or Superbill allows patients to rate provider performance and post coded ratings on an Internet site.
9. _____ Encounter forms are not used by offices implementing an EHR. The EHR directly links the patient visit with the corresponding charges.
10. _____ Medical necessity ensures that the appropriate diagnosis is linked to the proper procedure.

Workplace Applications

1. Daniel Miller (DOB 03/21/2012) is in the office for left ear pain. His father states he has been pulling at his ear for the past 3 days and is not sleeping through the night, but he denies any fever or runny nose. Daniel has no known allergies and is not on any medications. His vital signs are Wt: 28 lb, T: 97.9°F taken on the forehead, R: 20, and P: 112, regular. Dr. Martin determines that Daniel's lungs are clear to auscultation. The examination on the neck is supple with no lymphadenopathy noted, and there are no other significant findings. Dr. Martin determines a diagnosis of otitis media. The plan of care is over-the-counter pain medications and antihistamines, and Dr. Martin instructs Daniel's father to bring him back to Walden-Martin in 1 week if his condition does not improve. Create an urgent care visit for Daniel and document the following information in the Progress Notes.
   S: C/O left ear pain. Father states child is pulling at his ear for the past 3 days and is not sleeping through the night. Denies fever or runny nose. NKA. Not taking any current medications.
   O: Vital signs: Weight 28 lb, T: 97.9°F (forehead), Pulse: 112 and regular, R: 20. LUNGS: Clear to auscultation. NECK: Supple, no lymphadenopathy. No significant findings.
   A: otitis media
   P: OTC pain medications and antihistamines. RTC 1 week if not better.
2. Complete the Superbill and Ledger for Daniel Miller's established problem-focused visit today.
3. Post the charge to Daniel Miller's ledger.
3. Create a claim for Daniel Miller's visit today.
4. Dr. Able has asked you to be in charge of a new compliance team for the prevention of fraud and abuse practices. What types of employees would you ask to be part of the team? The agenda of the first meeting will be to define fraud and abuse and provide examples of each. Once you have compiled a list, discuss solutions and proper ways to handle these situations. Define for your team the penalties for fraudulent activities.

EHR in Review

1. Dr. Walden's patient, Aaron Jackson (DOB 10/17/2011), presents for an appointment today. He is being seen for a wellness examination. The provider ordered an MMR vaccine, which the medical assistant administered. Create a Wellness encounter and document the MMR in the immunization record.
   Immunization: MMR 0.5 mL given IM in the left vastus lateralis. The manufacturer is Hospira Laboratory, and the lot number is 4578T. The expiration date is 01/16/2020. No reaction is noted.
2. Complete a Superbill for Aaron Jackson's MMR injection. There is no copay for the service. Use the Fee Schedule to obtain the fees for both the MMR and administration fee.
3. Update the Ledger for Aaron's injection today.
4. Complete a Claim for Aaron's service today.
5. Results of a radiology examination ordered by Jean Burke, NP, came in today for Tai Yan (DOB 04/07/1956). Use the Diagnostics/Laboratory Results tab in the left Info Panel of the Patient Dashboard to document the results of the lumbar spine x-ray performed last Tuesday: Impression; Moderate Degenerative Disk Disease.

7

The Personal Health Record and Patient Portals

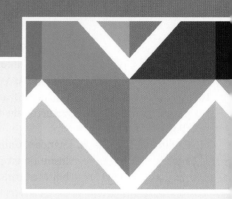

CHAPTER OBJECTIVES

1. Define and explain the purpose of keeping a personal health record (PHR).
2. Describe the three ways of storing PHR data, and outline the advantages and drawbacks of each.
3. Describe how a PHR can be synchronized with medical devices, such as blood pressure cuffs, blood glucose meters for patients with diabetes, and peak flow meters for patients with asthma.
4. Discuss the need for interoperability between PHR systems, electronic health records (EHRs) systems, and related systems.

5. Explain how direct-to-consumer laboratory services can help protect a patient's privacy.
6. Discuss the benefits of creating a PHR for consumers and for providers.
7. Identify steps in setting up a PHR.
8. Identify steps in maintaining the PHR.
9. Define and explain patient portals.

KEY TERMS

advance directive A binding legal document prepared and signed by a competent individual outlining the person's wishes should the person become incapacitated; for example, a medical power of attorney and a living will.

caregiver A person responsible for providing physical care and emotional support, usually in a home-care setting, to a person who is ill, disabled, or dependent.

host A server that provides data transfer, storage space, and other services to users at remote locations; a host has a unique domain name and is, in effect, the point at which a website originates.

living will The part of an advance directive that specifies which life-sustaining treatments (for example, mechanical ventilation and tube feeding) should be administered or withheld if the person becomes incapacitated.

medical power of attorney (also called durable power of attorney for healthcare or healthcare proxy) The part of an

advance directive naming a trusted person to make medical decisions on the patient's behalf should he or she become unable to make such decisions independently.

online community A virtual meeting space where like-minded people with common interests or concerns interact and build relationships using real-time chat rooms, asynchronous threaded discussions, discussion groups, social media, news groups, web conferencing, and other technologies.

patient-controlled health record The portion of a patient portal that contains data loaded by the patient and to which he or she alone may grant or deny access.

patient portal A website that serves as an information transfer hub between patient and physician and that provides information and services, such as secure email, search capabilities, access to an online appointment book, and limited access to patient records.

personal health record (PHR) A secure, comprehensive record of health information that is controlled by the individual, creating a confidential electronic or paper-based file that is easy to access, manage, and share.

populate To complete a template or create a record by filling in a set of predetermined fields with information ranging from demographic data to values and measurements (for example, vital signs) to entire documents (such as correspondence and operative reports).

social networking The practice of using online communities to expand one's social or business contacts and to exchange content, such as images and instant messages; the term also refers to the broader phenomenon of this practice, which has created virtual communities with millions of members.

Wi-Fi (short for Wireless Fidelity, a technologic certification body) A means of connecting wirelessly to the Internet using a local area network or router.

WHAT IS A PERSONAL HEALTH RECORD?

A **personal health record (PHR)** is a comprehensive electronic or paper-based record of health information controlled by the individual, through which he or she can access, manage, and share confidential health information. As society becomes increasingly mobile, easier access to patients' health information can contribute to better health and care. PHRs also get patients more actively involved in their healthcare.

PHRs may be maintained by the patient or stored elsewhere, such as part of an electronic health record (EHR) or with an insurance carrier. Many employers, such as Walmart and Intel, have arranged for their employees to have access to a PHR. The PHR is a means of keeping health information current, safe, and in a single location. The Centers for Medicare & Medicaid Services support such initiatives as a way of reducing medical errors and cutting costs. Military veterans have access to a PHR system (Box 7.1).

Recall from Chapter 1 that continuity of care encompasses the planning and coordination of care, which requires accessible healthcare information that can be shared with specialists and others during medical emergencies. Continuity of care also requires good communication between the patient and his or her providers and healthcare staff. A PHR improves continuity of care, particularly for those who move or switch providers frequently and for those who see multiple specialists, by consolidating health information. Like an EHR, it can also help the patient save time and money by keeping various specialists from ordering duplicate tests and procedures.

It's easy for patients to get lost in the many details of medication refills, appointment schedules, symptoms, diagnoses, and treatment instructions. Keeping a PHR may allow patients to stay on top of their healthcare, perhaps spotting important trends. Many PHRs allow for the patient to confidentially contact his or her provider with concerns. This provides the opportunity for a discussion of the issue and for the creation of a plan of care.

The Personal Health Record vs. the Medical Record

A PHR may sound like an EHR. Both are a means of keeping health information up to date. Both offer some protection against loss of, or damage to, records that are stored elsewhere. And both aggregate data from physicians, hospitals, and allied health professionals into a single record.

The primary difference between a PHR and an EHR or a paper medical chart is who controls the data. Some observers have compared the concept of a PHR to that of a bank.

BOX 7.1 Selected Web-Based Personal Health Records

HealthVault
www.healthvault.com
HealthVault is Microsoft's foray into the PHR arena. It is also in beta testing, although it appears to be further along in the development process than the comparable Google product. HealthVault emphasizes health promotion tools, such as weight loss and blood pressure management. Microsoft has partnered with the manufacturers of several medical devices so that measurements can be downloaded from the devices and recorded directly into HealthVault.

My Health*e*Vet
www.myhealth.va.gov
This site, which is password protected after the patient registers, offers an online PHR tailored to the needs of veterans; it includes a medical library, podcasts, many health assessment and health promotion tools, and a place in which to record military medical history.

Web MD Health Manager
www.webmd.com/phr
Web MD offers a free PHR at this site. It includes A to Z disease information, drug guides, nutrition advice, and pregnancy and parenting information, as well as a template in which patients can store their health information. Some users may sign up for the Health Manager through their employers.

SyncChart
www.synchart.com
SyncChart is an online personal health record management system in which users can enroll themselves and up to seven family members for a small subscription fee (at time of print $9.95 per year). Elements of SyncChart include emergency access, health report printing, medication summary, advance directives, living will, and immunizations.

Just as a bank account holder uses a PIN and ATM card for security, makes deposits, and writes checks, the PHR user accesses a password-protected account, populates the PHR with data, and decides to whom the data may be distributed and for what purposes. The patient can even specify that information from the PHR be disclosed only in emergency situations. Some systems, such as My Health*e*Vet, give users the option of printing emergency access information on a customized wallet card. Such information could be important in the event of a pandemic or a mass-casualty event such as a terrorist attack.

Because an individual is not a covered entity, the patient-controlled PHR is not subject to Health Insurance Portability and

Accountability Act (HIPAA) privacy protection; nor does it necessarily constitute a legal document. However, if a provider, hospital, or other covered entity incorporates data from the PHR, the information becomes subject to HIPAA regulations. In addition, if a covered entity hosts a patient portal, it is required to provide the patient with a notice of privacy practice (NPP) that explains to the patient how the health information stored in it can be kept secure and confidential.

Researchers have found a closer connection between PHR systems and EHR systems than just their functionality, however (Trends and Applications 7.1). Physicians who have implemented EHR systems are aware of the benefits patient portals can offer the busy medical office, but many physicians are not convinced patient-controlled PHR systems can help the medical office yet. They are aware that patients use them and say that their patients' PHR systems were stored on some form of electronic media, such as a website or mobile application (app). However, the percentages of positive responses were low across the board. For example, only 7% of physician EHR adopters report that they actually use the information in their patient-controlled PHR systems.

TRENDS AND APPLICATIONS 7.1   The Personal Health Record: New Technology, New Questions

Relevance. Time-strapped practitioners worry that when patients share their PHR systems, providers will be expected to sift through heaps of clinically irrelevant information that patients have entered into their own records. Will providers be held legally responsible if, for instance, they did not read in paragraph 14 that Mrs. Verbosa was having occasional episodes of chest pain?

Communication. Many physicians are concerned that PHR systems or patient portals with messaging capabilities give the patient too much access to their providers. Studies have found, to the contrary, that patients tend to use email instead of calling, leaving practitioners with about the same workload as before.

Security. How can a patient's identity be authenticated once the PHR becomes interoperable with the EHR and other systems? What about the identities of caregivers authorized to view the patient's information? Patient portals will require usernames and passwords, but it's up to the patient to keep that information secure.

Access. A question closely related to security is that of access. If a patient portal or gateway is used rather than a PHR, how much information should the practitioner give the patient, and which information should the patient be allowed to modify? Can patients be trusted to modify, if they wish, their allergy list, blood type, and other data for which accuracy is critical? So far, most patient portals are used to update demographics, schedule appointments, request medication refills, and pay bills.

Fragmentation. If a patient is using a PHR, the physician is unlikely to benefit from it if the patient chooses not to share the data. The problem is compounded if the data are not electronically compatible with the EHR used by the medical practice. Incompatible PHR systems make it more difficult to convey information to the provider and may serve to delay the implementation of nationwide interoperability standards for EHR systems and PHR systems.

Upkeep. Maintenance is critical if a PHR is to remain useful to patients and their providers. Yet physicians and hospitals are still getting into the habit of sending copies of progress notes, laboratory reports, and similar documents to patients. When patients fail to receive or obtain copies of parts of their records, the PHR becomes incomplete and less useful, especially to emergency personnel and others not familiar with the patient's medical history. As upkeep is becoming easier, the meaningful use program requires eligible providers to make visit summaries available to a patient within 3 days of the encounter.

CRITICAL THINKING EXERCISE 7.1

How do you explain the connection between EHR adoption by the medical physician and PHR use by the patient? Does EHR use encourage patients to participate in their own healthcare? Or are proactive patients just more likely to patronize cutting-edge practices to begin with?

CRITICAL THINKING EXERCISE 7.2

Review the items in Box 7.2 and then name three items not listed in the box that may be useful to store in a PHR.

What Information Is Stored in a Personal Health Record?

The PHR should be a comprehensive collection of health information. Much like the EHR maintained by a medical office, the PHR should include information regarding patient demographics and past medical, family, and social history. It should provide ICE (in case of emergency) contact information for loved ones who should be notified if the patient is transported to a hospital and is unable to communicate.

A PHR is also used to store information about a patient's allergies, current medications, and previous hospital and physician visits. In addition, a PHR may provide resources for managing patient illness and disease. For example, a patient with diabetes may include a link to the American Diabetes Association to stay updated on the disease, or a recently discharged soldier might complete a screening tool to gauge his or her risk for posttraumatic stress disorder. Finally, patients sometimes store insurance information and claims payment history to keep a record of claims paid or denied. Box 7.2 lists information that a typical comprehensive PHR might contain.

In Chapter 3 we met Ellen, a 37-year-old, who has multiple sclerosis. After a recent flare-up of her disease, Ellen had decided to take a more active role in her healthcare. She began requesting copies of her records from her physicians, including her neurologist, ophthalmologist, gastroenterologist, and general practitioner. In addition to receiving copies of these records, Ellen generated quite a bit of paperwork of her own, such as records requests, opt-out notices specifying to whom her health information can be disclosed, and a request for correction of erroneous information she discovered in her file.

Ellen was soon overwhelmed with operative summaries, authorization forms, and other documents, so she decided to organize it into a PHR. She wants her husband, Kent, who is her caregiver during her long periods of convalescence, to be able to find the information he needs if she isn't able to help him locate it, and she thinks a PHR will be a useful tool for doing so. In this chapter, we follow Ellen again as she creates and uses her new PHR.

Types of Personal Health Records

A patient like Ellen who has made the important decision to create a PHR must further decide whether to use a paper record,

BOX 7.2   What Does a PHR Contain?

Some PHR systems are created entirely by the patient, whereas others start with an online template at a web-hosting site. As a result, the information that a PHR might contain varies widely. It might consist of no more than a bare-bones summary of the individual's health history and emergency information. Other PHR systems comprise a detailed health record as well as a broad array of continually updated health promotion tools and information about diseases and conditions. Below are listed many of the items you might find in a comprehensive PHR:

Emergency Information
Patient's name, address, birth date, phone number, and Social Security number
Contact information for loved ones who should be notified if the patient is injured or killed or if the patient suddenly becomes ill
List of allergies to medications, foods, or other substances (latex, intravenous contrast solution, and so on)
Contact information for the patient's pharmacy
List of current medications, dosages, and prescribing physicians
Organ donor authorization

Contact Information and Legal Documents
Health insurance information
Life insurance designation of beneficiary form
Contact information for physicians with whom the patient is established
Advance directive (including living will and medical power of attorney)
Contact information for dentists, therapists, or other healthcare providers

Family History
Health status or age and cause of death of first-degree relatives (mother, father, and siblings)
History of genetic or inherited diseases

Medical History
Chronologic list of surgical procedures and hospitalizations, including specific dates and treatment locations
List of acute illnesses and chronic diseases, including dates diagnosed, treatment received, providers' names, comments or notes to explain the event or condition, and correspondence with providers
List of accidents and injuries, including dates, treatment received, providers' names, and an explanation of the event and any residual problems linked to it, such as pain syndromes

History of exposure to toxic chemicals in the workplace or elsewhere
Documentation of physician visits
Results of laboratory, pathology, or imaging studies
Immunizations received, including dates and any adverse reactions
Vaccinations received, such as those for pneumonia and flu, and any adverse reactions

Social History
Occupation
Nutritional habits and physical activity regimen
Use of tobacco in any form
Use of alcohol or illegal drugs

Health Logs
Physical activity logs
Food journal
Blood glucose readings (especially for patients with diabetes or prediabetic conditions)
Blood pressure measurements
Cholesterol
Body temperature
Weight and body mass index (BMI)
Heart rate
Respiratory rate
Pain scale self-reports

Health Promotion Tools
Smoking cessation information and tools to track progress
Caregiver assistance, including lists of local resources
Advice for healthy eating, including logs to track food intake, weight, and physical activity
Self-care information about healthy sleep habits, including information on how to beat insomnia and when to visit a sleep clinic
Emergency preparedness resources, such as instructions for assembling a disaster preparedness kit and a first aid kit
Mental health resources, such as information about stress and depression, numbers for suicide hotlines, and self-care advice for improving coping skills
Substance abuse resources, such as screening tools and links to information and help for those who may be abusing alcohol, prescription drugs, or illegal drugs

a stand-alone software program, or an online web-based PHR. Cost, portability, privacy, and other factors should be considered in making this decision.

CRITICAL THINKING EXERCISE 7.3

What type of person or patient is most likely to benefit from creating a PHR? What type of person or patient is most likely to create one? Are they the same?

Paper-Based Personal Health Records

Traditionally the PHR has been paper based. This method is inexpensive and secured as the patient's property. Paper-based PHR systems are generally organized into three-ring binders so that documents can easily be added or removed. Tabbed dividers, like those used in patient records kept in medical offices, can be used to organize and identify documents.

Of course, paper PHR systems have all the disadvantages of paper charts in a medical office. The chief drawback is the difficulty of sharing information. If the patient is ever crushed by a falling piano, say, or if he suddenly falls ill after eating tainted sushi, that tidy little three-ring binder sitting on a shelf in his home office won't do the emergency medical technicians much good. In addition, paper-based PHR systems require more work to maintain than an electronic version. The user must remember to gather the data and organize it in a timely manner. Patients who frequent a medical office or have a series of testing on a regular basis might find this overwhelming.

Personal Health Record Software

Patients who want to have their health information in electronic form but do not wish to store their private information online may decide to purchase a stand-alone software product. These

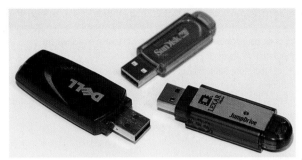

FIG. 7.1 USB drives, also called *thumb drives* or *flash drives*.

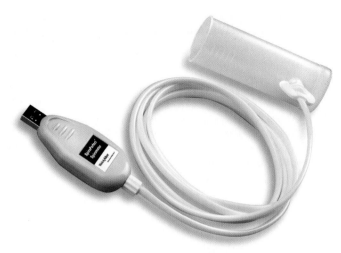

FIG. 7.2 A spirometer with a USB connection capable of linking directly to a computer. (Courtesy of Welch Allyn.)

programs allow the individual to create and save health information to a computer. The files can also be made portable if they are saved to a USB drive (also called a *thumb drive* or a *flash drive*), a small device that contains a digital memory chip on which electronic data can be stored and easily moved from one computer to another. A USB drive can be attached to a keychain and plugged in to most computers (Fig. 7.1). Still, the files are not fully functional when the software is not available.

Online Personal Health Record

Many of us find it tough to imagine how we got by without computers to manage our lives. We use accounting software to compute our taxes, we check our credit card and bank balances on secure websites, we make dinner reservations and buy theater tickets online, and we even order stamps online when we need to send mail. Maintaining a web-based PHR, then, seems like a natural extension of the things we're already doing online.

Keeping a PHR in cyberspace means that it's accessible from any computer in the world that has an Internet connection. That's a big plus for patients like Ellen. She sometimes travels to a hospital in another state to see one of her specialists, and she likes the idea of being able to pull up her PHR from her laptop. The hospital offers free **Wi-Fi**, so Ellen can even access her PHR from the lobby.

Many websites have been established at which a patient can create a free PHR; the websites are even offered as apps installed in the patient's mobile device for quick reference and use. Sites with advanced services and security generally charge a subscription fee. Another advantage of a web-based PHR is that it usually gives the patient easy access to a database of health information. Just as a medical assistant or provider using an EHR can quickly look up medication dosages, disease signs and symptoms, and evidence-based screening and treatment guidelines, the user of a web-based PHR can do so as well. Databases of information are not simply limited to medication, either. Apps like MyFitnessPal offer users nutritional information on just about every food you can think of to create food diaries and document physical activity.

Careful research is a good idea before choosing a PHR. Dozens of choices are available, some of which are listed in Box 7.1. In addition, several Medicare Advantage or Part D drug plans offer PHR systems to their members. Ellen selected an online PHR with an extensive library of health information and a suite of health promotion tools. She also joined a free **social networking** site for people with MS. The sharing of personal health information through **online communities** is a great way for people like Ellen to feel connected with other individuals who share the same health concerns.

INNOVATIVE FEATURES OF PERSONAL HEALTH RECORDS

As you might imagine, PHR systems are capable of doing a great deal more than just storing personal health data and linking to medical and drug information. However, many of these features, some of which are described below, are fee-based add-ons that require a monthly or annual subscription. For some patients, especially those with chronic conditions and their caregivers, this may be money wisely spent. For others the money may be wasted because the features don't work if the patient doesn't use them.

Synchronization with Medical Devices

Some PHR systems are capable of linking directly to medical devices, such as scales, blood pressure cuffs, blood glucose meters for patients with diabetes, peak flow meters for patients with asthma, pedometers, and heart rate monitors. Using a USB connection, measurements taken by the device can be downloaded directly into a tracking template on the PHR (Fig. 7.2).

ICE Notification

Other applications allow the user to preselect which pieces of information from the PHR to make available to emergency personnel in the event of an accident or acute illness. The data can then be downloaded to a mobile device. Mobile apps like ICE, My Medical, and Emergency Contact are available for iPhone, Android, and iPad and are available for free or at low cost to download. A wallet card can also be printed to give first responders instructions for accessing the information.

Ellen's PHR gave her the option of printing a summary of her essential medical information, along with login instructions for emergency personnel. She now carries the printed summary and a wallet card with her wherever she goes.

Drug Alerts

Just as a practitioner using an EHR receives a warning if he or she tries to prescribe a drug to which the patient is allergic or one that may cause an adverse reaction with another drug the patient takes, patients themselves can link their PHR systems to online software apps that will generate such alerts. The programs usually offer suggested alternatives to the medication being prescribed and send email alerts to the patient's provider. Mobile apps that focus on drug alerts such as Dosecast, Davis Mobile High Alert Drug, and MedCoach can help patients maintain and understand medication usage.

Limited Interoperability

Throughout this text we've discussed the concept of interoperability, the ability of separate systems to share information in compatible formats. Thus far, interoperability of PHR systems with EHR systems, pharmacy systems, and so on has proved elusive. Tang and colleagues warn that interoperability is critical if PHR systems are to avoid becoming "information islands" on which selected health data are isolated from the patient's main health record.

Parts of certain EHR systems are interoperable with certain external systems, though. For instance, urgent care clinics called MinuteClinic have entered into a strategic alliance with Microsoft's HealthVault to make all data from a patient's visit immediately downloadable to the patient's HealthVault PHR. If the patient goes to another urgent care clinic or chooses a different PHR, he or she loses this advantage (thus giving the patient an incentive to use both MinuteClinic and HealthVault).

Even without interoperability PHRs can allow the patient to share information with their providers. Some PHR systems have a feature that allows patients to email their information to their physicians ahead of time. Practices that use paper charts can print the information and place the sheets right into the patient's chart. For a fee the information can be transferred to the actual forms used by a particular office. Patients can also scan documents, such as correspondence and **advance directives** (including **living wills**), into their records. The physician can return information to the patient through the PHR as well by using secure email.

Direct-to-Consumer Laboratory Services

In the past, a patient nearly always had to visit a physician to have a blood test ordered. Direct-to-consumer, web-based laboratory testing takes out the middleman. Let's say Chris, a 49-year-old man, is paying higher-than-average rates for life insurance because of his high cholesterol. He's been working out and watching his diet, using the PHR to track his progress, but Chris's insurance company will reassess his rates only once every 3 years. Chris wants to be sure his cholesterol has dropped before he requests a reassessment. Using a PHR that links him to a network physician who can submit the laboratory order and refer him to an approved facility, he can have the cholesterol test performed and have the results sent to his PHR account.

Telephone Consults

Worried parents, business travelers, and others with frequent need of a physician, or with a temporary lack of access to one, will appreciate the convenience of being able to share their PHR with a physician by telephone. There are fees attached to this service, but it may be less expensive and faster than paying for a visit to an urgent care center, assuming one is available. Patients should consider hidden charges, though, such as registration fees, that may be billed in addition to a monthly subscription fee and a flat-rate consultation fee.

Satellite and MP3 Technology

The satellite folks who can read our license plates from space continue to find creative uses for global positioning system (GPS) technology. Technology like Fitbit allows users to monitor daily activities through a small bracelet worn daily. Susie Smith can map out a biking or walking route that's exactly 3.2 miles or whatever length she specifies. Or she can enter her current route to find out whether four laps around the dog park is really a whole mile. Then, drawing on the health goals and physical activity preferences she's outlined, the PHR can design a personal training session for her. When she's finished her workout, she can upload data from her heart rate monitor or pedometer into her PHR to find out and record how far she walked or rode, whether she reached her target heart rate, and how many calories she burned.

CRITICAL THINKING EXERCISE 7.4

Do you think a PHR or other health apps have the power to change an individual's health behavior? Why or why not?

Why Create a Personal Health Record?

In the introduction to this text and elsewhere, we reported that most physicians who adopt EHR systems say they'll never go back to paper. A similar point might be made about individuals who create PHR systems: They'll never go back to relying solely on their physicians to keep their health records for them.

Studies indicate that even though PHR systems haven't been around long, users already indicate a high rate of satisfaction with them. The PHR seems to have hopscotched over that bumpy period during which the bugs are worked out of a new technology. Perhaps that's because PHR systems are really just a novel application of many existing technologies. Little is known yet, say Tang and colleagues, about how people select PHR technology and integrate it into their lives. But the biggest implementation will come with physicians offering patient portals as a means to monitor healthcare.

For Ellen it made sense to create a PHR to help her keep track of information from multiple specialists and to gain more control over her healthcare decision making. She showed her PHR to Keira, one of her home health aides. Keira, whose physician had recently warned her that she showed signs of developing type 2 diabetes, decided to create a PHR for herself in order to monitor her weight, body mass index, heart rate, and physical activity. A Harris poll indicates that, like Keira and Ellen, more than half of Americans keep some sort of PHR. It stands to reason that the numbers will continue to grow.

Benefits to Individuals, Patients, and Caregivers

In this chapter we've tossed about the terms "individual," "consumer," "patient," and "PHR user" interchangeably, but a PHR isn't just for sick people. It's a powerful health promotion tool for those with no health problems, and it can help those with chronic conditions stay as healthy as possible by taking charge of their health. Keira, for example, discovered that keeping a PHR gave her additional motivation to stick to her fitness goals. She tracked her progress in her PHR and showed the encouraging results to her physician during her next visit.

Most PHR systems are more than just repositories of health information. They offer patients and caregivers the opportunity to do the following:

- Take an active role in a loved one's healthcare, particularly when those involved in care decisions—children of elderly parents, for instance—live in different parts of the country. (Remember, though, that the individual maintains control of the PHR if he or she is competent to do so. That means that he or she must give permission to any family member who wants to access the information. Many PHR systems allow the patient to set up a separate password for others authorized to access the information in the record. A more permanent step is to grant **medical power of attorney** to a loved one and then file this information in the PHR.)
- Get a big-picture view that helps in planning and coordinating care.
- Learn about the diseases and conditions that affect them or their loved ones.
- Build friendships with and derive support from others who have the same condition.
- Lessen the likelihood that duplicate tests and procedures will be ordered.
- Monitor medications and potential drug interactions.
- Reduce the likelihood of medication errors and other medical errors.
- Follow physician self-care instructions for nutritional plans, postoperative self-care, and so on.
- Ensure that first responders can gain quick access to information in a medical emergency.
- Access data from anywhere (if an online PHR is chosen).
- Protect against unforeseen damage to or loss of information in the medical records maintained by healthcare providers.
- Promote open communication among patients, providers, and staff.
- Improve continuity of care by consolidating health information from multiple specialists.
- Participate in researchers' tracking of population health trends.

CRITICAL THINKING EXERCISE 7.5

Aside from security concerns, what reasons might there be for an individual not to create a PHR?

Benefits to Providers

Practitioners who view patients as partners in making healthcare decisions will appreciate the advantages a PHR offers. From a provider's perspective, PHR systems improve patients' compliance with instructions and medication regimens and generally improve patients' recall of health-related events. In addition, PHR systems give clinicians an alternative means of communicating with patients if secure email can be exchanged through the PHR.

CRITICAL THINKING EXERCISE 7.6

How do PHR systems benefit health insurance carriers?

STEPS IN CREATING THE PERSONAL HEALTH RECORD

Creating the PHR can seem like an overwhelming job, but patients should keep in mind that information does not need to be collected all at once. An easy way for patients to approach this task is to request copies of records during each of their next scheduled appointments with their healthcare providers and specialists. Users planning to implement web-based PHR systems should ask their physician how to log in to the patient portal and obtain a username and password. Patients should also remember the payoff: Proper organization of the information will make it easy to locate when it's needed. There are three main steps users should follow in creating a PHR:

1. Decide which type of information to store in the PHR, and explore the methods of storing it.
2. Request copies of medical records from physicians' offices by signing records release forms, and be prepared to pay a fee for them. The patient may ask about the fee and time frame before making the request. It should include only the cost of copying supplies and labor and may take 60 to 90 days to complete. Inquire whether the office stores records in electronic format as an alternative to copying.
3. Begin collecting and organizing the health information. A three-ring binder may be the best way initially to organize the documents. Tabbed, color-coded dividers help separate the different types of information. Once the health information has been organized, it can be transferred to another method of storage, such as a web page or software application, according to the patient's preference. Some health forms may be downloaded from free PHR sites to aid the organization of patient health information. Fig. 7.3 shows a sample of one such form. To download the complete form, visit www.myphr.com.

MAINTAINING THE PERSONAL HEALTH RECORD

Although the patient may spend a great deal of time up front to populate and organize the PHR, that time will be wasted if maintenance isn't a top priority. An outdated PHR is useless. Smolij and Dun, who studied various models of managing health information, believe that patients' lack of diligence in updating the PHR and their questionable judgment about what to include in it make the PHR "highly unreliable and its validity and value questionable." Being diligent about keeping the PHR updated will make a valuable tool for patients and providers.

Health Information Form *for Adults*

AHIMA
American Health Information
Management Association®

A. IDENTIFICATION

Name (Last)   (First)   (Middle)

Maiden Name

Primary Address

City	State	Zip Code	Country

Alternate Address

City	State	Zip Code	Country

Home Phone   Work Phone

Cell Phone   E-mail Address

Date of Birth   ☐ Male   ☐ Female

Height   Weight   Eye Color   Hair Color

Ethnicity/Race   Birthmarks/Scars

Blood/RH Type   Special Conditions   Marital Status

Occupation

Company Name

Address

City	State	Zip Code	Country

Phone Number   Languages Spoken—Primary and Secondary

Primary Health Insurance Carrier   Policy Number

Secondary Health Insurance Carrier   Policy Number

B. EMERGENCY CONTACTS

In Case of Emergency, Notify: Primary Contact

Name (Last)   (First)   (Middle)

Relationship

Address

City	State	Zip Code	Country

Home Phone   Work Phone

Cell Phone   E-mail Address

In Case of Emergency, Notify: Secondary Contact

Name (Last)   (First)   (Middle)

Relationship

Address

City	State	Zip Code	Country

Home Phone   Work Phone

Cell Phone   E-mail Address

In Case of Emergency, Notify: Medical Contact

Physician (Indicate Specialty)

Phone

Dentist   Phone

Pharmacy   Phone

FIG. 7.3 Sample health forms that may be used in a PHR. (From www.myPHR.com; © 2006 by the American Health Information Management Association. All rights reserved.)

CRITICAL THINKING EXERCISE 7.7

One might argue that any patient who takes the initiative to create a PHR and spends at least several hours populating it probably has a good grasp of what information is important to include and what may safely be excluded. Do you agree with this line of reasoning? Why or why not?

Each time patients are seen by a healthcare provider, they may need to sign a specific authorization for the medical office to release their records. (Some PHR systems offer, for a fee, conversion of a patient's existing medical records and health-related documents into a PHR by a trained nurse-abstractor.

The patient can purchase a monthly subscription to have new information added as it is generated, ensuring that the record stays up to date.) Ellen used the records release offered as a free download in her PHR. Each time she had an appointment with a physician, she simply opened the file and changed the date on the request before printing and signing it. Then she took the request with her to the visit.

Patients should be sure to log their weight, any immunizations or vaccinations given, laboratory results, results of imaging studies (for instance, colon and breast cancer screenings), vital signs, medication changes, and the findings of physical examinations. The information entered should

Health Information Form *for Adults*

AHIMA
American Health Information
Management Association®

Page No.

C. HEALTHCARE PROVIDERS

Healthcare Provider Speciality | Primary Care Physician ☐ Yes ☐ No | Phone | Emergency Phone No. (after hours)

Name | E-mail Address

Group or Association | Fax

Address | Web Address/URL

City | State | Zip Code | Country

Healthcare Provider Speciality | Primary Care Physician ☐ Yes ☐ No | Phone | Emergency Phone No. (after hours)

Name | E-mail Address

Group or Association | Fax

Address | Web Address/URL

City | State | Zip Code | Country

Healthcare Provider Speciality | Primary Care Physician ☐ Yes ☐ No | Phone | Emergency Phone No. (after hours)

Name | E-mail Address

Group or Association | Fax

Address | Web Address/URL

City | State | Zip Code | Country

Healthcare Provider Speciality | Primary Care Physician ☐ Yes ☐ No | Phone | Emergency Phone No. (after hours)

Name | E-mail Address

Group or Association | Fax

Address | Web Address/URL

City | State | Zip Code | Country

© 2006, American Health Information Management Association

FIG. 7.3, cont'd

always be accompanied by a date. Many PHR systems provide templates in which such information can be logged and easily retrieved.

PATIENT PORTALS

Part of Stage 2 of Meaningful Use is to increase health information exchange between providers and to promote patient engagement by giving patients secure online access to their health information. With this requirement we have seen the development of patient portals, sometimes referred to as a tethered PHR because it is "tethered" to a specific healthcare organization and its EHR. These portals differ from a PHR in that they are provider-controlled gateways to an EHR and other services at the healthcare facility. Patients can view their health information, request prescription refills, schedule appointments, pay bills, and send email to their healthcare providers. A part of Stage 1 of Meaningful Use requirements, providers must also provide access to problem lists, medication lists, and allergy records within 4 business days of the information being available to the provider. Within the patient portal, the **patient-controlled health record** is the part of the site that contains data loaded by the patient and to which he or she alone may grant or deny access.

Like PHRs, patient portals get patients more involved in their healthcare. As long as they are seeing providers at the same healthcare facility, all of their laboratory work and diagnostic testing is available to them. Chronic conditions can be tracked; blood glucose levels and $A1_c$ levels can be tracked and graphed, so a diabetic patient can easily see the changes over time.

Patient portals can become that one place that patients go to for health information and services. For those busy patients, having online access for prescription refills, appointment requests, and even provider communication available 24/7 are a tremendous benefit. The fact that a patient portal is provider tethered means that the patient does not have to use his or her time to maintain the record. The patient always has the right to disagree with the information in the patient portal, and the healthcare facility must follow HIPAA guidelines for updating the patient record with that information.

PHRs and patient portals are both amazing tools to get patients more involved in their own healthcare. If a patient is seeing multiple providers at multiple healthcare facilities, a PHR can become the central repository for all of his or her health information. This repository can be useful for all of the providers involved in the patient's care, as they can easily see what treatment is being provided. For those patients who do not want to take the time to create and maintain a PHR, patient portals would be a way for them to stay informed and involved in their healthcare.

CHAPTER SUMMARY

- The PHR is a comprehensive collection of patient health information maintained in one central location and controlled by the patient. A PHR and an EHR both keep health information current, offer some insurance against damage to records stored elsewhere, and consolidate data from physicians, hospitals, and allied health professionals into a single record. The primary difference between a PHR and an EHR or a paper medical chart is who controls the information in the record. Because an individual is not a covered entity, the PHR is not subject to HIPAA privacy protection and does not necessarily constitute a legal document, although it may be accepted as evidence in some court cases. Information about medication allergies, a list of current medications, immunization records, loved ones' contact information, organ donor and living will instructions, and a brief medical, social, and family history are essential information in any PHR. Detailed documents supporting this information, such as scans of correspondence and full laboratory results, help to confirm accuracy but are not essential. Health promotion tools, such as smoking cessation logs, are other optional additions to the PHR.

- Traditionally the PHR has been a paper-based document kept in a simple three-ring binder. This method is inexpensive, easy to maintain, and secure. Its chief drawback is the difficulty of sharing information. Patients who want to have their health information in an electronic format but do not wish to store their private information online may decide to purchase a stand-alone software product. The files, but not the full functionality of the PHR, can be made portable by saving them to a USB drive. Creating a PHR online means the patient's health record is accessible from any computer in the world that has an Internet connection, and the online PHR offers the bonus of easy access to health information. Although a basic web-based PHR may be free, for a PHR with advanced services and security, a subscription fee is generally charged.

- Using its advanced health promotion features, a patient can synchronize the PHR with a variety of medical devices, such as blood pressure cuffs and heart rate monitors. Doing so allows, for example, patients with hypertension to monitor their blood pressure and fitness over time, easily tracking the data in their EHR and, if they choose, sharing it with their physician.

- Interoperability of PHR systems with EHR systems and other systems, such as hospital and pharmacy networks, is critical if PHR systems are to become a viable means of sharing patients' health data, rather than isolating it.

- Direct-to-consumer laboratory services can allow patients to control who sees the results of their blood tests.

- Having a PHR can help individuals who create it to get a big-picture view of their healthcare, learn about diseases and conditions, build relationships with others who have the same condition, save money on duplicate tests and procedures, communicate openly with healthcare personnel, take an active role in a loved one's healthcare, monitor medications, reduce the likelihood of medication errors and interactions, follow self-care instructions, give first responders quick access to information in a medical emergency, access data from anywhere, protect against unforeseen loss of information, improve continuity of care, and participate in researchers' tracking of population health trends. From a provider's perspective, PHR systems do all of the above as well as improve patients' compliance with instructions and medication regimens, improve patients' recall of health-related events, and give the clinician an alternative means of communicating with patients.

- Selecting a storage device, obtaining medical records, submitting records release forms, and organizing health information are all important steps in establishing a PHR.

- The time spent initially populating and organizing a PHR will be wasted if patients don't make maintenance a top priority. To do so, they must collect copies of progress notes, prescriptions, and other documents on each visit to a healthcare provider.

- Patient portals are the provider-tethered options for patients to view their health information, contact providers, request prescription refills, and schedule appointments. Patients can also view and track various laboratory tests and diagnostic studies.

CHAPTER REVIEW ACTIVITIES

Key Terms Review

Match the term in column A to the definition in column B.

1. Medical power of attorney

2. Advance directive

3. Host

4. Caregiver

5. Populate

6. Patient portal

7. Personal health record

8. Living will

9. Personally controlled health record

10. Wi-Fi

11. Social networking

a. The *part* of an advance directive naming a trusted person to make medical decisions on the patient's behalf should he or she become unable to make such decisions independently

b. Legal document outlining a person's wishes regarding which treatments should be administered or withheld if the person becomes incapacitated

c. To complete a template or create a record by providing the missing information for a set of predetermined fields

d. Provides information and services, such as secure email; access to an online appointment book; and limited access to patient records

e. Secure, comprehensive record of health information that is controlled by the individual

f. A person who provides physical care and emotional support to a person who is ill, disabled, or dependent

g. The *part* of an advance directive that specifies which life-sustaining treatments should be administered or withheld if the person becomes incapacitated

h. The point at which a website originates or resides

i. The practice of using online communities to expand one's contacts and exchange content

j. A means of connecting wirelessly to the Internet using a local area network or router

k. The portion of a patient portal to which the patient has access and may grant or deny access

True/False

Indicate whether the statement is true or false.

1. _____ A PHR may be paper based or electronic.
2. _____ The primary difference between a PHR and an EHR or a paper medical chart is its storage location.
3. _____ The PHR is a legal health record with the same legal standing as an EHR under HIPAA.
4. _____ A list of current allergies and medications should be included in the PHR.
5. _____ Patients may use the PHR to share health information with caregivers in order to better understand their medical treatments and manage disease.
6. _____ The information in stand-alone PHR systems created with software programs is not portable into other systems.
7. _____ An online PHR is accessible from any computer in the world that has an Internet connection.
8. _____ All PHR systems require membership and setup fees in addition to purchase of a monthly subscription.
9. _____ Some PHR systems integrate satellite technology to help users plan biking or walking routes.
10. _____ Patient portals are more present than ever in medical offices because of the meaningful use requirement.

Workplace Applications

1. Visit www.webmd/phr.com and register for a free PHR. What type of health assessments are used in this free service? Describe the advantages and disadvantages of using this site to maintain a patient PHR.

2. Using a search engine, identify four different websites and apps (other than those given in this chapter) for creating and maintaining a PHR and other health-related information. What are the strengths and weaknesses of each site? What kinds of resources and tools are provided to users? What security measures are taken to ensure confidentiality? Are the sites free, or do they have charges associated with them?

3. Your office is implementing a patient portal to its EHR. This transition will occur next month, and patients will be given login information at regular office visits. There will be all-staff training for the patient portal on next Tuesday from 4 to 5 PM in the meeting room. Use SimChart for the Medical Office (SCMO) to set the training in the Calendar. Then use the email Correspondence tool to create an Office Memo informing staff of this training and agenda.

4. Mora Siever (DOB 01/24/1964) is in the process of collecting data for her PHR. She comes to the office today to complete a patient records access request form to review the contents of her health record as part of this goal. She is interested in accessing all progress notes, immunizations, and radiology and laboratory reports from 2005 to the present for the creation of her PHR. Complete the Medical Record Release form in SCMO.

EHR in Review

1. Ken Thomas (DOB 10/25/1961) had a form completed by Dr. Walden for a life insurance policy. The fee for form completion is $20. Update the patient's ledger to reflect this charge.

2. The following office expenses were incurred during the month of November. Complete the Petty Cash journal. The amount of Petty Cash on hand at the start of the month is $200. Enter "date reconciled" as today. Once the posting is complete, what is the amount of Petty Cash on Hand? (Subtract expenses from starting amount)

Date	Description	Expense
11/02/20XX	Postage	21.80
11/08/20XX	Shuttle to hospital	8.00
11/16/20XX	Facial tissue	35.00
11/21/20XX	Napkins and plates for Thanksgiving luncheon	27.08

3. Jean Burke, NP, has ordered an electrolyte panel for Tai Yan (DOB 04/07/1956) for chronic kidney disease (CKD). Create a laboratory requisition for the patient using Form Repository and update the patient's Problem list to include CKD. (You may need to create an encounter to document the Problem List if one does not already exist.)

4. Norma Washington (DOB 08/01/1944) calls the office today. She cannot remember when her next appointment is scheduled. Use the Calendar search to located Norma's next appointment.

Review of Paper-Based Office Procedures

When working in a paper-based healthcare facility, staff members use very similar procedures but different tools. Let's take a look at how a patient would progress through a paper-based healthcare facility.

When a patient calls to make an appointment, the medical assistant must have access to the appointment book. The times that the providers are not available would have been blocked out previously. This is called setting up the appointment matrix. Using the scheduling procedures for the healthcare facility, the medical assistant would find the appropriate day and time and write in the patient's name, DOB, and the reason for the visit.

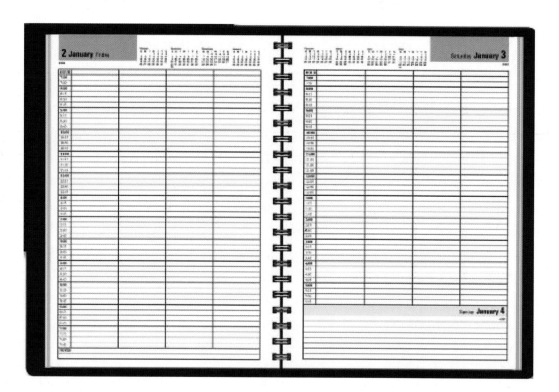

If this is a new patient, the medical assistant may have sent the patient the Patient Registration Form to complete before arriving at the healthcare facility. Another option is for the patient to complete this form upon arrival. The medical assistant should review the form for completeness and also obtain a copy of the patient's insurance card, both the front and back. This form is then placed in the patient's medical record.

ACCOUNT # _____

PATIENT # _____

NEW PATIENT INFORMATION   DATE _____

PATIENT'S NAME (PLEASE PRINT)	S.S. #	MARITAL STATUS	SEX	BIRTH DATE	AGE
		S M W D SEP	M F		

STREET ADDRESS PERMANENT TEMPORARY	CITY AND STATE	ZIP CODE	HOME PHONE#
PATIENT'S EMPLOYER	OCCUPATION (INDICATE IF STUDENT)	HOW LONG EMPLOYED	BUS. PHONE # EXT. #
EMPLOYER'S STREET ADDRESS	CITY AND STATE		ZIP CODE
DRUG ALLERGIES, IF ANY	PHARMACY		PHARMACY PHONE #
SPOUSE OR PARENT'S NAME	S.S. #		BIRTH DATE
SPOUSE OR PARENT'S EMPLOYER	OCCUPATION (INDICATED IF STUDENT)	HOW LONG EMPLOYED	BUS. PHONE #
EMPLOYER'S STREET ADDRESS	CITY AND STATE		ZIP CODE
*SPOUSE'S STREET ADDRESS, IF DIVORCED OR SEPARATED	CITY AND STATE	ZIP CODE	HOME PHONE #

PLEASE READ: ALL CHARGES ARE DUE AT THE TIME OF SERVICES. IF HOSPITALIZATION IS INDICATED, THE PATIENT IS RESPONSIBLE FOR FURNISHING INSURANCE CLAIM FORMS TO THE OFFICE PRIOR TO HOSPITALIZATION.

REFERRED BY	STREET ADDRESS, CITY, STATE	ZIP CODE	PHONE #
☐ BLUE SHIELD (GIVE NAME OF POLICYHOLDER)	☐ ALLIANCE ☐ OTHER ☐ ALLIANCE SELECT	BIRTH DATE	POLICY #
☐ OTHER (WRITE IN NAME OF INSURANCE COMPANY)	NAME OF POLICYHOLDER	BIRTH DATE	POLICY #
☐ OTHER (WRITE IN NAME OF INSURANCE COMPANY)	NAME OF POLICYHOLDER	BIRTH DATE	POLICY #

☐ MEDICARE #	☐ RAILROAD RETIREMENT #	☐ MEDICAID #

☐ INDUSTRIAL	WERE YOU INJURED ON THE JOB? ☐ YES ☐ NO	DATE OF INJURY	INDUSTRIAL CLAIM #
☐ ACCIDENT	WAS AN AUTOMOBILE INVOLVED? ☐ YES ☐ NO	DATE OF ACCIDENT	NAME OF ATTORNEY

WERE X-RAYS TAKEN OF THIS INJURY OR PROBLEM? ☐ YES ☐ NO	IF YES, WHERE WERE X-RAYS TAKEN? (HOSPITAL, ETC.)	DATE X-RAYS TAKEN

HAS ANY MEMBER OF YOUR IMMEDIATE FAMILY BEEN TREATED BY OUR PHYSICIAN(S) BEFORE? INCLUDE NAME OF PHYSICIAN AND FAMILY MEMBER.

NEAREST RELATIVE OR FRIEND NOT RESIDING WITH YOU	STREET ADDRESS, CITY, STATE	ZIP CODE	PHONE #

ALL PROFESSIONAL SERVICES RENDERED ARE CHARGED TO THE PATIENT. NECESSARY FORMS WILL BE COMPLETED TO HELP EXPEDITE INSURANCE CARRIER PAYMENTS. HOWEVER, THE PATIENT IS RESPONSIBLE FOR ALL FEES, REGARDLESS OF INSURANCE COVERAGE. IT IS ALSO CUSTOMARY TO PAY FOR SERVICES WHEN RENDERED UNLESS OTHER ARRANGEMENTS HAVE BEEN MADE IN ADVANCE WITH OUR OFFICE BOOKKEEPER.

INSURANCE AUTHORIZATION AND ASSIGNMENT

Name of Policy Holder_____   HIC Number _____

I request that payment of authorized Medicare/Other Insurance company benefits be made either to me or on my behalf to _____ for any services furnished me by that party who accepts assignment/physician. Regulations pertaining to Medicare assignment of benefits apply.

I authorize any holder of medical or other information about me to release to the Social Security Administration and Health Care Financing Administration or its intermediaries or carriers any information needed for this or a related Medicare claim/other Insurance Company claim. I permit a copy of this authorization to be used in place of the original, and request payment of medical insurance benefits either to myself or to the party who accepts assignment. I understand it is mandatory to notify the health care provider of any other party who may be responsible for paying for my treatment. (Section 1128B of the Social Security Act and 31 U.S.C. 3801-3812 provides penalties for withholding this information.)

Signature_____   Date_____

Accounts past 60 days will accrue an interest charge.   NEW PATIENT INFORMATION

(From Beik J: Health Insurance Today, ed 5, St. Louis, 2015, Saunders.)

Another form that can be sent to the patient to complete before arrival is the health history form. This form should also be reviewed by the medical assistant for completeness and for clarification of any information that the patient has documented on the form. This form also is placed in the patient's medical record.

PATIENT HEALTH HISTORY

A   IDENTIFICATION DATA   Please print the following information.

Today's date _____

Name _____   ___ Male ___ Female

Address _____   ___ Married ___ Separated ___ Divorced ___ Widowed ___ Single

_____   Date of Birth _____

Telephone _____
Home number   Work number

B   PAST HISTORY

Have you ever had the following: (Circle "no" or "yes", leave blank if uncertain)

Measles ___ no yes	Heart Disease ___ no yes	Diabetes ___ no yes	Hemorrhoids ___ no yes
Mumps ___ no yes	Arthritis ___ no yes	Cancer ___ no yes	Asthma ___ no yes
Chickenpox ___ no yes	Sexually Transmitted Disease ___ no yes	Polio ___ no yes	Allergies ___ no yes
Whooping Cough ___ no yes	Anemia ___ no yes	Glaucoma ___ no yes	Eczema ___ no yes
Scarlet Fever ___ no yes	Bladder Infections ___ no yes	Hernia ___ no yes	AIDS or HIV+ ___ no yes
Diphtheria ___ no yes	Epilepsy ___ no yes	Blood or Plasma Transfusions ___ no yes	Infectious Mono ___ no yes
Pneumonia ___ no yes	Migraine Headaches ___ no yes	Back Trouble ___ no yes	Bronchitis ___ no yes
Rheumatic Fever ___ no yes	Tuberculosis ___ no yes	High Blood Pressure ___ no yes	Mitral Valve Prolapse no yes
Stroke ___ no yes	Ulcer ___ no yes	Thyroid Disease ___ no yes	Any other disease ___ no yes
Hepatitis ___ no yes	Kidney Disease ___ no yes	Bleeding Tendency ___ no yes	Please list: _____

MAJOR HOSPITALIZATIONS: If you have ever been hospitalized for any major medical illness or operation, write in your most recent hospitalizations below.

Hospitalizations	Year	Operation or illness	Name of hospital	City and state
1st Hospitalization				
2nd Hospitalization				
3rd Hospitalization				
4th Hospitalization				

TESTS AND IMMUNIZATIONS: Mark an X next to those that you have had.

Tests: Immunizations:

☐ TB Test   ☐ Electrocardiogram   ☐ Influenza

☐ Rectal/Hemoccult   ☐ Chest x-ray   ☐ Hepatitis B

☐ Sigmoidoscopy   ☐ Mammogram   ☐ Tetanus

☐ Colonoscopy   ☐ Pap Test   ☐ MMR

☐ Polio

ALLERGIES: List all allergies (foods, drugs, environment). ☐ None

_____
_____
_____

CURRENT MEDICATIONS: List the following that you are currently taking: Prescription medications, over-the-counter (OTC) medications, vitamin supplements, and herbal supplements. ☐ None

Medication   Frequency

_____
_____
_____

ACCIDENTS/ INJURIES: Describe all serious accidents, severe injuries, head injury, or fractures. Include the date each occurred. ☐ None

Accident/Injury: Date:

_____
_____
_____

C FAMILY HISTORY

For each member of your family, follow the purple or blue line across the page and check boxes for:
1. His or her present state of health
2. Any illnesses he or she has had

	Good Health	Poor Health	Deceased	If deceased, write in age and cause of death.	Allergies or Asthma	Diabetes	Heart Disease	Stroke	Cancer	High Blood Pressure	Glaucoma	Arthritis	Ulcer	Kidney Disease	Mental Health Problems	Alcohol/Drug Abuse	Obesity	High Cholesterol	Thyroid Disease
Father:																			
Mother:																			
Brothers/Sisters:																			

D SOCIAL HISTORY

EDUCATION _____ High school   _____ College   _____ Postgraduate

Occupation _____   Years _____

Previous occupations _____   Years _____

_____   Years _____

Have you ever been exposed to any of the following in your environment?

☐ Excess dust (coal, lime, rock)   ☐ Cleaning fluids/solvents   ☐ Radiation   ☐ Other toxic materials

☐ Sand   ☐ Hair spray   ☐ Insecticides

☐ Chemicals   ☐ Smoke or auto exhaust fumes   ☐ Paints

Please answer the follwing questions by placing an X in the box in front of the word Yes or No, except where you are asked for specific information. This information is obviously highly confidential and will be released to other healthcare professionals or insurance carriers ONLY with your consent.

DIET:

Do you eat a good breakfast? ☐ Yes ☐ No

Do you snack between meals (soft drinks, chips, candy bars)? ☐ Yes ☐ No

Do you eat fresh fruits and vegetables each day? ☐ Yes ☐ No

Do you eat whole grain breads and cereals? ☐ Yes ☐ No

Is your diet high in fat content? ☐ Yes ☐ No

Is your diet high in cholesterol content? ☐ Yes ☐ No

Is your diet high in salt content? ☐ Yes ☐ No

Are you allergic to any foods? ☐ Yes ☐ No

How many glasses of water do you drink each day? _____

How would you describe your overall eating habits? ☐ Excellent ☐ Good ☐ Fair ☐ Poor

PERSONAL HISTORY:

Do you find it hard to make decisions? ☐ Yes ☐ No

Do you find it hard to concentrate or remember? ☐ Yes ☐ No

Do you feel depressed? ☐ Yes ☐ No

Do you have difficulty relaxing? ☐ Yes ☐ No

Do you have a tendency to worry a lot? ☐ Yes ☐ No

Have you gained or lost much weight recently? ☐ Yes ☐ No

Do you lose your temper often? ☐ Yes ☐ No

Are you disturbed by any work or family problems? ☐ Yes ☐ No

Are you having sexual difficulties? ☐ Yes ☐ No

Have you ever considered committing suicide? ☐ Yes ☐ No

Have you ever desired or sought psychiatric help? ☐ Yes ☐ No

EXERCISE:

Do you exercise on a regular basis? ☐ Yes ☐ No

Does your job require strenuous, sustained physical work? ☐ Yes ☐ No

SLEEP PATTERNS:

Do you seem to feel exhausted or fatigued most of the time? ☐ Yes ☐ No

Do you have difficulty either falling asleep or staying asleep? ☐ Yes ☐ No

USE OF TOBACCO/ALCOHOL/CAFFEINE/DRUGS: Amt:

How much do you smoke per day? ☐ Cigarettes ___

☐ Don't smoke   ☐ Cigars/pipes ___

Do you take two or more alcoholic drinks per day? ☐ Yes ☐ No

Do you drink six or more cups of coffee or tea per day? ☐ Yes ☐ No

Are you a regular user of sleeping pills, marijuana, tranquilizers, pain killers, etc? ☐ Yes ☐ No

Have you ever used heroin, cocaine, LSD, PCP, etc? ☐ Yes ☐ No

List any country outside the USA you have visited in the past six months. _____

When did you have your last physical examination? _____

(From Bonewit-West K: Today's Medical Assistant, ed 3, St. Louis, 2016, Elsevier.)

If the patient needs to have the records from his or her previous provider sent to your facility, the patient would need to complete a Release of Information form. A copy of this form is placed in the medical record, and the original is sent to the patient's previous provider. This form should be reviewed to make sure that the patient has provided all of the pertinent information.

Central Texas Dermatology Clinic • 102 Westlake Drive • Austin, Texas 78746

AUTHORIZATION TO DISCLOSE HEALTH INFORMATION

I hereby authorize the use or disclosure of information from the medical record of:

Patient Name: _____   Date of Birth: _____

Social Security# _____   Daytime Phone: _____

I authorize the following individual or organization to disclose the above named individual's health information:

_____   Address: _____

This information may be disclosed TO and used by the following individual or organization:

_____   Address: _____

Please release the following:

____ Progress Notes   ____ Pathology Reports   ____ Lab Reports   ____ Any and all Records

____ Other Diagnostic reports (specify _____

____ Other (specify) _____

   Including Information (if applicable) pertaining to:

   ____ Mental Health   ____ Drug/Alcohol   ____ HIV/AIDS   ____ Communicable Treatment

Purpose or Need for Disclosure:

____ Continued Patient Care   ____ Personal Use

____ Attorney/Legal   ____ Insurance Claim/Application

____ Disability Determination   ____ Other (specify) _____

I understand that the information in my health record may include information relating to sexually transmitted disease, acquired immunodeficiency syndrome (AIDS), or human immunodeficiency virus (HIV). It may also include information about behavioral or mental health services, and treatment for alcohol and drug abuse.

I understand that the information released is for the specific purpose stated above. Any other use of this information without the written consent of the patient is prohibited.

I understand that I have the right to revoke this authorization at any time. I understand that if I revoke this authorization I must do so in writing and present my written revocation to the individual or organization releasing information. I understand that the revocation will not apply to information already released in response to this authorization. I understand that the revocation will not apply to my insurance company when the law provides my insurer the right to contest a claim under my policy. Unless otherwise revoked, this authorization will expire on following date, event or condition: _____

If I fail to specify an expiration date, event or condition, this authorization will expire in six months.

I understand that authorizing the disclosure of this health information is voluntary. I can refuse to sign the authorization. I need not sign this form in order to ensure treatment. I understand that I may inspect or copy the information to be used or disclosed, as provided in CFR 164.524. I understand that any disclosure of information carries with it the potential for an unauthorized re-disclosure and the information may not be protected by federal confidentiality rules. If I have questions about disclosure of my health information, I can contact Theresa Farren at 512-327-7779.

_____   _____
Signature of Patient or Legal Representative   Date

_____   _____
Relationship to Patient (If Legal Representative)   Witness

+--+
| **COMPLETE ONLY IF INFORMATION IS TO BE RELEASED DIRECTLY TO PATIENT:** |
| I understand that my medical record may contain reports, test results, and notes that only a |
| physician can interpret. I understand and have been advised that I should contact my physician |
| regarding the entries made in my medical record to prevent my misunderstanding of the |
| information contained in these entries. I will not hold Central Texas Dermatology liable for |
| any misinterpretation of the information in my medical record as a result of not contacting my |
| physician for the correct interpretation. |
| |
| _____   _____ |
| Signature of Patient or Legal Representative   Date |
| |
| _____   _____ |
| Relationship to Patient (If Legal Representative)   Witness |
+--+

Dr. review/signature/date _____

Date request completed _____   # of pages copied _____

Staff Signature _____

PHI Log completed _____

(From Proctor D: Kinn's The Medical Assistant, ed 13, St. Louis, 2016, Elsevier.)

The medical record will be created and a Superbill prepared with the patient demographic information and date of service. The Superbill will then be clipped to the front of the medical record so that it is available for the provider to complete.

When the patient is called in from the reception area, the chief complaint, vital signs, height, and weight are taken. All of this information needs to be documented in the patient's medical record. This is done in the progress notes, and generally it is done using SOAP charting. The chief complaint will be documented in the S, subjective, section; vital signs, height, and weight will be documented in the O, objective, section. The provider will document in the A, assessment, and P, plan, sections of the progress note. During the billing process the medical assistant may review the progress note to determine what services were provided and the diagnosis (found in the assessment section).

PROGRESS NOTES:

PROBLEM ORIENTED - PROGRESS NOTES

Date	Time	Problem Number	FORMAT: Problem Number and TITLE: S = Subjective O = Objective A = Assessment P = Plan
			S: Mother states that her child has had a runny nose and her throat has been
			sore for 2 days.
			O: Vital signs: T 98.8 P 96 R 24
			Weight: 42 lb.
			General: alert and active. HEENT: sclera clear. TMs negative. Positive clear rhinorrhea.
			Pharynx benign. Heart: regular without murmur.
			Lungs: clear to auscultation and percussion. Abdomen: negative tenderness.
			Positive bowel x 4. GU: negative. Neuro: good tone.
			A: Upper respiratory tract infection.
			P: 1. A prescription for Rondec DM, 1/2 tsp q6h prn cough and congestion.
			2. Instructed mother to contact office if child does not improve.

NAME–Last	First	Middle	Attending Physician	Record No.	Room/Bed
Michaels	Jessica	L	Frank Edwards, MD	1	24

Form 663/25 © BRIGGS, Des Moines, IA 50306 (800) 247-2343 www.BriggsCorp.com PRINTED IN U.S.A.   **PROBLEM ORIENTED - PROGRESS NOTES**

Medications must be reviewed with the patient, including prescriptions, over-the-counter products, herbal and mineral supplements, and vitamins. All new medications must be documented.

Stephen Damiani D.O., INC.
Medication List

Patient Name: _____   Allergies: _____

_____

Date	Medication	Dosage	Frequency	Refills	Pharmacy

A problem list may be used in a paper-based Problem-Oriented Medical Record. This is updated by the medical assistant based on the provider's diagnosis.

PROBLEM LIST:

MASTER PROBLEM LIST
For use of this form, see AR 40-66; the proponent agency is the Office of The Surgeon General

MAJOR PROBLEMS

PROBLEM NUMBER	DATE ONSET	DATE ENTERED	PROBLEM	DATE RESOLVED
1.				
2.				
3.				
4.				
5.				
6.				
7.				
8.				
9.				
10.				
11.				
12.				

TEMPORARY (MINOR) PROBLEMS

PROBLEM LETTER	PROBLEM	DATES OF OCCURRENCES					
A.							
B.							
C.							
D.							
E.							
F.							
G.							
H.							

PATIENT'S IDENTIFICATION (Use mechanical imprint if available; for typed or written entries give: Name, SSN, Unit, Sex, Birthdate, and Duty Phone)	SUMMARY OF PROBLEMS, ALLERGIES, MEDICATIONS, SURGERIES AND TRAUMAS:
	NOTE: DO NOT DISCARD FROM CHART

DA FORM 5571, OCT 86   USAPA V2.00

The next step in the patient visit is the completion of the Superbill. The top portion of the Superbill was completed when the patient checked in (for new patients) or the night before (for established patients). The provider should check off the services provided and indicate the diagnosis. The medical assistant then determines the fees for the services by consulting the fee schedule. That amount is then recorded on the Superbill, and any previous balance is added to the new charges to come up with the new balance. If the patient makes a payment at the time of service, this is also indicated on the Superbill. If the provider has written in a diagnosis but has not indicated the ICD-10 code, the medical assistant would look that up using the most current ICD-10-CM manual. If services were provided that are not listed on the Superbill, the medical assistant would look them up using the most current CPT manual.

Tri-State Medical Group   008112

400 North 4th Street • Anytown, Iowa 50622
Phone: 319-555-5734 • Fax: 319-555-5758
Fed. Tax I.D. # 42-1435XXX

ACCOUNT NO.	DOB	DATE OF SERVICE
PATIENT NAME		PROVIDER
INSURANCE ID #-PRIMARY		SECONDARY

DESCRIPTION	CODE		FEE	DESCRIPTION	CODE	FEE	DESCRIPTION	CODE	FEE
OFFICE VISIT	NEW	ESTAB.		DT, Pediatric	90702		Removal Skin Tags up to 15 Lesions	*11200	
Minimum	99201	99211		MMR	90707		Exc. Malignant Lesion, Trunk, Arm or Leg		
Brief	99202	99212		Oral Polio	90712		Exc. Malignant Lesion, Face, Ear, Eyelid, Nose		
Limited	99203	99213		IVP Polio	90713		Exc. Malignant Lesion, Scalp, Hand, Neck, Feet		
Extended	99204	99214		Varicella	90716		Lacer, Repair 2.5cm or Less/Location:	*12001	
Comprehensive	99205	99215		Td, Adult	90718		Scalp, Nk, Axille, Ext. Genitalia, Trk, Hands/Feet		
Prenatal Care		59400		DTP & HIB	90720		Lacer, Repair 2.5cm or Less/Location:	*12011	
Global		99024		Influenza	90659		Face, Ears, Eyelids, Nose, Lips & Mucous Mem.		
PREVENTIVE	NEW	ESTAB.		Hepatitis B, Newborn to 11 Years	90744		Burn w/Dressing, w/o Anesth. Small	16020	
Infant	99381	99391		Hepatitis B, 11-19 Years	90747		Wart Removal	*17110	
Age 1-4	99382	99392		Hepatitis B, 20 Years & Above	90746		Removal FB Conjunct. Ext. Eye	*65205	
Age 5-11	99383	99393		Pneumococcal	90732		Removal FB Ext. Auditory Canal	69200	
Age 12-17	99384	99394		Hemophilus Infl. B	90645		Ear Lavage	69210	
Age 18-39	99385	99395		Therapeutic:	90782		Tympanometry	92567	
Age 40-64	99386	99396		Allergy Inject Single	95115		EKG Tracing Only w/o Interp. & Rept	93005	
Age 65 & Over	99387	99397		Allergy Inject Multiple	95117		Nebulizer Therapy (x)	94640	
OFFICE CONSULTATION				B-12	J3420		Pulse Oximetry	94760	
Limited		99241		Injection / Aspiration	20600		Cryosurgery		
Intermediate		99242		Small joint-Finger, Toes,Ganglion			Debridement	11041	
Extended		99243		Injection / Aspiration	20605		Excise Ingrown Toenail	11730	
Comprehensive		99244		Intermediate jt-Wrist, Elbow, Ankle			Colposcopy w/Biopsy	57454	
Complex		99245		Injection / Aspiration	20610		Leep	57460	
LABORATORY PROCEDURES				Major jt. - Shoulder, Hip, Knee			Endometrial Bx	58100	
Venipuncture		36415		Inject Tendon/Ligament	20550		Cryotherapy	57511	
Routine Urinalysis w/o Microscopy		81002		Aristacort	J3302		Peak Flow Measurement	94160-52	
Hemoccult		82270		Depo Provera	J1055		Intradermal Tests CMI # Doses =	95025	
Glucose Blood Reagent Strip		82948		Rocephin	J0696		Intradermal Tests/Allergens	95024	
Wet Mount		87210		OFFICE PROCEDURE / MINOR SURGERY			Intravenous Access	36000	
PAP Smear		88155		I & D Abscess	10060		Immunotherapy/Single Injection	95120	
Urine Pregnancy		81025		Removal FB Subcutaneous	*10120		Immunotherapy/Double Injection	95125	
Other:		99000		I & D Hematoma	10140		Regular Spirometry	94010	
X-RAY				Puncture Aspiration Abscess	10160		Spirometry Read by Physician	94010-26	
X-ray Cervical Spine		75052		Exc. Ben. Lesion #:			Spirometry w/pre & Post Bronchodilator	94060	
X-ray Thoracic Spine		72070		Location:			Spirometry/Bronchodilator read by Doctor	94060-26	
X-ray Lumbar Spine (2)		72100		Exc. Ben. Lesion #:			Skin Prick Test: # of Tests =	95004	
X-ray Lumbar Spine (Comp)		72110		Location:			Vial Preparation	95165	
X-ray Pelvis (1 view)		72170					HOSPITAL ORDERS		

X-ray Sacrum & Coccyx	72220
X-ray Clavicle (Complete)	73000
X-ray Shoulder (2) or	73030
X-ray Humerus (2 views)	73060
X-ray Elbow (AP & LATE)	73070
X-ray Forearm (AP & LA)	73090
X-ray Wrist (AP & LATE)	73100
X-ray Wrist (3 Views)	73110
X-ray Hand (2 Views)	73120
X-ray Hand (3 Views)	73130
X-ray Finger (2 Views)	73140
X-ray Hip (2 Views)	73510
X-ray Hips (Bilateral)	73520
X-ray Scoliosis (2 AP & LA)	72069
X-ray Femur (AP & LATE)	73550
X-ray Knee (AP & LATE)	73560
X-ray Knee (3 Views)	73564
X-ray Tibia & Fibula	73590
X-ray Ankle (3 Views)	73610
X-ray Foot (AP & LATER)	73620
X-ray Foot (AP. LA.,)	73630
X-ray Calcaneus (2 Views)	73650
X-ray Toes	73660
X-ray Pelvis & Hip Inf	73540
Elbow, Minimum of 3 Views	73080

IMMUNIZATIONS & INJECTIONS	
PPD Intradermal TB Tine	86580
DTaP	90700

Hospital orders:
OB Non-Stress Test
OB Ultrasound-Diagnostic
OB Ultrasound-Routine
Biophysical Profile
Mammogram-Diagnostic
Mammogram-Routine
Ultrasound _____
Gallbladder Ultrasound
Pelvic Ultrasound
Doppler Studies _____
IVP
Upper GI
Lower GI
Barium Enema
Barium Swallow

Cystogram
MRI
CT Scan _____
Chest X-ray
X-ray _____
Bone Densitometry
EKG
Holter Monitor
Echocardiogram
Treadmill
Thallium Stress Test
Doppler Studies _____
PFT-Partial
PFT-Complete
Cardiac Rehab

Physical Therapy

Diet Consultation

Laboratory
_____
_____
_____
_____
_____
_____

AUTHORIZATION TO PAY BENEFITS AND RELEASE INFORMATION TO TRI-STATE MEDICAL GROUP: I hereby authorize payment directly to the undersigned Physician of all Surgical and / or Medical Benefits, if any, otherwise payable to me for his / her services as described above. I have read and understand the Financial Policy and that I am financially responsible for charges not covered by this insurance. I also authorize the undersigned Physician to release any information acquired in the course of my examination or treatment.

Signed: _____
Date: _____

Provider's Signature _____   Date _____

PREVIOUS BALANCE	
CHARGES TODAY	
TOTAL	
AMOUNT PAID	
BALANCE DUE	

DX or Other Information

Samples:

Your next appointment is:

BILLING COPY

(From Beik J: Health Insurance Today, ed 5, St. Louis, 2015, Saunders.)

After the Superbill is completed, the charges and payments should be posted to the patient's ledger. As payments are made to the patient's account from the insurance company, any adjustments would also be posted to the patient's ledger. A copy of the ledger can be used as a patient statement and mailed.

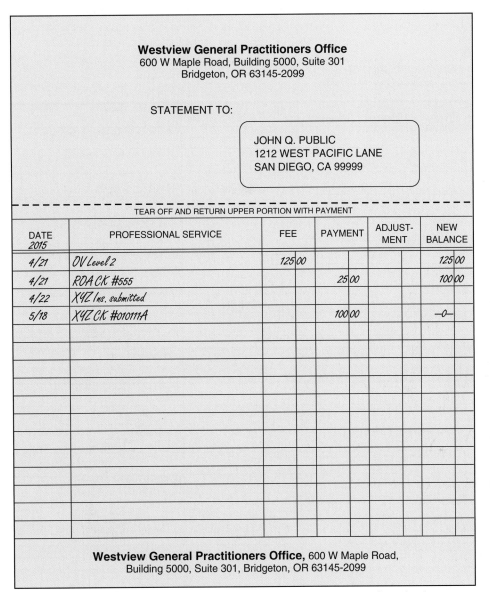

(From Beik J: Health Insurance Today, ed 5, St. Louis, 2015, Saunders.)

The final step in the billing process would be to submit the claim to the patient's insurance carrier. In a fully paper-based system, this would be done using a CMS-1500 claim form. The information from the Superbill and patient record would be used to complete the form accurately.

(From Beik J: Health Insurance Today, ed 5, St. Louis, 2015, Saunders.)

If the provider has determined that the patient needs some further diagnostic services, such as an MRI, a preauthorization form will need to be completed. The medical assistant should be able to get the needed information from the patient record, but if there is any question the provider should be consulted.

Tri-State Medical Group

PREAUTHORIZATION REQUEST FORM

PATIENT INFORMATION

Last Name: _____   First Name: _____

DOB: _____   Member #: **R** _____   Group #: _____

PREAUTHORIZATION REQUEST INFORMATION

Please list *both* procedure/product code <u>and</u> narrative description:

CPT / HCPCS Code(s): _____   Durable Medical Equipment: ☐ Rental ☐ Purchase

Description: _____

_____

Date of Service: _____   Length of Stay (if applicable): _____

Place of Service or Vendor Name: _____

Assistant Surgeon Requested? ☐ Yes ☐ No   **Please list *both* diagnosis(es) code <u>and</u> narrative description:**

1. ICD-10 Code: _____

    Description: _____

2. ICD-10 Code: _____

    Description: _____

Ordering Physician/Provider: _____   Office Location: _____
                              FIRST <u>AND</u> LAST NAMES PLEASE

Referring Physician/Provider: _____
                                FIRST <u>AND</u> LAST NAMES PLEASE; REQUIRED FOR PRIME PLANS

Date: _____   Contact Person: _____   Phone: _____

> ***Please Note: Incomplete forms will delay the preauthorization process.***
> ***Requests received after 3:00 PM are processed the next working day.***
>
> **PacificSource responds to preauthorization requests within 2 working days.**
> **A determination notice will be mailed to the requesting provider, facility, and patient.**
>
> **Please attach pertinent chart notes as appropriate.**

FOR INTERNAL OFFICE USE ONLY:

STATUS: APPROVED / DENIED / PENDING / EXPLANATION

DATE: _____   **ACUITY:** _____   **INITIALS:** _____

Reason/Status _____

_____

Field 11 Notes _____   LOS Approved _____

☐ Chart notes filed with preauthorization

Notes _____

Field 10 Facility Copy _____

PO Box 5555 • Somewhere OR 00908 • (541) 555-5584 • (800) 555-6052 x 2584

MEDICAL AFFAIRS DEPARTMENT CONFIDENTIAL FAX: (541) 555-2051

9/8/2003

(From Beik J: Health Insurance Today, ed 5, St. Louis, 2015, Saunders.)

As you can see, the paper-based system looks very much like an electronic system, and the information needed is the same. An electronic system can easily generate the forms using the information in the EHR database. In a paper-based system the medical assistant needs to know where in the paper-based chart to find the information.

CMS Documentation Guidelines

Accurate medical record documentation is important not only for quality healthcare but also for reimbursement purposes. The Centers for Medicare & Medicaid Services (CMS) have established some specific guidelines to facilitate both patient care and reimbursement. According to CMS:

"Documentation is an important aspect of patient care and is used to:
- Coordinate services among medical professionals
- Furnish sufficient services
- Improve patient care
- Comply with regulations
- Support claims billed
- Reduce improper payments"
https://www.cms.gov/Medicare-Medicaid-Coordination/Fraud-Prevention/Medicaid-Integrity-Education/Downloads/docmatters-presentation-handout.pdf accessed 10/1/2016

GENERAL PRINCIPLES OF MEDICAL RECORD DOCUMENTATION

Some of these principles may seem like common sense, but it is important to review and implement these principles when documenting in the medical record. The documentation for each patient encounter should include:
- The reason for the encounter (chief complaint)
- Relevant history
- Physical examination findings and prior diagnostic results
- Assessment, clinical impression, or diagnosis

- Medical plan of care
- Date and legible identity of observer

The above items sound very much like SOAPE noting as discussed in Chapter 5.

The following items should also be clearly stated:
- Rationale for ordering diagnostic and other ancillary services
- Past and present diagnoses
- Health risk factors
- Patient progress, treatment changes, and response
- Support for diagnostic and treatment codes reported on the health insurance claim form or billing statement

The medical record should be complete and legible (if using paper medical records and handwritten notes). While we strive for conciseness in the medical record, all details for the patient encounter should be documented.

EVALUATION AND MANAGEMENT CODES

The evaluation and management (E&M) codes in CPT are used to document the patient encounter with the provider. This could be an office visit, an inpatient hospital visit, emergency department visit, nursing home visit, etc. The three components used to determine the correct E&M code are:
- History
- Examination
- Medical decision making

The documentation in the medical record is used to determine and/or support the E&M code choice. The tables below will demonstrate how the correct level for all three components can be determined.

Key Component – History

Type of history	Chief Complaint	History of Present Illness	Review of Systems	Past, Family, and/ or Social History
Problem Focused	Required	Brief	N/A	N/A
Expanded Problem Focused	Required	Brief	Problem Pertinent	N/A
Detailed	Required	Extended	Extended	Pertinent
Comprehensive	Required	Extended	Complete	Complete

Key Component – Physical Examination

Type of Examination	Description
Problem Focused	A limited examination of the affected body area or organ system
Expanded Problem Focused	A limited examination of the affected body area or organ system and any other symptomatic or related body area(s) or organ system(s)
Detailed	An extended examination of the affected body area(s) or organ system(s) and any other symptomatic or related body area(s) or organ system(s)
Comprehensive	A general multisystem examination or a complete examination of a single organ system (and other symptomatic or related body area[s] or organ systems[s])

Key Component – Medical Decision Making

Type of decision making	Number of diagnoses or management options	Amount and/or complexity of data to be reviewed	Risk of significant complications, morbidity, and/or mortality
STRAIGHTFORWARD	Minimal	Minimal or None	Minimal
LOW COMPLEXITY	Limited	Limited	Low
MODERATE COMPLEXITY	Multiple	Moderate	Moderate
HIGH COMPLEXITY	Extensive	Extensive	High

https://www.cms.gov/Outreach-and-Education/Medicare-Learning-Network-MLN/MLNProducts/Downloads/eval-mgmt-serv-guide-ICN006764.pdf accessed 10/1/2016

These guidelines can be used when reviewing the documentation to determine the correct E&M code for reimbursement purposes. When the documentation fully supports the code choices, the reimbursement will be at the highest level possible, and the risk of having an unfavorable audit is reduced.

Not only must all of the services be documented in the medical record, but the record also must be signed. According to CMS this can be a handwritten signature, as long as it is legible, or an electronic signature. When EHRs are used the signature will be electronic. Below are the CMS's guidelines for using an electronic signature:

- Systems and software products must include protections against modification, and you should apply administrative safeguards that correspond to standards and laws.
- The individual whose name is on the alternate signature method and the provider bear the responsibility for the authenticity of the information being attested to.

- Physicians are encouraged to check with their attorneys and malpractice insurers in regard to the use of alternative signature methods.
- Part B providers use a qualified electronic prescribing (e-prescribing) system.
- Prescriptions for drugs incident to durable medical equipment (DME) must be made via a qualified e-prescribing system.

https://www.cms.gov/Outreach-and-Education/Medicare-Learning-Network-MLN/MLNProducts/downloads/Signature_Requirements_Fact_Sheet_ICN905364.pdf accessed 10/1/2016

Although EHRs have made documentation more standardized and efficient, it is still important to make sure that the documentation is complete and accurate. By following the CMS documentation guidelines, you can be assured that quality patient care has been provided and that all of the billing information is supported.

Front Office, Clinical Care, and Coding and Billing Application Exercises

Let's follow a new patient all the way through his or her visit to Walden-Martin Family Medical Clinic. These activities can be completed in the Simulation Playground of SimChart for the Medical Office (SCMO).

FRONT OFFICE

Dr. Angela Perez and Dr. David Kahn have both recently joined Walden-Martin Family Medical Clinic as providers. You will need to set up the appointment matrix for these providers so that the appointment calendar will show when they are available to see patients.

SET UP APPOINTMENT MATRIX

Dr. Perez:
- Lunch break from 11:30 AM until 12:30 PM
- Hospital rounds from 8:00 AM until 9:00 AM
- Catch-up time from 2:30 PM until 3:00 PM

Dr. Kahn:
- Lunch break from 12:00 PM until 1:00 PM
- Hospital rounds from 8:30 AM until 9:30 AM
- Nursing home visits on Tuesdays from 3:00 PM until 5:00 PM

1. Within the Front Office Calendar, click on the Add Appointment button.
2. Select Block as the Appointment Type, Lunch as the Block Type, and Angela Perez, MD, in the For field.
3. Using the calendar picker select today's date in the Date field.
4. For the Start Time select 11:30 AM, and for the End Time select 12:30 PM.
5. Click in the box next to Recurrence, select Daily as the Recurrence Pattern, and select End By and, using the calendar picker, select the date 6 months from today.
6. Click on the Save button, and the appointment will display on the calendar.
7. Click on the Add Appointment button.
8. Select Block as the Appointment Type, Other as the Block Type, and Angela Perez, MD, in the For field.
9. Using the calendar picker select today's date in the Date field.
10. For the start time select 8:00 AM, and for the End Time select 9:00 AM.
11. Click in the box next to Recurrence, select Daily as the Recurrence Pattern, and select End By and, using the calendar picker, select the date 6 months from today.

12. Click on the Save button, and the appointment will display on the calendar.
13. Click on the Add Appointment button.
14. Select Block as the Appointment Type, Hold as the Block Type, and Angela Perez, MD, in the For field.
15 Using the calendar picker select today's date in the Date field.
16. For the Start Time select 2:30 PM, and for the End Time select 3:00 PM.
17. Click in the box next to Recurrence, select Daily as the Recurrence Pattern, and select End By and, using the calendar picker, select the date 6 months from today.
18. Click on the Save button, and the appointment will display on the calendar.
19. Click on the Add Appointment button.
20. Using the steps described above, enter the Block appointments for Dr. Kahn.

A new patient has called in and would like an appointment with Dr. Perez for next Tuesday at 1:00 PM to talk about recurrent migraine headaches. Schedule this appointment.

SCHEDULING A NEW PATIENT APPOINTMENT

Patient Name: Megan E. Casper
Date of Birth: 01/14/1984
Home Phone: 123-123-6065
Primary Insurance: MetLife
Policy Holder: Megan E. Casper
SSN: 987-66-5544
ID Number: 3467JP098
Group Number: DC8301

1. Within the Front Office, Calendar, click the Add Appointment button.
2. Within the New Appointment window, select Patient Visit as the appointment type.
3. Select New Patient Visit as the visit type.
4. Document Migraine headaches as the Chief Complaint.
5. Select the Create New Patient radio button.
6. Enter "Casper" in the Last Name field and enter "Megan" in the First Name field.
7. Change the year to 1984 in the calendar picker and go to January 1984 and select the 14th.
8. Click on the radio button next to Female.
9. Enter 123-123-6065 in the Home Phone field.
10. Select Angela N. Perez, MD, as the provider.
11. Select MetLife from the Primary Insurance drop-down menu.

12. Enter "Megan E. Casper" in the Name of Policy Holder field.
13. Enter "987-66-5544" in the SSN of Policy Holder field.
14. Enter "3467JP098" in the ID Number field.
15. Enter "DC8301" in the Group Number field.
16. Click the Save button.
17. Use the calendar picker to select next Tuesday as the appointment date.
18. Select a start time of 1:00 PM and an end time of 1:30 PM.
19. Click the Save button, and the appointment will be displayed on the calendar.

Megan shows up at Walden-Martin for her appointment, and you must complete the registration process.

COMPLETING PATIENT DEMOGRAPHICS

Megan Casper demographic information:
Address: 8301 Waldorf Blvd.
   Anytown, AL 12345-1234
SSN: 987-66-5544
Emergency Contact: Zach Casper
Emergency Contact Phone: 123-789-6547
Employer: Anytown Clinic
Work Phone: 123-567-8765
Insurance: MetLife
   1234 Insurance Avenue
   Anytown, AL 12345-1234
Claims Phone: 800-123-0412

1. Click on the Patient Demographics icon.
2. On the Patient tab enter "Casper" in the Last Name field and click on the Search Existing Patients button.
3. Click on "Megan" in the First Name column.
4. Enter "8301 Waldorf Blvd" in the Address 1 field.
5. Enter "Anytown" in the City field.
6. Select "United States" from the Country drop-down menu.
7. Select "AL" from the State/Province field.
8. Enter "12345-12344" in the ZIP/Postal Code field.
9. Enter "Zach Casper" in the Emergency Contact Name field.
10. Enter "123-789-6547" in the Emergency Contact Phone field.
11. Click on the Guarantor tab.
12. Click on the Self radio button in the Relationship of Guarantor to Patient field.
13. Enter "Anytown Clinic" in the Employer Name field and "123-567-8765" in the Work Phone field.
14. Select Angela N. Perez, MD, from the Primary Provider drop-down menu.
15. Click on the Insurance tab.
16. Enter "1234 Insurance Avenue" in the Claims Address field and "Anytown" in the City field.
17. Select "United States" from the Country drop-down menu and "AL" from the State/Province drop-down menu.
18. Enter "12345-1234" in the ZIP/Postal Code field and "800-123-0412" in the Claims Phone field.
19. Click on the Save Patient button.

In addition to entering demographic information for new patients, it is often the responsibility of the medical assistant to update the demographic information for established patients as their addresses or insurance information changes.

UPDATING PATIENT DEMOGRAPHICS

Amma Patel has called Walden-Martin to inform you of an address change. Her new address is 1029 Hudson Lane, Anytown, AL 12345-1234.
1. Click on the Patient Demographics icon.
2. Enter "Patel" in the Last Name field and click on the Search Existing Patients button.
3. Click on "Amma" in the First Name Column.
4. Enter "1029 Hudson Lane" in the Address 1 field.
5. Click on the Save Patient button.

Now that Megan is all checked in for her appointment and her patient demographics have been completed, it is time for the clinical medical assistant to take over.

The first thing that must occur so that documentation in the EHR can start is the creation of an encounter. This will open up the clinical care areas of the EHR.

Creating an Encounter:
1. Click the tab for the Clinical Care module or click on the Find Patient icon.
2. Perform a patient search for Megan Casper (DOB 01/14/1984) and confirm her date of birth.
3. Select Office Visit from the left Info Panel.
4. Use today's date as the Date and select New Patient Visit from the Visit Type drop-down menu.
5. Click the Save button.

Once the encounter has been created the medical assistant can start the documentation process. The first screen visible in SCMO is the Allergies screen.

DOCUMENT ALLERGIES

Megan states that she is allergic to ibuprofen tablets. She becomes nauseous when she takes them and describes this as a moderate reaction. She is also allergic to nuts and develops hives and itching when she eats them; this is also a moderate reaction.

1. Within the Allergy record section, click the Add Allergy button. An Add Allergy window will appear.
2. Select the Medication radio button in the Allergy Type field.
3. Document "Ibuprofen" in the Allergen field. Begin typing "Ibuprofen" in the Allergy field and select "Ibuprofen Tablet (Motrin, Motrin IB)" from the drop-down menu.
4. Select the Nausea check box to indicate the reactions.
5. Select the Moderate radio button to indicate the reaction severity.
6. Select the Self radio button to indicate that the patient is reporting her own allergy.
7. Select the Very Reliable radio button to indicate the confidence level.
8. Click Save to add ibuprofen to the patient's allergy grid.
9. Click the Add Allergy button.
10. Select the Food radio button in the Allergy Type field.

11. Document "Nuts" in the Allergen field. Begin typing "Nuts" in the Allergy field and select "Nuts" from the drop-down menu.

12. Select the Hives and Itching check boxes to indicate the reactions.

13. Select the Moderate radio button to indicate the reaction severity.

14. Select the Self radio button to indicate that the patient is reporting her own allergy.

15. Select the Very Reliable radio button to indicate the confidence level.

16. Click Save to add nuts to the patient's allergy grid.

The next step with a patient is to go over the health history. The patient may have filled out a patient history form before arriving for the appointment, or the medical assistant may use an interview to collect the information from the patient.

ENTER PATIENT HEALTH HISTORY

The following information was obtained from Megan:
Medical History:
  Chicken Pox; February 10, 1987
  Broken collarbone; June 16, 1993
Social History:
  Lives with Zach Casper, 36 years old, husband
  Feels safe in her home
  Father is alive and well at 56 years old. Current medical conditions include hypertension and type 2 diabetes.
  Mother is alive and well at 56 years old. Current medical conditions include hypercholesterolemia.
  Married and employed full time
  No tobacco use, never smoked
  Occasionally drinks alcohol, a glass of wine with dinner
  Does not use illegal drugs or substances
  Exercises regularly, goes to the gym 3 times a week
  No special diet
  Drinks 3 to 4 cups of coffee per day

1. Within the Medical History tab, click the Add button beneath the Past Medical History grid.

2. In the Add Past Medical History window, use the calendar picker to find February 10, 1987. First select "1987" from the year drop-down menu; then use the arrows to move to February and then click on the 10. Document "chicken pox" as the medical issue. Click the Save button and repeat this work flow to document Ms. Casper's past medical history of a broken collarbone.

3. Within the Social and Family History tab, click the Add New button beneath the Family History grid.

4. In the Add Family History window, document "Zach" as the name, "36" as the age, and "Husband" as the relationship. Click the Save button.

5. Select the Yes radio button to indicate that Megan does feel safe in her home.

6. Click the Add button beneath the Paternal section.

7. In the Add Paternal Family Member window, document "Father" as the relationship, "56" as the age, and "Hypertension and type 2 diabetes" as current medical conditions.

Click the Save button and repeat this work flow for Megan's mother in the Maternal section.

8. Use the Marital Status drop-down menu to indicate that Megan is married.

9. Use the Employment drop-down menu to indicate that Megan is satisfied with her job.

10. Within the Tobacco section, select the Never radio button to indicate Megan's tobacco use.

11. Within the Alcohol/Drugs section, select the Occasionally radio button to indicate how frequently Megan drinks alcohol and document "Wine with dinner" in the Comments field. Select the Never radio button to indicate Megan's usage regarding illegal drugs or substances.

12. Within the Activities/Exposures/Habits section, select the Yes radio button to indicate that Megan does exercise regularly. Document "Goes to the gym 3 times/week" in the Comments field.

13. Within the Nutrition section, select the No radio button to indicate that Megan does not follow a special diet but does consume caffeine. Document "3-4 cups per day" to indicate the amount of caffeine Megan consumes.

14. Click the Save button.

The next step in the interview process is to obtain the chief complaint. In the appointment schedule you see that Megan made the appointment for migraines. Now is the opportunity to collect more information about her migraines. Using an open-ended question like "What brings you here today?" will give the patient the opportunity to expand on what has been happening with him or her. You may need to use follow-up questions to get all of the information needed. Below is the information Megan provided related to her chief complaint. You will be documenting this information in SCMO.

DOCUMENTING CHIEF COMPLAINT

In response to your question Megan states that she has been having migraine headaches for many years, starting in the fifth grade, and that they seem to be getting worse. They seem to affect the left side of her head, and the pain is excruciating. She would put it at 9 out of 10 at the peak of the headache. She sees flashing lights and is very light sensitive when she has a headache. Megan will lie down in a dark room until the worst of it passes. She also experiences nausea with the migraines.

1. Select Chief Complaint from the Record drop-down menu.

2. Document the reason for Megan's visit in the Chief Complaint field.

3. Document symptoms associated with the chief complaint in the History of Present Illness section.

4. Within the Review of Systems section, in the HEENT section, select the Yes radio button for HA (headache) and Vision Changes. In the GI section select the Yes radio button for N/V (nausea and/or vomiting).

5. Document your name in the Entry By field and click the Save button.

You will now move on to the medication section of the medical record. It is important to document all prescription medications as well as over-the-counter products that the patient is using regularly.

DOCUMENTING MEDICATIONS

Below is the medication information provided by Megan:
Prescription Medication:

Maxalt tablets, 5 mg, orally, 1 dose may repeat ×1 in 2 hours; was not very effective, so she stopped taking them March 3, 2015

Over-the-Counter Product:

Multivitamin, 1 tablet orally daily.

1. Within the Prescription Medications tab, click the Add button.
2. Within the Add Prescription Medication window, document "Maxalt" in the Medication field or select it from the drop-down by starting to type in "Maxalt" in the Medication field and then selecting "Rizatriptan Tablet – (Maxalt)."
3. Select 5 from the Strength drop-down.
4. Select Tablet from the Form drop-down.
5. Select Oral from the Route drop-down.
6. Select "1 dose may repeat ×1 in 2 hours" from the Frequency drop-down.
7. Select the Discontinued radio button to indicate the status of the medication.
8. Use the calendar picker to find March 3, 2015 for the Discontinued Date.
9. Document "Wasn't working for migraines" in the Reason field.
10. Click the Save button to update Megan's Medication record.
11. Click on the Over-the-Counter Products tab to document the multivitamin.
12. Click on the Add Medication button.
13. Document "multivitamin" in the Generic Name field (you will not be using the drop-down menu).
14. Document "1 tablet" in the Dose field.
15. Document "once daily" in the Frequency field.
16. Select "Oral" from the Route drop-down menu.
17. Select the Active radio button in the Status section.
18. Click on the Save button to update Megan's Medication record.

After interviewing the patient to collect the history, chief complaint, and medication information, the medical assistant collects the height, weight, and vital signs data.

DOCUMENT VITAL SIGNS, HEIGHT, AND WEIGHT

Below are the data for Megan:

Temperature: 98.9 Forehead
Pulse: 72, regular
Respirations: 18, regular
Blood Pressure: 124/82, right arm, sitting, manual with cuff
Height: 5 feet 6 inches
Weight: 136 pounds

1. Select "Vital Signs" from the Record drop-down box. The Vital Signs record is organized into a Vital Signs tab and a Height/Weight tab.

2. Within the Vital Signs tab, click Add button.
3. Document "98.9" as the temperature in the Fahrenheit field. Select Forehead from the Site drop-down menu. Notice that the temperature is also displayed in Celsius after it is entered as Fahrenheit.
4. Document "72, regular" as the pulse and select Radial from the Site drop-down menu.
5. Document "18, regular" as the Respiration.
6. Document "124" as the systolic blood pressure and select Right arm from the Site drop-down menu. Document "82" as diastolic blood pressure and select Manual with cuff from the Mode drop-down menu. Select Sitting from the Position drop-down menu.
7. Click Save button.
8. Within the Height/Weight tab, click the Add button.
9. Document the Height as "5 ft, 6 in" using the individual Height fields. Document the Weight as "136" in the lb field. The BMI will auto-calculate.
10. Click the Save button.

After the physical examination Dr. Perez determined that Megan truly does suffer from migraines. This will need to be added to the Problem List.

Maintaining Problem List:

1. Select Problem List from the Record drop-down menu and click the Add Problem button.
2. Select "Migraine headache" as the diagnosis.
3. Select the ICD-10 Code radio button and document "G43.909" as the code.
4. Document today's date as the date identified using the calendar picker.
5. Select the Active radio button to indicate that this is a current diagnosis.
6. Click the Save button. Megan's Problem List will update to reflect her diagnosis of migraine headaches.

Now that the clinical care has been provided and documented, the reimbursement process must start. The first step in this process is the completion of the Superbill. The provider is ultimately responsible for indicating the services provided and the diagnosis. If these are not indicated on the Superbill itself, they can be obtained from the medical record. The medical assistant may be responsible for assigning the fee for the services provided. The fees are taken from the healthcare facility's fee schedule.

COMPLETING A SUPERBILL

Dr. Perez has indicated that a new patient, expanded office visit was provided to Megan with a diagnosis of migraine headaches. Megan has a $10 office visit copay that she made while she was at Walden-Martin.

1. Click the tab for the Coding and Billing module.
2. Select Superbill from the left Info Panel.
3. Perform a patient search for Megan Casper and confirm her date of birth.
4. Select the correct encounter in the Encounters Not Coded table.
5. Select the ICD-10 radio button.

6. Document "Migraine headaches, G43.909" in the Rank 1 Diagnosis box.
7. Use the Fee Schedule link to determine the fee and CPT code for a detailed office visit for a new patient.
8. Document "1" in the Rank column for Detailed in the Office Visit box, followed by "89.00" in the Fee column and "99204" in the Est column. Click the Fee Schedule link in the top right corner for reference.
9. Click the Save button.
10. Because this was the only service provided, click the Next button three times to progress to the fourth page of the Superbill.
11. Document "$10.00" in the Copay field.
12. Document "$0.00" in the Previous Balance field.
13. Document "$79.00" in the Balance Due field.
14. Click the Same Name as Patient check box, under Insured's Name.
15. Click the Same Address as Patient check box.
16. Select the Self radio button for the Patient Relationship to Insured field.
17. Select the Married radio button for the Patient Status field.
18. Select the No radio button to indicate that there is no other health benefit plan.
19. Select the No radio buttons to indicate that the patient condition is not related to employment, an auto accident, or other accident.
20. Click the check box to indicate that you are ready to submit the Superbill.
21. Select the Yes radio button to indicate that a signature is on file.
22. Enter today's date in the Date field.
23. Click Save button.
24. Click the Submit Superbill button.

After the Superbill has been submitted, the information needs to be documented on the patient ledger. The ledger is used to track all services and procedures provided to the patient as well as payments and adjustments made to the account. The information on the Superbill will be used to complete the ledger.

COMPLETING A PATIENT LEDGER

Superbill information:
    Date of Service: Today's date
    Services provided: 99204
    Charges: $89.00
    Patient paid: $10.00
1. Select Ledger from the left Info Panel.
2. Perform a patient search for Megan Casper and confirm her date of birth.
3. Click on the arrow on the right side of the screen, across from Megan's name.
4. Document the today's date in the Transaction Date and DOS using the calendar picker.
5. Select Angela N. Perez, MD, from the Provider drop-down menu.
6. Document "99204" in the Service column.
7. Document "89.00" in the Charges column.

8. Document "10.00" in the Payment column.
9. The Balance of $79.00 is auto-populated based on the amounts listed in the previous columns.
10. Click the Save button.

Now that the services and fees have been documented, we need to submit a claim to the insurance carrier so that Walden-Martin can be reimbursed for the services provided to Megan. Again the information from the Superbill will be used to complete the claim. SCMO uses the HIPAA 5010 (electronic claim format).

PREPARE A CLAIM

Superbill information:
    Date of Service: Today's date
    Services provided: 99204
    Diagnosis: Migraine headaches, G43.909
    Charges: $89.00
    Patient paid: $10.00
1. Select Claim from the left Info Panel.
2. Perform a patient search for Megan Casper and confirm her date of birth.
3. The submitted Superbill appears under the Encounter Type in the List of Superbills for Megan Casper.
4. Click the icon (paper and pencil) under the Action column to progress to the Claim.
5. Review the information auto-populated in the Patient Info, Provider Info, and Payer Info tabs.
6. Within the Encounter Notes tab, select the Yes radio button to indicate the HIPAA form is on file, and document the date. Note that the diagnosis entered in Superbill is in the DX1 field under Encounter Diagnosis.
7. Click the Save button.
8. Within the Claim Info tab, select the No radio buttons to indicate that Megan's condition is not related to employment or an auto accident.
9. Select the Yes radio button in the Release of Info field.
10. Select the Yes radio button in the Assignment field.
11. Select the Yes radio button to indicate that the signature is on file.
12. Click the Save button.
13. Click the Charge Capture tab.
14. Document today's date in the DOS From and DOS To columns.
15. Document "99204" in the CPT/HCPCS column.
16. Document "11" in the POS column. Click the Place of Service link in the top right corner for reference.
17. Document 1 in the DX column to link the procedure code to the diagnosis listed in the Encounter Notes tab.
18. Document "89.00" in the Fee column. This amount will auto-populate in the Total Charges field below the table.
19. Document "1" in the Units column.
20. Document "10.00" in the Amount Paid field below the table. The $79.00 the balance will auto-populate in the Balance Due field.
21. Click the Save button.
22. Click the Submission tab.

23. Select the check box to indicate that you are ready to submit the Claim.
24. Select the Yes radio button to indicate that there is a signature on file.
25. Document the date in the Date field.
26. Click the Save button.
27. Click the Submit Claim button to submit the Claim electronically.

Two weeks have now passed, and we have received a payment from MetLife for Megan's services. MetLife has paid $63.20 of the $79.00 balance, and because Walden-Martin is a participating provider with MetLife, the remaining balance of $15.80 will have to be written off (as an adjustment).

Posting Payments and Adjustments:
1. Select Ledger from the left Info Panel.
2. Perform a patient search for Megan Casper and confirm her date of birth.

3. Click on the arrow on the right side of the screen, across from Megan's name.
4. Click on the Add Row button.
5. Document the today's date in the Transaction Date and DOS using the calendar picker.
6. Document "INSPYMT" in the Service column.
7. Document "63.20" in the Payment column.
8. Document "-15.80" in the Adjustment column. Be sure to include the minus sign in front of the dollar amount so that the amount is subtracted from the balance.
9. Click the Save button.
10. The Balance and Total Ledger Balance will be auto-calculated.

We have just taken a patient from scheduling an appointment through the clinical care and finally to getting her bill paid, all by using an electronic health record. The use of EHRs has made this whole process much more efficient for providers as well as patients.

SimChart Supplement

To the Instructor

SimChart for the Medical Office: Learning the Medical Office Workflow was developed to provide step by step guidance in utilizing all of the features of SimChart for the Medical Office. Utilizing all of the helpful materials provided within the program, this text will walk you and your students through the three modules of the product as well as provide practice with the TruCode encoder feature.

Organization

The text is organized into four units:
1. **Navigating SimChart for the Medical Office.** This unit introduces the student to the product and provides background on the three modules, the simulation playground, the encoder, and some of the typical workflow steps that medical assistants will encounter.
2. **Front Office.** This unit introduces students to the front office module of the product and concludes with 20 related assignments for students to complete in SimChart for the Medical Office.
3. **Clinical Care.** This unit introduces students to the clinical care module of the product and concludes with 41 related assignments for students to complete in SimChart for the Medical Office.
4. **Coding & Billing.** This unit introduces students to the coding & billing module of the product and concludes with 49 related assignments for students to complete in SimChart for the Medical Office.

Quick Tips

The following are some tips that will help you to utilize SimChart for the Medical Office to the fullest.

Familiarize Yourself with Instructor Resources

Access Instructor Resources as often as needed; whenever you have a question regarding a process or where to locate a particular feature. Watch *A Guided Tour of SimChart for the Medical Office* before logging in to SimChart for the Medical Office for the first time.

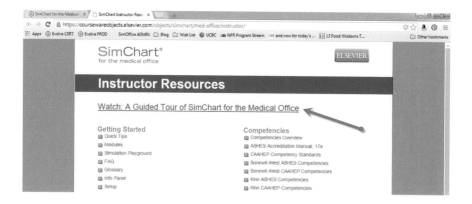

Refer to the Lesson Plan Index

The *Lesson Plan Index* in the Implementation and Lesson Plan folders provides suggested activities to incorporate SimChart for the Medical Office in lectures and labs. *The Lesson Plan Index* is organized by week with details on the level of activity, the forum for delivery, and the use of setting.

Review the Assignments and Grading Features

The instructor view is comprised of Assignments and Grading. When you log in to SimChart for the Medical Office, you land within the **Assignments** module.

- Select a Course Name from the Course List to review selected assignments. Within the **Grading** module, follow the same path to review the auto-graded questions and simulation work for an assignment.

Release Assignments to Your Course

Elsevier provides 110 pre-built, peer-reviewed assignments. In the **Assignments** module, you can **Assign All** or **Review & Select** assignments. Keep in mind that assignments cannot be retracted once assigned to the class.

- **Assign All** is a quick and easy way to give students access to all of the assignments for practice and completion. Daily or weekly assignments can be provided to students by way of syllabus or in-class discussion to keep students on task.
- **Review & Select** gives you the ability to time your assignment releases using the selection assignment function.

Create Your Own Folder Structure

- After selecting a course in the Assignments module, select the Organize tab to review and organize assignments into folders. For example, categorize assignments by the week you wish to release them to students or archive any assignments not needed. Refer to *Assigning Assignments* in the Assignments folder for more information.

Review a Graded Assignment

Students cannot make additional changes after submitting an assignment. The application automatically generates a preliminary grade based on a student's quiz performance. Once a student clicks the Submit Assignment button, the assignment moves from the Open Assignments tab to the Graded Assignments tab in the student view and the quiz results are immediately available for student review. An instructor can then manually review a student's simulation work, enter a grade for the simulation work, and use the Grading Rubric to approve or adjust the automatically generated grade.

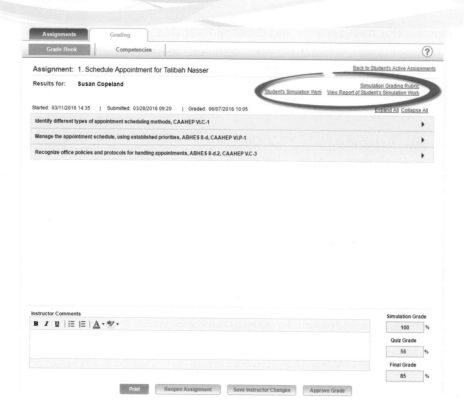

Allow Students to Reattempt an Assignment

Clicking the **Reopen Assignment** button sends a student's assignment back to the Open Assignments tab in the student view and labels it as **REOPENED**. This allows a student to continue the simulation exercise of an assignment and make changes to the post-case quiz. The student can resubmit the assignment for grading when finished.

Students Review and Print Graded Assignments

Once a student submits an assignment, the assignment moves from the Open Assignments tab to the Graded Assignments tab in the student view and the automatic grade displays. If an instructor changes a grade based on a student's simulation work, the Grade column in the Graded Assignments grid displays the percentage for that assignment in bold. Students can print assignments and add them to a portfolio.

10 Ways to Implement SimChart for the Medical Office

1. Register a Patient and Schedule an Appointment

Conduct contests to see which student can register a patient and schedule a new patient appointment the quickest, ensuring that all information is entered correctly.

2. Correspondence

Have students create appointments and then complete Appointment Reminder letters to confirm upcoming patient appointments. As students progress through the modules, have them complete additional communication using the templates in Correspondence.

3. Review Legal Documents

When discussing advance directives, have students access and complete the document in the simulation. Although most forms are electronic, some forms such as the Advance Directive must be printed and completed by hand in order to demonstrate office workflow. In a medical office, a medical assistant would hand an Advance Directive to a patient for them to fill out by hand. The medical assistant would then upload the completed form to the patient record

4. Document Vital Signs

Instruct students to take each other's vital signs and document that information in the patient record.

5. Differentiate Between Medication Types

Give students a list of various medication types, including prescriptions, over-the-counter products, and herbal supplements. Have students document each medication in the patient record.

6. Request Orders and Lab Requisitions

Role-play scenarios in which one student acts as the medical assistant and the other acts as a patient who needs a procedure.

7. Code Diagnoses and Procedures

Give students a list of ICD and CPT codes and have them determine which codes are correct for a patient encounter.

8. Explain How a Superbill is Connected to a Claim

Group students into pairs. Have each student complete a Superbill, then have them switch patients to complete the Claim.

9. Discuss Accounts Receivable Principles

Have each student complete a Superbill and Ledger for a different patient. Then, complete the Day Sheet as a class using each student's patient information.

10. Complete a Patient Visit from Beginning to End

Demonstrate how medical assisting is connected to an electronic health record by walking students through a patient visit. Begin with scheduling an appointment, then move to documenting clinical care, and end by submitting a Superbill and Claim.

To the Student

SimChart for the Medical Office: Learning the Medical Office Workflow will provide you with unique, hands-on learning of the simulated medical office. The assignments in this text provide realistic practice of all of the tasks you will encounter in a real medical office—from front office (administrative) skills to clinical skills to practice management skills (billing, coding, and insurance).

Completing a medical assistant program is a rigorous undertaking. The medical assistant profession is complex and requires a student to gain a complete understanding of how a medical office functions, from the time the patient makes an appointment until the insurance carrier pays for the services provided in the encounter. Follow these tips to become a successful medical assistant student.

Quick Tips

Familiarize Yourself With Student Resources

Review all of the resource materials before class and refer to them whenever you have a question regarding a particular process or feature in SimChart for the Medical Office.

Review the Assignments

The student homepage is comprised of an **Open Assignments** tab and a **Graded Assignments** tab. All available assignments appear in the Open Assignments tab. As you complete and submit assignments, they move to the Graded Assignments tab for review.

Although student performance within the **Quiz** of an assignment generates a grade that is automatically visible, an instructor can still modify this grade based on simulation work. The grade is not final until your instructor approves the automatically generated score and the Grade column in the grid displays the percentage for that assignment in bold.

Follow Your Instructor's Lead

Instructors can incorporate SimChart for the Medical Office into the classroom several ways. Follow instructions regarding how and when to use the application.

Access the Simulation

The **Simulation Playground** button above the list of assignments directs you to a practice version of the medical office. Within this environment, you can practice common medical office tasks such as registering patients, scheduling appointments, documenting patient care, and completing the coding and billing for a patient encounter.

Information documented in the Simulation Playground remains saved but is not submitted for grading. However, your instructor can access your Simulation Playground in order to review your practice.

If desired, you can erase your work in the Simulation Playground and begin a new session by selecting the 'Start new simulation session and clear all previously saved patient information' radio button upon entry.

Save Your Work

Almost every screen has a **Save** button. Be sure to save your work in all screens before progressing or exiting. You can even save work within an assignment before submitting, making it easy to return and continue.

Review Assignment Details and Complete Simulation

- Click the **Open Assignments** tab and then click the title of the assignment to complete. Review the assignment description, objectives, and competencies before clicking the **Start Assignment** button in the **Description** tab to enter the simulation. After completing the simulation, click the **Back to Assignment** link and the **Quiz** tab to answer the questions tied to the assignment.

Answer All Quiz Questions to Submit Assignment

All assignments include questions tied to a specific competency that is reinforced by the simulation tasks. Answer all questions before submitting an assignment.

Check Your Work

- An assignment cannot be edited once it is submitted, so check all answers to quiz questions and ensure that your simulation work is accurate and complete before clicking the **Submit Assignment** button.

Review Graded Assignment Upon Completion

The system automatically grades quiz questions upon submission and moves the assignment from the **Open Assignments** tab to the **Graded Assignments** tab.
- Select the title of the graded assignment to review the automatically generated grade. Once you submit an assignment, your instructor can evaluate the simulation work manually.
  After reviewing the simulation portion of an assignment, your instructor can provide comments and approve or adjust the automatically generated grade. After your instructor approves a grade, the Grade column in the Graded Assignments grid displays the percentage for that assignment in bold. You can then print the graded assignment.

Use Available Resources

Instructors are the best resource, but they can't answer questions if students don't ask them. If one student has a question, another student probably does too, so you will be doing everyone a favor by asking.
- Ask your instructor questions after class or during office hours if you are uncomfortable asking during class.
- Email your instructor if questions arise outside of class.
  Fellow students are another great resource. Social networking sites can also be a great way to stay in contact outside of class.
- Form study groups to review content on an ongoing basis or prepare for exams.
- Create a Facebook group for a specific class and post questions and/or study tools for everyone to access.
  Textbooks are the basis for most class content. Glossaries, indexes, and online resources can provide additional details about unfamiliar terms and topics.
- List questions from the chapter before class and ask the instructor if your questions are not answered during class.
- Make notes and highlight important content.

Teamwork

The ability to work well with others is an invaluable tool in the workforce. Group projects are a great opportunity to develop interpersonal skills that will make you an asset to any team.
- Volunteer to be the leader of the group or use your people skills to bring out the quiet one in the group.
- If you are typically the quiet member of a group, offer at least one suggestion during every group meeting.

- Practice active listening and do not interrupt. Avoid distractions. Give the person you are speaking with your undivided attention so you process the message.
- Body language can sometimes convey more than words. Observing the body language of others while you are delivering a message will help you to determine if they are receiving the intended message.
- Respect diversity. Understanding that people come from different backgrounds will facilitate collaboration. Team players are respectful of everyone's opinion.
- Gossiping is destructive to a productive learning and work environment. The impact of gossiping can hurt feelings and induce anger, neither of which help to create a positive environment.

Be Considerate

Group projects can also serve as an opportunity to develop skills that help you cooperate with all types of personalities. Remember that practicing consideration will not go unnoticed. Your instructor will remember the example you set, which will come in handy when you ask them to provide a referral letter.

- Be considerate of all classmates in and out of class.
- Do not interrupt your teacher or your classmates as this is rude and disruptive.
- Remember that everyone comes from different backgrounds, so keep an open mind and learn from what others share in class.
- Do not gossip. Gossip damages relationships and is unprofessional.

Be Professional

Approaching school as if it were a job allows you to start developing your professionalism skills the moment you start your medical assistant program. Consistent attendance helps you retain more information, participating in class demonstrates that you are engaged in class discussion, balancing priorities helps you to be prepared for any unexpected scheduling complications, and adhering to established policies will all help you succeed.

- Participate in class. You do not have to raise your hand to answer every question, but you should always be engaged in class discussion.
- Determine daycare details in advance and establish a backup plan in case your transportation falls through.
- Keep a calendar to track all of your commitments and be realistic about how long activities really take.
- Contact your instructor immediately if absence is unavoidable.
- Follow the dress code. If you are not already required to follow a dress code while in school, you will certainly have a dress code for practicum.
- Make sure scrubs are in good condition. Pants should not drag on the floor, and tops should be an appropriate length.
- Cover tattoos and remove visible body piercings.
- Always behave professionally when dressed in scrubs and avoid going out socially in scrubs because it could reflect poorly upon healthcare professions.

Work Ethic

Taking responsibility for your education and seeking clarification when you don't understand something in class will help you develop the habit of ensuring comprehension in the workplace. This will ultimately help you to provide the best patient care possible.

- Do your own work and credit your sources. Understand plagiarism and its consequences. Allowing others to use your work is still considered cheating.
- Complete all assignments before the due date and remember that you receive the grade you earn; instructors do not "give" grades.
- Always clean up after yourself. Whether you are in the lab or in a lecture, make sure that your workspace is as clean as or cleaner than when you sat down.

Job Readiness Skills

Many of the skills needed to obtain and maintain a job can be developed while a student is still in a Medical Assistant program.

Positive Mental Attitude

Nobody wants to work with someone who always has a negative outlook. Those who tend to see the worst should use this time as an opportunity to start changing their mindset.

- Keep your self-talk positive. When presented with a difficult situation, identify an aspect of the situation that will benefit the patient, organization, or staff.
- Smile, even when you don't feel like it. Smiling can help create positive interactions which contribute to a positive environment overall.
- Embrace change. Change is inevitable, especially in healthcare. Viewing change as an opportunity to learn and improve rather than a chore can also contribute to a positive environment. Try to identify how change can benefit the patient, organization, and staff.

Time Management

Time management is a skill needed for school as well as work. Figuring out how to balance priorities while in school can carry over to your work.

- Determine daycare details in advance. Having a plan in place when your child or daycare provider is sick can help to minimize schedule complications. Investigate the options available in your area. Is there a center that accepts sick children? Can a close friend or family member care for your child?
- Secure reliable transportation or establish a backup plan if you have car trouble. Know the bus routes and ask other students or co-workers about carpooling.
- Keep a calendar to track all of your commitments and prevent double-booking. Most cellular phones provide a calendar function and paper agendas are also available. Whichever version you prefer, keep it current with your work schedule, personal activities, and family activities.
- Be realistic about how long activities really take. For example, if you don't have more than one hour available for a dentist appointment and you know that traffic is always hectic, you should choose another day for the appointment.

Lifelong Learning

Change occurs frequently in healthcare and developing tools to help with staying current in your field will make you a better medical assistant.

- Join your national and local professional organization.
- The American Association of Medical Assistants (CMA (AAMA)) provides continuing education opportunities including an annual national convention, CMA Today magazine, membership in the state organization that provides opportunities at a more local level, and online and paper-based CEUs.
- The American Medical Technologists (RMA) provides an annual national meeting, AMT State Society meetings, and online and paper-based CEUs.
- Find workshops and seminars that promote new skill development or update existing skills. For example, diagnostic and procedural coding manuals are updated every year. Attending a workshop regarding this topic will ensure that you are using current coding criteria. Requesting information and demonstrations from manufacturers when they release laboratory tests or equipment is another good way to remain current.

Dressing for Success

Since healthcare is a conservative field, follow the dress code policy at all times.

- Cover tattoos and remove visible body piercings. Some dress code policies even go so far as to state that there can only be one earring in each ear.

- If scrubs are required, make sure they are in good condition. Pants should not drag on the floor and tops should be an appropriate length.
- Some positions require business casual attire. If unsure as to what clothes are allowed, be sure to ask. Business casual is not the same as casual clothing worn at home. Sweatpants, yoga pants, shorts, midriff baring tops, flip flops, shirts with logos or statements, and halter tops are not appropriate.

Resume Building

All of the skills obtained in school help to build a resume that will attract potential employers. Welcome every opportunity to learn a new skill and showcase these skills in your resume.

- Create a portfolio with examples of different skills learned, such as a business letter written using Microsoft Word, a project organized using Microsoft Excel, samples of EHR documentation using an application such as SimChart for the Medical Office, and a checklist of clinical and administrative skills gained during practicum. Refer *Appendix A* for more information.
- List experience using software programs such as SimChart for the Medical Office, Microsoft Word, Microsoft Excel, Microsoft PowerPoint, or Microsoft Access. Include extracurricular activities such as tutoring or involvement in any student or professional organizations. This type of background demonstrates a willingness to expand beyond the basics required in school.

Navigating SCMO

About SimChart for the Medical Office

Modules

SimChart for the Medical Office is organized within three modules which contain the main aspects of the medical office workflow: Front Office, Clinical Care, and Coding & Billing (Figure 1-1). The default landing page upon entering the simulation is the Front Office Calendar to represent opening the medical office for the day. From that point, users can navigate freely throughout all of the modules of the medical office workflow in order to practice or accomplish the specific tasks of an assignment.

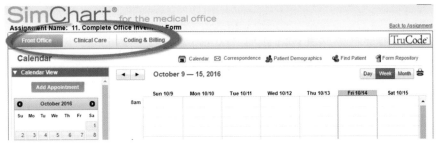

Figure 1-1 The three modules of SimChart for the Medical Office: Front Office, Clinical Care, and Coding & Billing.

- The **Front Office** module features the Calendar, which is the most frequently referenced aspect of daily medical office workflow. (See workflow items 1- 6 at the end of this unit for some typical front office tasks.)
- The **Clinical Care** module features all of the clinical charting for a patient record. (See workflow items 7-20 at the end of this unit for some typical clinical care tasks.)
- The **Coding & Billing** module contains all practice management functionality necessary to complete an encounter. (See workflow items 21-24 at the end of this unit for some typical coding & billing tasks.)

Simulation Playground

The Simulation Playground is the practice environment of SimChart for the Medical Office. Although the same functionality is available in assignments, the Simulation Playground is meant to serve as an opportunity for students to familiarize themselves with simulation features prior to completing assignments.

Simulation Playground Access for Students

In the Simulation Playground, students can practice aspects of clinical documentation, office workflow, and practice management. Encourage students to collaborate by registering each other as new patients, documenting vital signs, and coding Superbills. Students can even review an assignment description and practice the assignment in the Simulation Playground before beginning the graded assignment. This practice can help students become familiar with identifying the steps necessary to complete an assignment.

- Upon entry, continue work or clear previous work to begin a new session. Select the first radio button, unless you want to clear your work (Figure 1-2).

Simulation Playground Access for Instructors

- Instructors can access the simulation by clicking the **Simulation Playground** button within the Assignments tab (Figure 1-3).

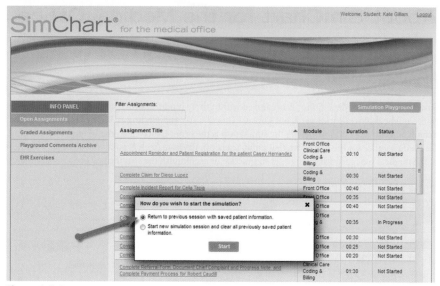

Figure 1-2 Simulation Playground radio buttons: return to previous session or start new simulation session.

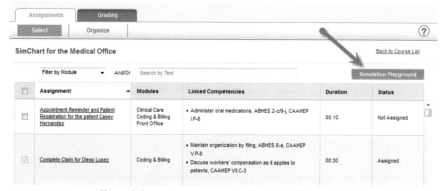

Figure 1-3 Instructor access to the Simulation Playground.

- To review a student's Simulation Playground, click the **Student's Playground** link at the top of an individual student's Active Assignments screen.

Encoder

The TruCode Encoder tool is an electronic medical coding resource to use when documenting diagnoses or procedures in SimChart for the Medical Office. Since SimChart for the Medical Office is intended for educational use, a limited set of CPT codes are available within the tool. There are two ways to access the encoder:

1. Clicking the TruCode button in the top right corner opens the tool in a new tab to use as reference while navigating throughout the application. This button is always visible throughout the application (Figure 1-4).
2. Placing a cursor in a field that requires coding will reveal an additional TruCode button. Accessing the tool this way will auto-populate the selected code where the cursor is placed in the simulation (Figure 1-5).

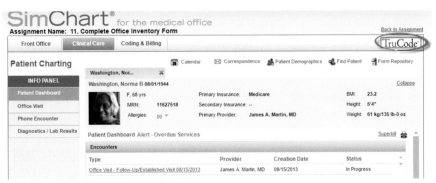

Figure 1-4 TruCode Encoder.

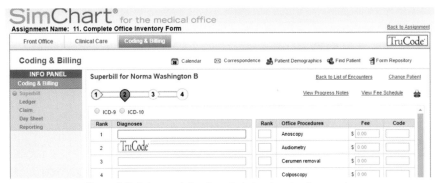

Figure 1-5 Auto-populating the selected code using the encoder.

Performing a Search

Use the CodeBooks control (the search field at the top of the screen) to search for codes by terms or code (Figure 1-6). The following code books are included:

- **ICD-10-CM Diagnosis** and **External Cause** – These books consist of an alphabetic index where you can look up terms and a tabular of codes, which includes all instructional notes.
- **ICD-10-PCS Procedure** – This book consists of an alphabetic index where you can look up terms and a table where you choose the specifics of the procedure to construct the ICD-10-PCS procedure code.
- **ICD-9-CM Diagnosis**, **E Code**, and **Procedure** – These books consist of an alphabetic index where you can look up terms and a tabular of codes, including all instructional notes.
- **CPT** and **HCPCS** – In these books, both the index and tabular are searched simultaneously and tabular results are displayed based upon the search.

Search Results

When searching a code book by terms (except for CPT and HCPCS), the alphabetic index appears in the control. The Search Results pane displays all index entries from the alphabetic index that match the search terms (Figure 1-7).

If a code has an instructional note, the **I** symbol appears to the left of the code when the code is highlighted. Instructional notes contain Includes, Excludes, and Notes from the chapter, section, and category levels.

- To view the note, click the symbol (Figure 1-8).

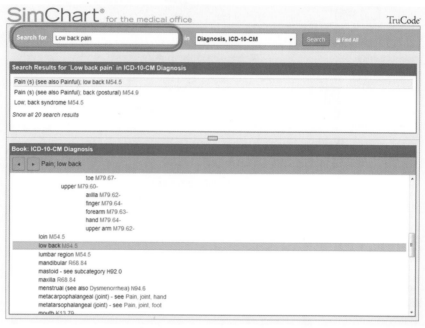

Figure 1-6 Searching by code type.

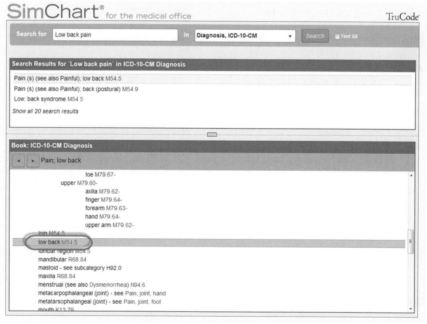

Figure 1-7 The Search Results pane.

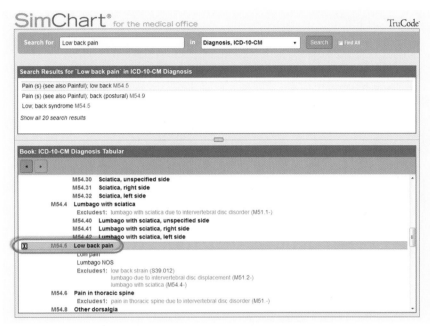

Figure 1-8 Clicking the symbol to view instructional notes.

Documentation

Documentation options vary depending on access point.
- Accessing the Encoder tool by clicking the TruCode button in the top right corner opens the tool in a new tab to use as reference while navigating throughout the application. In order to document this way, copy the desired code and paste it into the correct field within the simulation.
- Accessing the Encoder tool by placing a cursor in a field requiring coding reveals an additional TruCode button and will auto-populate the selected code where the cursor is placed in the simulation (Figure 1-9).

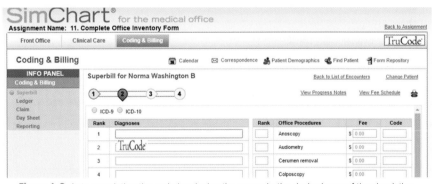

Figure 1-9 Auto-populating the code by placing the cursor in the desired area of the simulation.

- Expand the list of codes beneath the desired code by clicking the code associated with a diagnosis (Figure 1-10).
- After expanding a diagnosis to confirm that it is the most specific code available, click the code that appears in red in order to auto-populate it within the simulation and continue documenting (Figures 1-11 and 1-12).

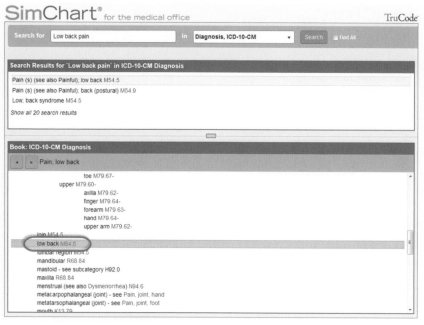

Figure 1-10 Expanding the list of codes.

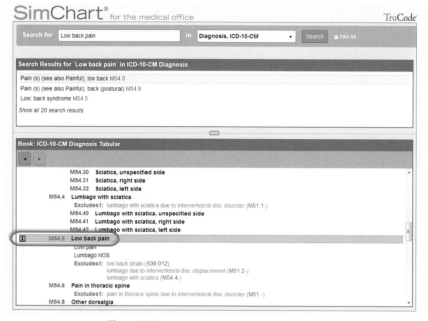

Figure 1-11 Click on the code that appears in red.

Info Panel

Navigating the Info Panel

The Info Panel is visible on the left side of the screen in all modules and contains tasks specific to the workflow of that particular module.

Navigating SCMO

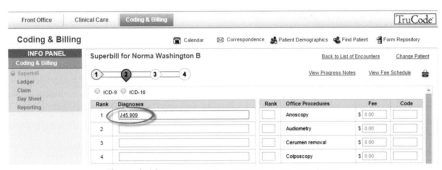

Figure 1-12   The code auto-populated in the simulation.

Front Office

The Front Office module defaults to the calendar view. Form Repository or Correspondence sections can be selected by clicking on the icons at the top of the screen.

- Selecting the **Form Repository** icon displays patient and office form templates to use in the medical office (Figure 1-13). Performing a patient search after selecting a form unlocks a form for editing and saves any changes to that patient's record.

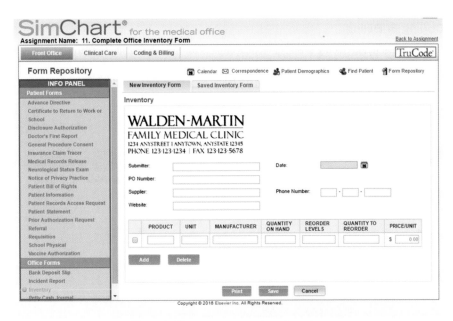

Figure 1-13   Templates in the Form Repository.

- Selecting the **Correspondence** icon displays the email, letter, and phone communication templates available for use in the medical office.

Clinical Care

The Info Panel in the Clinical Care module displays patient visit options. Selecting a patient displays the Patient Dashboard for that patient. Before documenting in the patient record, a student must create a patient encounter in order to tie documentation to a specific date and time (Figure 1-14).

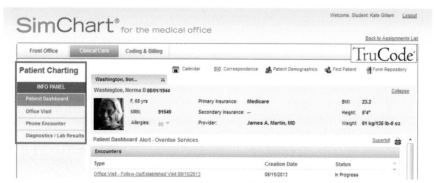

Figure 1-14 The Info Panel in the Clinical Care module.

Coding & Billing

The Info Panel in the Coding & Billing module displays the **Superbill**, **Ledger**, **Claim**, **Day Sheet Reporting** and **Auditing** (Figure 1-15). You must perform a patient search and select an encounter before coding a Superbill. After submitting a Superbill, you may progress to the Claim.

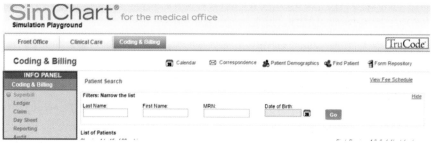

Figure 1-15 The Info Panel in the Coding & Billing module.

Assignment Overview

Assignment Components

The assignments available in SimChart for the Medical Office have been authored and peer-reviewed by medical assisting instructors. An assignment is comprised of a description, objectives, competencies, a simulation exercise, and quiz questions.

- Access assignments after logging in to SimChart for the Medical Office. All assignments are located in the **Open Assignments** tab of the Info Panel. Click the assignment title to enter and view the components of an assignment (Figure 1-16).

Navigating SCMO

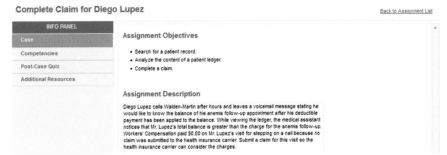

Complete Claim for Diego Lupez   Back to Assignment List

| INFO PANEL |
| Case |
| Competencies |
| Post-Case Quiz |
| Additional Resources |

Assignment Objectives

- Search for a patient record.
- Analyze the content of a patient ledger.
- Complete a claim.

Assignment Description

Diego Lupez calls Walden-Martin after hours and leaves a voicemail message stating he would like to know the balance of his anemia follow-up appointment after his deductible payment has been applied to the balance. While viewing the ledger, the medical assistant notices that Mr. Lupez's total balance is greater than the charge for the anemia follow-up. Workers' Compensation paid $0.00 on Mr. Lupez's visit for stepping on a nail because no claim was submitted to the health insurance carrier. Submit a claim for this visit so the health insurance carrier can consider the charges.

Figure 1-16   Click the assignment title to enter and view the components of an assignment.

- The **Case** tab displays the objectives and description for an assignment. You can also enter the simulation portion of an assignment from within this tab by clicking the **Start Assignment** button at the bottom of the screen.
- The **Competencies** tab lists the competencies tied to the assignment, including competency name, accrediting body, and competency number. Competencies addressed in the simulation are reinforced with quiz questions. Since some competencies speak to general practices, the application incorporates quiz questions that address general best practices any medical office should adopt.
- The **Post-Case Quiz** tab contains review questions that complement the concepts addressed in the simulation exercise. As mentioned above, quiz questions address general best practices any medical office should adopt.
- The **Additional Resources** tab lists additional content such as texts or articles to refer to when completing an assignment. If there are no resources listed, none have been provided.

Reopened Assignments

If you are disappointed with your simulation work and your instructor lets you start over, or your instructor believes that retaking an assignment would benefit your development, your instructor can reopen a submitted assignment.

If an instructor has reopened an assignment, that assignment moves back to the Open Assignments tab with a status of REOPENED.

- When your instructor reopens an assignment, you may continue working on the simulation as well as make changes to your post-case quiz. Review the **Description** and **Competencies** tabs to ensure that you understand what tasks you are expected to perform within the assignment.
- Click the Reopen Assignment button to continue working.
- When you finish documenting in the EHR, click the **Back to Assignment** link. Click the Post-Case Quiz tab to modify any quiz questions. Click the **Resubmit Assignment** button when finished.

The resubmitted assignment moves back to the **Graded Assignments** tab. Your grade will remain the same as your previous attempt until your instructor reviews your reattempted simulation work and adjusts your grade. Final grades appear in bold within the Grade column.

Student Workflow

- Students should review the **Case** and **Competency** tabs before clicking the **Start Assignment** button to begin the simulation portion of an assignment. Within the simulation, clicking the **Assignment Details** tab on the right side displays the assignment objectives and description in case you need a reminder. Once you complete the simulation portion, clicking the **Back to Assignment** link returns to the assignment overview.

- Next, answer the quiz questions before clicking the **Submit Assignment** button. Review questions for each assignment generate an automatic initial grade an instructor can approve or adjust after reviewing a student's simulation work. Although the auto-graded assignment is immediately available for your review from within the **Graded Assignments** tab, an instructor can still modify this grade, so you should understand that this automatically generated grade is not final. Final grades are displayed in bold in the **Graded Assignments** tab.

Workflow Steps

1. Review Case and Competencies tabs.
2. Click the Start Assignment button within the Case tab.
3. Complete the simulation work.
4. Click the Back to Assignment button.
5. Complete the review questions within the Post-Case Quiz tab.
6. Click the Submit Assignment button within the Post-Case Quiz tab.
7. Review the auto-graded assignment within the Graded Assignments tab.

Medical Office Workflow Tasks

SimChart for the Medical Office assignments enforce workflows medical assistants will encounter in most medical offices. The general steps required to complete assignment tasks are provided in this guide. These steps, along with information provided in the Assignment Description or simulation, provide students with all of the information necessary to successfully complete assignments.

The amount of information provided within the simulation is determined by the purpose of the assignment. For example, the Assignment Description for an assignment titled, *Document the Patient Visit and Submit the Superbill for Celia Tapia,* should contain all of the information necessary to complete that assignment. On the other hand, the simulation for an assignment titled, *Submit the Superbill for Celia Tapia,* should contain all of the information necessary to complete that assignment. Students must determine where to navigate within the simulation to locate the necessary information in this case. Following, you will find 24 workflow steps that are typical to the medical assistant workflow.

1. Register a Patient

1. Click the **Patient Demographics** icon.
2. Perform a patient search to confirm that a record does not already exist.
3. Click the **Add Patient** button.
4. Using the patient information form provided with an assignment as reference, complete the required fields (*) within the **Patient, Guarantor,** and **Insurance** tabs. Click the **Save Patient** button before moving to a different tab.
5. After providing information in all of the three tabs, click the **Save Patient** button to save the demographic information.
6. Click the X to close out of the Patient Demographics. You will automatically be directed to the new patient record, where you can create an encounter and begin documenting patient care.

2. Schedule an Appointment

1. Click the **Add Appointment** button or anywhere within the calendar to open the New Appointment window.
2. Select the appointment type using the **Appointment Type** radio buttons.
3. Select the visit type using the **Visit Type** dropdown.
4. Document the reason for the patient visit in the **Chief Complaint** text box.

Navigating SCMO

5. Select the **Search Existing Patients** radio button to determine if the patient requesting the appointment is an established patient. If the patient is not an established patient, select the **Create New Patient** radio button to gather necessary patient data prior to the patient's first office visit.

6. If the patient is an established patient, confirm the patient's date of birth to ensure you have located the correct patient record. Select the radio button next to the patient name and click the **Select** button. Confirm the auto-populated details.

7. Select the correct provider by using the Provider dropdown menu.

8. Use the calendar picker to confirm or select the appointment day in the **Date** field.

9. Select a start and end time for the appointment using the **Start Time** and **End Time** dropdown menus.

10. Click the **Save** button. The patient's appointment will display in the calendar.

3. Prepare Patient and Office Communication

1. Click the **Correspondence** icon to access email, letter, and phone message templates.

2. Select the correct template from the Correspondence Info Panel.

3. For patient communication, click the **Patient Search** button to perform a patient search and save the communication to the patient record. Performing a patient search before preparing a letter will help to ensure accurate documentation in the patient record.

4. Using the Patient Search fields, locate the correct patient record. Once you locate the correct patient in the List of Patients, confirm the date of birth to ensure you have located the correct patient record.

5. Select the radio button next to the patient name and click the **Select** button. Confirm the auto-populated details and provide any additional details needed.

6. Click the **Send** button.

7. All patient correspondence is saved in the Correspondence section of the Patient Dashboard. Within the Clinical Care module, select the letter from the **Correspondence** section of the Patient Dashboard. The letter will open in a new browser tab for reference or printing.

4. Prepare Patient and Office Forms

1. Click the **Form Repository** icon to access patient and office form templates.

2. Select the correct template from the Form Repository Info Panel.

3. For patient forms, click the **Patient Search** button to perform a patient search to auto-populate patient demographic information and save the form to the patient record. Performing a patient search before preparing a form will help to ensure accurate documentation in the patient record. Confirm the auto-populated details and enter any additional information needed.

4. Using the Patient Search fields, locate the correct patient record. Once you locate the correct patient in the List of Patients, confirm the date of birth to ensure you have located the correct patient record.

5. Select the radio button next to the patient name and click the **Select** button. Confirm the auto-populated details and provide any additional details needed.

6. Complete the necessary information and click the **Save to Patient Record** button.

7. Within the Clinical Care module, select the form from the **Forms** section of the Patient Dashboard. The letter will open in a new browser tab for reference or printing.

 HELPFUL HINT

Although most forms are electronic, some forms such as the Inventory form and the Advance Directive must be printed and completed by hand in order to demonstrate office workflow. For example, a medical assistant would give an Advance Directive to a patient for them to fill out by hand. The medical assistant would then upload the completed form to the patient record.

5. Create a Phone Encounter

1. Click the **Find Patient** icon.
2. Using the Patient Search fields, locate the correct patient record. Once you locate the correct patient in the List of Patients, confirm the date of birth to ensure you have located the correct patient record.
3. Select the radio button next to the patient name and click the **Select** button. Confirm the auto-populated details and provide any additional details needed.
4. Create a phone encounter for the patient by clicking **Phone Encounter** in the Info Panel.
5. In the Create New Encounter window, document the name of the caller in the **Caller** field. The patient's provider will auto-populate.
6. Document the reason for call in the **Message** field.
7. Click the **Save** button and begin documenting within the encounter. The **Record** dropdown is expanded upon entering an encounter in order to communicate the record sections available for documentation. Refer to the following pages for instructions regarding the sections of Clinical Care.

6. Create a New Office Visit

Create a new office visit encounter to document patient care on a new day.
1. After performing a patient search and locating the correct patient, create an encounter by clicking **Office Visit** in the Clinical Care Info Panel.
2. Select the correct visit type from the **Visit Type** dropdown.
3. Select the correct provider from the **Provider** Dropdown.
4. Click the **Save** button and begin documenting within the encounter. The **Record** dropdown is expanded upon entering an encounter in order to communicate the record sections available for documentation. Refer to the following pages for instructions regarding the sections of Clinical Care.

7. Document in an Existing Office Visit

Document patient care for the same day within an existing encounter.
1. After performing a patient search and locating the correct patient, select the existing encounter from the Encounters section of the Patient Dashboard to begin documenting within the encounter.

8. Document an Allergy

1. Click the **Find Patient** icon.
2. Using the Patient Search fields, locate the correct patient record. Once you locate the correct patient in the List of Patients, confirm the date of birth to ensure you have located the correct patient record.
3. Select the radio button next to the patient name and click the **Select** button. Confirm the auto-populated details and provide any additional details needed. Create a new encounter or select an existing encounter to begin documenting. The Allergies section automatically appears upon entering the encounter.
4. Click the **Add Allergy** button to document patient allergies. An Add Allergy window will appear.
5. Select the correct radio button in the **Allergy Type** field. The Allergen dropdown options change based on the Allergen Type selected.
6. Complete all fields and click the **Save** button.
7. Use the icons in the Action column to edit or delete your documentation.

9. Document a Chief Complaint

1. Click the **Find Patient** icon.
2. Using the Patient Search fields, locate the correct patient record. Once you locate the correct patient in the List of Patients, confirm the date of birth to ensure you have located the correct patient record.
3. Select the radio button next to the patient name and click the **Select** button. Confirm the auto-populated details and provide any additional details needed. Create a new encounter or select an existing encounter to begin documenting.
4. Select **Chief Complaint** from the **Record** dropdown menu.
5. Document the reason for the patient visit in the **Chief Complaint** field. Use the patient's exact words if possible.
6. Document the site of the complaint (e.g., "near wrist") in the **Location** field.
7. Document symptom characteristics (e.g., "swollen") in the **Quality** field.
8. Document pain intensity in the **Severity** field. You may use a 0-10 scale with 0 being no pain (e.g., "6/10").
9. Document the length of time the complaint has been occurring (e.g., "four days") in the **Duration** field.
10. Document when the complaint occurs (e.g., "when walking") in the **Timing** field.
11. Document the circumstances of when the patient experiences symptoms (e.g., "with movement of the hand") in the **Context** field.
12. Document circumstances that change the nature of the complaint (e.g., "immobilizing wrist and applying ice") in the **Modifying Factors** field.
13. Document any additional symptoms (e.g., "numbness in fingers") in the **Associated Signs and Symptoms** field.
14. Click the **Save** button.

10. Document a Health History

1. Click the **Find Patient** icon.
2. Using the Patient Search fields, locate the correct patient record. Once you locate the correct patient in the List of Patients, confirm the date of birth to ensure you have located the correct patient record.
3. Select the radio button next to the patient name and click the **Select** button. Confirm the auto-populated details and provide any additional details needed. Create a new encounter or select an existing encounter to begin documenting.
4. Select **Health History** from the **Record** dropdown menu. Note the four tabs on the top of the screen: Medical History, Social and Family History, Pregnancy History (for a female patient), and Dental History.
5. Beginning within the **Medical History** tab, click the **Add New** button to document past medical history, past hospitalizations, or surgeries.
6. Use the icons in the Action column to edit or delete your documentation.
7. Continue to enter the rest of the history and click the **Save** button.

11. Document an Immunization

1. Click the **Find Patient** icon.
2. Using the Patient Search fields, locate the correct patient record. Once you locate the correct patient in the List of Patients, confirm the date of birth to ensure you have located the correct patient record.
3. Select the radio button next to the patient name and click the **Select** button. Confirm the auto-populated details and provide any additional details needed. Create a new encounter or select an existing encounter to begin documenting.
4. Select **Immunizations** from the **Record** dropdown menu.

5. Locate the row for the correct immunization in the **Vaccine** column and click on the green plus sign to the far right of that row. That row will become active to document an immunization.
6. Document the specific vaccine administered in the **Type** column.
7. Document the amount administered in the **Dose** column.
8. Document the date administered in the **Date** column.
9. Document the physician ordering the immunization in the **Provider** column.
10. Document how the immunization is administered (e.g., "SubQ, IM") and where the immunization is administered (e.g., "right deltoid") in the **Route/Site** column.
11. Document the manufacturer and lot number of the immunization in the **Mfr/Lot#** column.
12. Document the expiration date of the immunization in the **Exp** column.
13. Document any reactions to the immunization in the **Reaction** column.
14. Complete all fields and click the **Save** button.

12. Document a Medication

1. Click the **Find Patient** icon.
2. Using the Patient Search fields, locate the correct patient record. Once you locate the correct patient in the List of Patients, confirm the date of birth to ensure you have located the correct patient record.
3. Select the radio button next to the patient name and click the **Select** button. Confirm the auto-populated details and provide any additional details needed. Create a new encounter or select an existing encounter to begin documenting.
4. Select **Medications** from the **Record** dropdown menu. Note the three tabs on the top of the screen: Prescription Medications, Over-the-Counter Products, and Herbal and Natural Remedy Products. It is important to document all three types.
5. Within the tab of the type of medication you wish to document, click the **Add** button below the medication grid. An Add Medication window will appear.
6. Select the correct medication from the **Medication** dropdown menu or start typing the medication in the field.
7. Document the strength of the medication (e.g., "20 mg") in the **Strength** field.
8. Document the structure of the medication when consumed (e.g., "tablet") in the **Form** field.
9. Document how the medication is consumed (e.g., "oral") in the **Route** field.
10. Document how often the medication should be taken (e.g., "daily") in the **Frequency** field.
11. Document the reason for the medication in the **Indication** field.
12. Document the amount of the medication in the **Dose** field.
13. Document a Start Date for the medication in the **Start Date** field.
14. Indicate if a medication is current using the **Active** radio button, or if a patient has stopped taking the medication, using the **Discontinued** radio button.
15. Continue to document the rest of the medications and click the **Save** button.

13. Document an Out-of-Office Order

1. Click the **Find Patient** icon.
2. Using the Patient Search fields, locate the correct patient record. Once you locate the correct patient in the List of Patients, confirm the date of birth to ensure you have located the correct patient record.
3. Select the radio button next to the patient name and click the **Select** button. Confirm the auto-populated details and provide any additional details needed. Create a new encounter or select an existing encounter to begin documenting.
4. Select **Order Entry** from the **Record** dropdown menu.
5. Click the **Add** button below the Out-of-Office table to add an order.
6. Select the correct procedure from the **Order** dropdown and document any additional information needed. Fields vary based on the ordered procedure selected.
7. Click the **Save** button.

14. Prepare a Medication Prescription

If a patient calls for a medication refill, create a phone encounter. Refer to *Create a Phone Encounter* for more information.

1. Click the **Find Patient** icon. Using the Patient Search fields, locate the correct patient record. Once you locate the correct patient in the List of Patients, confirm the date of birth to ensure you have located the correct patient record.
2. Select the radio button next to the patient name and click the **Select** button. Confirm the auto-populated details and provide any additional details needed. Create a new encounter or select an existing encounter to begin documenting.
3. Select **Order Entry** from the **Record** dropdown menu and click the **Add** button below the Out-of-Office table to add an order.
4. Select **Medication Prescription** from the **Order** dropdown.
5. Document the disease the medication is treating in the **Diagnosis** field.
6. Document the complete name of the drug in the **Drug** field. Check the **Refill** checkbox if needed and provide the refill details.
7. Document the amount of the medication in the **Dose** field, the structure when consumed (e.g., "tablet") in the **Form** field, and how the medication is consumed (e.g., "oral") in the **Route** field.
8. Document physician directions to be printed on the label in the **Directions** field.
9. Document the amount of the medication in the **Quantity** field.
10. Document the timespan the medication should be taken (e.g., "10 days") in the **Days Supply** field.
11. Select the issue method using the **Electronic transfer** and **Paper** radio buttons.
12. Provide any additional information needed and click the **Save** button.
13. Use the icons in the Action column to edit or delete documentation. To print, click the edit icon in the Action column of the order and click the **Print** button.

15. Order a Requisition

1. Click the **Find Patient** icon.
2. Using the Patient Search fields, locate the correct patient record. Once you locate the correct patient in the List of Patients, confirm the date of birth to ensure you have located the correct patient record.
3. Select the radio button next to the patient name and click the **Select** button. Confirm the auto-populated details and provide any additional details needed. Create a new encounter or select an existing encounter to begin documenting.
4. Select **Order Entry** from the **Record** dropdown menu and click the **Add** button below the Out-of-Office table to add an order.
5. Select **Requisition** from the **Order** dropdown. Select the correct department from the **Requisition Type** field and complete any additional fields needed.
6. Click the **Save** button. Use the icons in the Action column to edit or delete your documentation.
7. Select the correct requisition type in the **Requisition** form of the Front Office **Form Repository**, then select the requisition from the **Requisition Type** dropdown menu. Click the **Patient Search** button and select the correct patient to auto-populate patient demographic information and save the form to the patient record.
8. Place the cursor in the **Diagnosis Code** field and click **TruCode** to access the encoder. The selected code will auto-populate where the cursor is placed in the simulation.
9. Enter the search terms in the Search field and select the source (**Diagnosis, ICD-9-CM or Diagnosis, ICD-10-CM**) from the dropdown menu. Click the **Search** button.
10. Click the code that appears in red next to the desired search result to expand this code and confirm that this is the most specific code available (Figure 1-17). Click the code that appears in the tree for the desired search result (Figure 1-18). This code will auto-populate in the **Diagnosis Code** field.
11. Complete any additional fields needed and click the **Save to Patient Record** button. The saved form will appear in the Forms section of the Patient Dashboard for reference and printing.

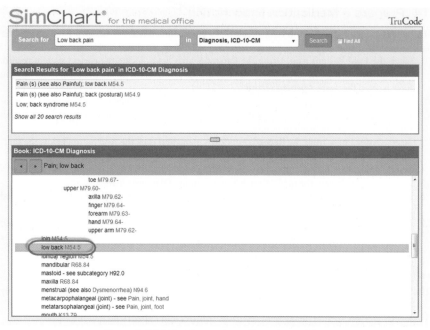

Figure 1-17 Select the most specific code possible.

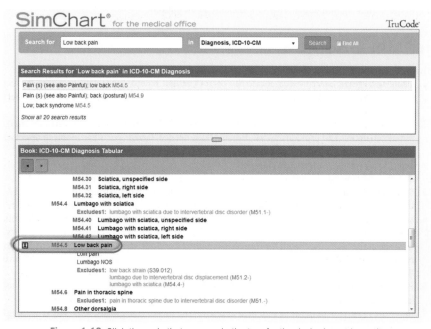

Figure 1-18 Click the code that appears in the tree for the desired search result.

16. Document Patient Education

1. Click the **Find Patient** icon.
2. Using the Patient Search fields, locate the correct patient record. Once you locate the correct patient in the List of Patients, confirm the date of birth to ensure you have located the correct patient record.

3. Select the radio button next to the patient name and click the **Select** button. Confirm the auto-populated details and provide any additional details needed. Create a new encounter or select an existing encounter to begin documenting.
4. Select **Patient Education** from the **Record** dropdown menu.
5. Select the correct category from the **Category** dropdown menu.
6. Select the correct subcategory from the **Subcategory** dropdown menu.
7. Select the teaching topic checkbox in the **Teaching Topics** field.
8. Click the **Save** button. This teaching topic will move from the **New** tab to the **Saved** tab. Expand the accordion of the saved patient education category to view and print the handout.

17. Document Preventative Services

1. Click the **Find Patient** icon.
2. Using the Patient Search fields, locate the correct patient record. Once you locate the correct patient in the List of Patients, confirm the date of birth to ensure you have located the correct patient record.
3. Select the radio button next to the patient name and click the **Select** button. Confirm the auto-populated details and provide any additional details needed. Create a new encounter or select an existing encounter to begin documenting.
4. Select **Preventative Services** from the **Record** dropdown menu.
5. Click the **Add** button below the grid of the correct category.
6. Select the correct recommendation from the **Health Recommendation** dropdown menu.
7. Document the date using the calendar picker.
8. Document any additional comments in the **Comments** field.
9. Click the **Save** button. The preventative service you added will display in the Preventative Services table.
10. Use the icons in the Action column to edit or delete your documentation.

18. Document Problem List

1. Click the **Find Patient** icon.
2. Using the Patient Search fields, locate the correct patient record. Once you locate the correct patient in the List of Patients, confirm the date of birth to ensure you have located the correct patient record.
3. Select the radio button next to the patient name and click the **Select** button. Confirm the auto-populated details and provide any additional details needed. Create a new encounter or select an existing encounter to begin documenting.
4. Select **Problem List** from the **Record** dropdown menu.
5. Click the **Add** button to add the correct problem as specified by the assignment.
6. In the Add Problem window, document the correct diagnosis in the **Diagnosis** field.
7. Select the ICD-9 or ICD-10 radio button (as specified by the instructor or assignment). Place the cursor in the corresponding text field and click **TruCode** to access the encoder. The selected code will auto-populate where the cursor is placed in the simulation.
8. Enter the search terms in the Search field and select the source (**Diagnosis, ICD-9-CM or Diagnosis, ICD-10-CM**) from the dropdown menu. Click the **Search** button.
9. Click the code that appears in red next to the desired search result to expand this code and confirm that this is the most specific code available (see Figure 1-17).
10. Click the code that appears in the tree for the desired search result (see Figure 1-18). This code will auto-populate in the Add Problem window. Review the *Using the Encoder* resource for additional information regarding the encoder.
11. Document the correct date in the Date Identified field.
12. Select the **Active** radio button in the Status field.
13. Click the **Save** button. The Problem List table will display the new problem.
14. Use the icons in the Action column to edit or delete your documentation.

19. Document Progress Notes

1. Click the **Find Patient** icon.
2. Using the Patient Search fields, locate the correct patient record. Once you locate the correct patient in the List of Patients, confirm the date of birth to ensure you have located the correct patient record.
3. Select the radio button next to the patient name and click the **Select** button. Confirm the auto-populated details and provide any additional details needed. Create a new encounter or select an existing encounter to begin documenting.
4. Select **Progress Note** from the **Record** dropdown menu.
5. Document the encounter date in the **Date of Service** field.
6. Document how the patient describes his or her symptoms in the **Subjective** field.
7. The physician completes documentation in the **Objective** field based on observations and completes documentation in the Assessment field based on the data provided in the Subjective and Objective fields. The physician then documents strategies for addressing the patient's symptoms in the Plan field and the effectiveness of the Plan in the Evaluation field.
8. Click the **Save** button.
9. Print the Progress Note by clicking the print icon in the top right corner.

20. Document Vital Signs

1. Click the **Find Patient** icon.
2. Using the Patient Search fields, locate the correct patient record. Once you locate the correct patient in the List of Patients, confirm the date of birth to ensure you have located the correct patient record.
3. Select the radio button next to the patient name and click the **Select** button. Confirm the auto-populated details and provide any additional details needed. Create a new encounter or select an existing encounter to begin documenting.
4. Select **Vital Signs** from the **Record** dropdown menu. Note the two tabs on the top of the screen: Vital Signs and Height/Weight. It is important to document in both tabs.
5. In the **Vital Signs** tab, click the **Add** button to document the patient's vital signs. The Position field below the Blood Pressure heading refers to the position of the patient.
6. Click the **Save** button. The table will display the vital signs documented.
7. In the **Height/Weight** tab, click the Add button to document height and weight.
8. Click the **Save** button. The table will display the height and weight documented.
9. Use the icons in the Action column to edit or delete your documentation.

21. Complete a Superbill

1. Click the **Find Patient** icon.
2. Using the Patient Search fields, locate the correct patient record. Once you locate the correct patient in the List of Patients, confirm the date of birth to ensure you have located the correct patient record.
3. After reviewing the patient encounter, click the **Superbill** link below the Patient Header. Select the correct encounter from the Encounters Not Coded table and confirm the auto-populated details. The View Progress Notes and View Fee Schedule links in the top right corner of the Superbill provide information necessary in completing the Superbill.
4. On page 1, select the ICD-9 or ICD-10 radio button (as specified by the instructor or assignment) and document the code.
5. Place the cursor in the Rank 1 **Diagnosis** field and click **TruCode** to access the encoder.
6. Enter the search terms in the Search field and select the source (**Diagnosis, ICD-9-CM or Diagnosis, ICD-10-CM**) from the dropdown menu. Click the **Search** button.
7. Click the code that appears in red next to the desired search result to expand this code and confirm it is the most specific code available (see Figure 1-17). Click the code that appears in the tree for the desired search result (see Figure 1-18). This code will auto-populate in the Diagnosis field and you can then document the associated diagnosis. Review the *Using the Encoder* resource for additional information regarding the encoder.

8. Document "1" in the Rank column for the correct service with the corresponding ICD-9 or ICD-10 code. Follow the steps outlined above to complete coding. Click the **Save** button. Then, click the **Next** button to progress through the Superbill.
9. On Page 4, document the copayment amount in the **Copay** field. The charges for today's visit will autopopulate in the **Today's Charges** field. Document the amount the patient owes in the Balance **Due field**.
10. Document any additional information needed and click the **Save** button.
11. Select the "I am ready to submit the Superbill" checkbox at the bottom of the screen. Select the **Yes** radio button to indicate that the signature is on file. Document the correct date in the Date field and click the **Submit Superbill** button.

22. Submit a Claim

1. Select **Claim** from the left Info Panel and perform a patient search to locate the claim.
2. Select the correct encounter and click the Edit button in the Action column. Confirm the auto-populated details. Seven tabs appear: Patient Info, Provider Info, Payer Info, Encounter Notes, Claim Info, Charge Capture, and Submission. Certain patient demographic and encounter information is auto-populated in the claim.
3. Review any auto-populated information in the **Patient Info**, **Provider Info**, and **Payer Info** tabs. Document any additional information needed and click the **Save** button.
4. Click the **Encounter Notes** tab. Review the auto-populated information and document additional information needed. Select the **Yes** radio button to indicate the HIPAA form is on file and provide the date. Document any additional information needed and click the **Save** button.
5. Click the **Claim Info** tab. Review the auto-populated information and document any additional information needed. Click the **Save** button.
6. Click the **Charge Capture** tab. Document the encounter date in the **DOS From** and **DOS To** columns. Place the cursor in the **CPT/HCPCS** column field and click **TruCode** to access the encoder. Enter the search terms in the Search field and select the source from the dropdown menu. Click the **Search** button.
7. Click the code that appears in red next to the desired search result to expand this code and confirm it is the most specific code (see Figure 1-17). Click the code that appears in the tree for the desired search result (see Figure 1-18). This code will auto-populate in the CPT/HCPCS field. Review the *Using the Encoder* resource for additional information regarding the encoder.
8. Document the place of service in the **POS** column. Click on the **Place of Service** link at the top of the screen for reference.
9. Document the diagnosis pointer from the Encounter Notes tab in the **DX** column and any modifiers needed in the **M1, M2,** and **M3** columns. Document the correct charge in the **Fee** column. Document the quantity used, if applicable, in the **Units** column. Click **Save**.
10. Click the **Submission** tab. Select the "I am ready to submit the Claim" checkbox. Select the Yes button to indicate the signature is on file and select the date. Click the **Save** button. Click the **Submit Claim** button.

23. Update a Ledger

1. Within the Coding & Billing tab, select **Ledger** from the left Info Panel.
2. Perform a patient search to locate the ledger for the correct guarantor.
3. Select the radio button for the correct patient and click the **Select** button. Confirm the auto-populated details in the header.
4. Select the arrow to the right of the patient's name to expand the ledger.
5. Document the correct date in the **Transaction Date** column using the calendar picker. Document the Date of Service in the **DOS** field.
6. Document the correct provider name in the **Provider** column.
7. Place the cursor in the Service column field and click **TruCode** to access the encoder. The **Service** column can also be used to enter a form of payment if only a payment is made.
8. Enter the search terms in the Search field and select the source (**Diagnosis, ICD-9-CM or Diagnosis, ICD-10-CM**) from the dropdown menu. Click the **Search** button.

9. Click the code that appears in red next to the desired search result to expand this code and confirm it is the most specific code available (see Figure 1-17). Click the code that appears in the tree for the desired search result (see Figure 1-18). This code will auto-populate in the Diagnosis field and you can then document the associated diagnosis. Review the *Using the Encoder* resource for additional information regarding the encoder.
10. Document the total charges in the **Charges** column.
11. Document the amount the patient paid in the **Payment** column.
12. Document the amount paid by insurance in the **Adjustment** column. The balance will auto-populate in the Balance column and the total will auto-populate in the **Total Ledger Balance** field below the table.
13. Click the **Save** button.

24. Complete a Day Sheet

1. Within the Coding & Billing tab, select **Day Sheet** from the left Info Panel.
2. Document the current date in the **Date** column using the calendar picker.
3. Document the correct patient name in the **Patient Name** column.
4. Document the correct provider in the **Provider** column.
5. Place the cursor in the **Service** column field and click **TruCode** to access the encoder. Enter the search terms in the Search field and select the source from the dropdown menu. Click the **Search** button.
6. Click the code that appears in red next to the desired search result to expand this code and confirm it is the most specific code (see Figure 1-17). Click the code that appears in the tree for the desired search result (see Figure 1-18). This code will auto-populate in the Service field. Review the *Using the Encoder* resource for additional information regarding the encoder.
7. Document the total charges in the **Charges** column.
8. Document the amount the patient paid in the **Payment** column.
9. Document the amount of any adjustments in the **Adjustment** column.
10. Document the new balance in the **New Balance** column.
11. Document the old balance in the **Old Balance** column.
12. Click the **Save** button.

abstracting Collecting data from a health record. Used when determining CPT, HCPCS, or ICD-10-CM codes; and for release of information.

abuse Unintentional deception in which a provider inappropriately bills for services that are not medically necessary, do not meet current standards of care, or are not medically sound.

account ledger Lists services provided, payments made by the patient, reimbursement received from the patient's insurance company, adjustments, and outstanding amount owed.

active patient An established patient who has seen the provider, or another provider in the billing group, within the past 3 years.

acute condition An illness or injury that is episodic (e.g., a seizure), has a sudden onset (such as a broken bone), is of limited duration (e.g., bronchitis), and generally responds well to prompt medical attention.

advance directive A binding legal document prepared and signed by a competent individual outlining the person's wishes should the person become incapacitated, e.g., a medical power of attorney and a living will.

anonymity The patient's right, which exists to varying degrees, to have private health data collected in a way that can never be linked or traced back to him or her.

anthropometric measurements Measurements of height, weight, and size used to compare the relative proportions of the human body in health and illness.

audit A review of employee activity within the EHR system, including an examination of which files were accessed or modified, as well as when and why.

audit trail A record that traces a user's electronic footsteps by recording activity and transactions, including unsuccessful attempts to view unauthorized screens, within the EHR system.

authentication The process of determining whether the person attempting to access a given network or EHR system is authorized to do so. User authentication can include password entry or use of biometric data (such as a digital fingerprint or voice signature) or a smart card (a data-laden microchip).

authorization A document giving a covered entity permission to use protected health information for specified purposes other than treatment, payment, or healthcare operations or to disclose protected health information to a third party specified by the patient.

business associates A person or entity that performs certain functions or activities that involve the use or disclosure of protected health information on behalf of a covered entity.

button An element of the user interface on which the user can click to execute a command, such as confirm, cancel, or exit.

caregiver A person responsible for providing physical care and emotional support, usually in a home-care setting, to a person who is ill, disabled, or dependent.

check box A specialized type of button that toggles on (checked) and off (unchecked). Check boxes are often used when more than one response might be appropriate (as in "Check all that apply"), but sometimes they should be interpreted to mean yes or no (as in a check box next to the caption "OK to mail?").

chief complaint (CC or cc) A brief statement of the problem, condition, or symptoms that prompted the patient to seek medical care. Sometimes referred to as chief concern.

chronic condition An illness that persists for a prolonged time (typically 3 months or longer), such as diabetes mellitus, emphysema, and arthritis.

clinical decision support (CDS) A set of patient-centered tools embedded within EHR software that can be used to improve patient safety, to ensure that care conforms to published protocol for specific conditions, and to reduce duplicate or unnecessary care and its associated costs.

closed patient record The record of a patient who will not be returning to the medical office or has not been seen in the past 10 years.

coding variance Medical coding mistakes caused by computer error or by various kinds of human error, from simple carelessness to incorrect application of coding guidelines and procedures.

compliance plan A written set of office policies and procedures intended to ensure compliance with laws regulating billing, coding, and third-party reimbursement.

computerized physician order entry (CPOE) An EHR function that allows a provider or provider-appointed licensed healthcare professional or credentialed medical assistant to enter the ordered medications and tests using an automated format; CPOE can reduce prescribing errors, delays, and duplication and can simplify inventory and billing processes.

confidentiality The obligation of professionals to keep a patient's information in confidence. The patient's right and expectation that individually identifiable health information will be kept private and not disclosed without the patient's permission. Confidentiality is protected by law to varying degrees.

consent Permission given to a covered entity for uses and disclosures of protected health information for treatment, payment, and healthcare operations.

consumer reporting agency An agency regulated by the Federal Trade Commission (FTC) under the Fair Credit Reporting Act (FCRA) that sells or cooperatively exchanges consumer information and history in areas such as credit and healthcare.

continuity of care A key aspect of quality that encompasses planning and coordination of care, communication among members of the healthcare team, and accessibility and transportability of information.

copayment A fixed sum of money, dictated by the insurance company, that is paid by the patient, usually at the time medical services are rendered.

covered entities Healthcare providers, health plans, and healthcare clearinghouses that transmit health information electronically.

CPT (Current Procedural Terminology) A comprehensive set of medical codes that describe procedures, treatments, and services for financial reimbursement and analytical purposes.

day sheet A register for all daily business transactions such as patient services, payments, and adjustments; also called a *day journal*.

default A preselected value or setting that will be used unless the user specifies a substitute by overriding the preselected choice.

disclosure Giving access to, releasing, or transferring information to a person or entity.

documentation The process of recording data about a patient's health history and status, including clinical observations and progress notes, diagnoses of illnesses and injuries, plans of care, patient education and self-care instructions given, vital signs taken, physical assessment findings, laboratory and imaging test results, medical treatments prescribed or administered, and surgeries performed and the outcomes; the term can also refer to the chronologic record that results from such data entry.

double-booking Giving two or more patients the same appointment slot with the same provider.

electronic data interchange (EDI) The standardized format used to transfer data from one computer system to another.

electronic health record (EHR) A computerized patient health record that allows the electronic management of a patient's health information by multiple healthcare providers and stores the patient's contact information, legal documents, demographic data, and administrative information; the term can also refer more broadly to a system that manages such records.

encounter A documented interaction or visit between a patient and healthcare provider.

encounter form A form generated to reflect the services and charges for a patient visit. It includes patient information and account balance. This may also be referred to as a Superbill.

encryption technology A system that keeps data secure by converting them to an unreadable code during transmission and then unencrypting the information when it reaches the recipient.

ethics Rules and standards of conduct that govern professional behavior and arise from our shared understanding of morality.

e-visit An evaluation and management service provided by a doctor or other qualified health professional to an established patient using a web-based or similar electronic-based communication network for a single patient encounter that occurs over safe, secure online communication systems.

fax machine A device capable of encoding documents and sending them over a telephone line; a secure fax sends fax transmissions via secure email, eliminating many of a fax's security risks.

field Space allocated on a form for specific numeric or text data.

fraud Presenting claims for services that an individual or entity knows or should know to be false resulting in a benefit to the presenting party.

guarantor The person who is legally responsible for a patient's account; the guarantor is usually the patient, but the guarantor for a minor or a person of decreased mental capacity may be a parent, trustee, or legal guardian.

high-alert medication A medication that poses a heightened risk of injury or death when administered improperly.

HIPAA 5010 The standard electronic claim format used by a noninstitutional provider or supplier to submit a claim electronically to Medicare and most other insurance carriers for covered services.

history of the present illness (HPI) Details about the duration, time, location, severity, context, associated signs and symptoms, quality, and modifying factors related to the patient's illness.

host A server that provides data transfer, storage space, and other services to users at remote locations; a host has a unique domain name and is, in effect, the point at which a website originates.

ICD-10-CM International Classification of Diseases, Tenth Revision, with Clinical Modification. A coding system used to describe inpatient and outpatient diagnoses.

inactive patient An established patient who has not been seen by his or her own provider or another provider in the billing group for 3 or more years.

interoperability The ability of separate EHR systems to share information in compatible formats.

laws Formal, enforceable rules and policies based on community standards of conduct.

letter templates Standardized, preconstructed documents that address specific topics but can be tailored to individual recipients.

living will The part of an advance directive that specifies which life-sustaining treatments (for example, mechanical ventilation and tube feeding) should be administered or withheld if the person becomes incapacitated.

Meaningful Use (MU) Part of the federal EHR Incentive program. If providers can show that they have implemented and are using EHRs in specified meaningful ways, they will receive financial incentives from the government.

medical coding The process of assigning standard numeric or alphanumeric codes to diagnoses, procedures, and treatments for research, disease tracking, and reimbursement purposes.

medical identity theft The unauthorized use of someone else's personal information to obtain medical services or to submit fraudulent medical insurance claims for reimbursement.

medical power of attorney (also called durable power of attorney for healthcare or healthcare proxy) The part of an advance directive naming a trusted person to make medical decisions on the patient's behalf should he or she become unable to make such decisions independently.

medication reconciliation The process of comparing the medication list in the patient's EHR with the patient's self-report of the medications he or she has been taking.

minimum necessary standard A key provision of the HIPAA Privacy Rule requiring that covered entities limit unnecessary or inappropriate access to and disclosure of protected health information. Disclosures should include only the minimum necessary amount of information to accomplish a given purpose.

no-show A patient who makes an appointment and neither shows up nor calls to cancel; the term also refers to the appointment itself (a "no-show appointment").

objective Readily seen, perceived, or measured by the clinician, not only by the patient.

Office of the National Coordinator for Health Information Technology (ONCHIT) Division of the Office of the Secretary, within the Department of Health and Human Services. Coordinates the effort to implement health information technology and the electronic exchange of health information.

off-label indication A use for a prescription drug other than that for which the U.S. Food and Drug Administration (FDA) has approved it.

online community A virtual meeting space where like-minded people with common interests or concerns interact and build relationships using real-time chat rooms, asynchronous threaded discussions, discussion groups, social media, newsgroups, web conferencing, and other technologies.

password A sequence of characters and sometimes spaces used to prevent unauthorized access to or disclosure of patient information contained in secure electronic files.

patient flow The efficient movement of patients through the medical office as a product of accurately estimated patient volume, a consistent provider pace, and efficient scheduling practices; the term generally refers to the overall flow of patients but can refer to the path of an individual patient.

patient information form A form used to gather data about the patient, including basic demographics, medical insurance data, and emergency contact.

patient portal A secure website where the patient can access personal health information, schedule appointments, and refill prescriptions 24 hours a day, using a username and password. Oftentimes it is part of the provider's EHR system.

patient-controlled health record The portion of a patient portal that contains data loaded by the patient and to which he or she alone may grant or deny access.

pay for performance (P4P) An outcomes-based payment model that offers providers financial incentives for meeting specific standards and electronically documenting compliance with them; punitive measures may be applied to providers who fail to comply.

personal health record (PHR) A secure, comprehensive record of health information that is controlled by the individual, creating a confidential electronic or paper-based file that is easy to access, manage, and share.

PFSH An abbreviation for past (medical), family, and social history.

populate To complete a template or create a record by filling in a set of predetermined fields with information ranging from demographic data to values and measurements (for example, vital signs) to entire documents (such as correspondence and operative reports).

practice management software Software used in a medical office to accomplish administrative (nonclinical) tasks, including entry of patient demographics, record keeping for insurance and other billing transactions, appointment scheduling, and advanced accounting functions.

privacy The patient's freedom to determine when, how much, and under what circumstances his or her medical information may be disclosed.

protected health information (PHI) Individually identifiable health information (i.e., demographic information, billing information, medical record numbers, account numbers, physical or mental condition, etc.) that is stored, maintained, or transmitted electronically.

purging The process of separating inactive patient health records from active ones.

radio button A specialized type of button on a software interface that toggles on (round button visible) and off (blank circle). Radio buttons tell the user that only one response is appropriate, because two radio buttons can't be depressed at the same time.

retention period The amount of time patient records must, by law, be maintained by the medical office.

review of systems (ROS) An organized inventory of each organ system, completed as part of the initial patient interview to pinpoint any unusual findings in the patient's history.

safeguards Measures taken to prevent interference with computer network operations and to avert security breaches involving the unauthorized use, disclosure, modification, erasure, or destruction of protected health information; these measures are specified by the HIPAA Security Rule, which applies only to data in electronic form.

screen saver A program that displays animation or an image on the screen if input (such as a keystroke) is not received for a given time period.

secondary use A use of health information that is not directly related to patient care. Such uses include statistical analysis; research, quality, and safety assurance processes; public health monitoring; payment; provider certification or accreditation; and marketing and other business activities.

secure electronic messaging A component of a patient portal or personal health record that allows for secure communication between the patient and the provider.

secure email An email system capable of transmitting an encrypted message and storing it in coded format until it is retrieved by the recipient via a secure web link.

show rate The percentage of patients in a practice who arrive for appointments as scheduled or call in advance to cancel or reschedule.

social networking The practice of using online communities to expand one's social or business contacts and to exchange content, such as images and instant messages; the term also refers to the broader phenomenon of this practice, which has created virtual communities with millions of members.

speech recognition A technology that converts speech into text.

structured data entry Documentation using controlled vocabulary via preloaded data, drop-down menus, radio buttons, and sentence builders.

subjective Perceived only by the patient and not evident to or measurable by the clinician.

telephone etiquette A polite, helpful response and respectful manner toward callers that shows patients they are cared for and valued.

template An electronic document that has a basic format in which the required information can be entered. Templates are often created for those documents that are needed over and over again, such as a new patient welcome letter.

third-party payer A party other than the patient, spouse, parent, or guardian who is responsible for paying all or part of the patient's medical costs, typically the insurance company.

views Different ways of displaying the same or similar information on a computer screen, usually with an increasing or decreasing level of detail (for example, looking at an electronic calendar in daily, weekly, and monthly views).

Wi-Fi (short for Wireless Fidelity, a technologic certification body) A means of connecting wirelessly to the Internet using a local area network or router.

INDEX

Page numbers followed by "*b*" indicate boxes; "*f*" figures; "*t*" tables.